Online Resources

Included with your purchase are multiple online resources. This includes the practice tests in an interactive format and a convenient study timer to help you manage your time.

Instructions for accessing these resources can be found on the last page of this book.

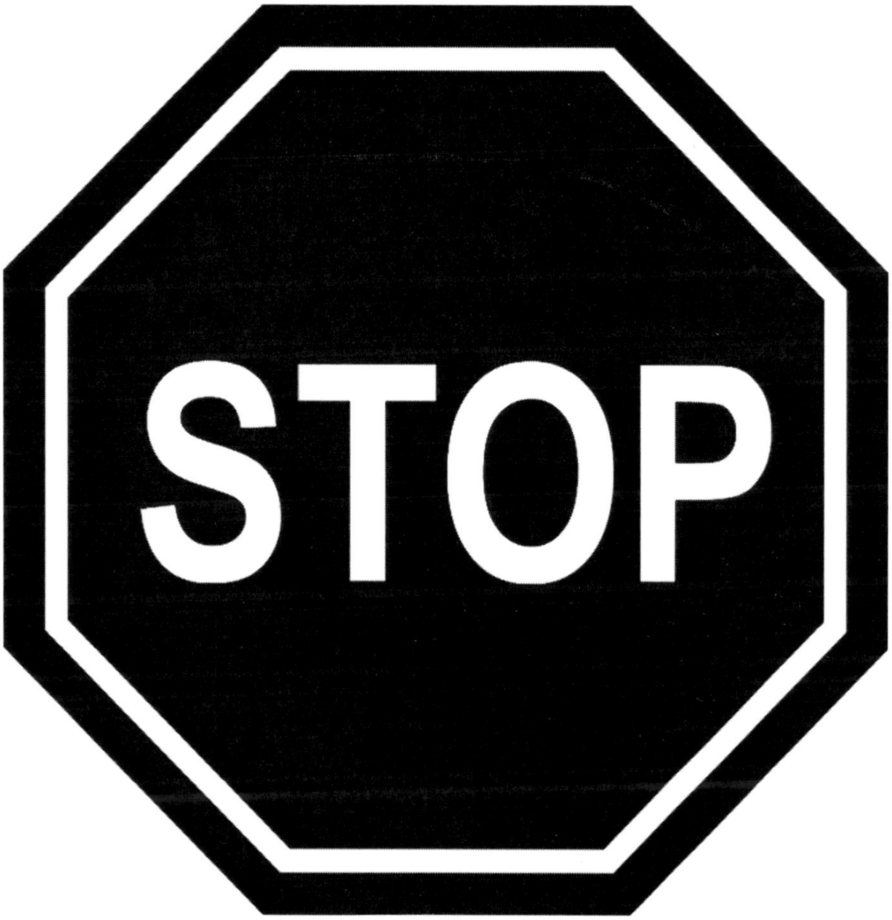

MCAT® Prep Book 2026-2027

20 Full-Length Practice Tests + MCAT Study Guide + Online Exam Simulator [10th Edition]

Lydia Morrison

Written and edited by TPB Publishing.

ISBN 13: 9781637756683

Table of Contents

Welcome

Dear Reader,

Welcome to your new Test Prep Books study guide! We are pleased that you chose us to help you prepare for your exam. There are many study options to choose from, and we appreciate you choosing us. Studying can be a daunting task, but we have designed a smart, effective study guide to help prepare you for what lies ahead.

Whether you're a parent helping your child learn and grow, a high school student working hard to get into your dream college, or a nursing student studying for a complex exam, we want to help give you the tools you need to succeed. We hope this study guide gives you the skills and the confidence to thrive, and we can't thank you enough for allowing us to be part of your journey.

In an effort to continue to improve our products, we welcome feedback from our customers. We look forward to hearing from you. Suggestions, success stories, and criticisms can all be communicated by emailing us at support@testprepbooks.com.

Sincerely,

Test Prep Books Team

Quick Overview

As you draw closer to taking your exam, effective preparation becomes more and more important. Thankfully, you have this study guide to help you get ready. Use this guide to help keep your studying on track and refer to it often.

This study guide contains several key sections that will help you be successful on your exam. The guide contains tips for what you should do the night before and the day of the test. Also included are test-taking tips. Knowing the right information is not always enough. Many well-prepared test takers struggle with exams. These tips will help equip you to accurately read, assess, and answer test questions.

A large part of the guide is devoted to showing you what content to expect on the exam and to helping you better understand that content. In this guide are practice test questions so that you can see how well you have grasped the content. Then, answer explanations are provided so that you can understand why you missed certain questions.

Don't try to cram the night before you take your exam. This is not a wise strategy for a few reasons. First, your retention of the information will be low. Your time would be better used by reviewing information you already know rather than trying to learn a lot of new information. Second, you will likely become stressed as you try to gain a large amount of knowledge in a short amount of time. Third, you will be depriving yourself of sleep. So be sure to go to bed at a reasonable time the night before. Being well-rested helps you focus and remain calm.

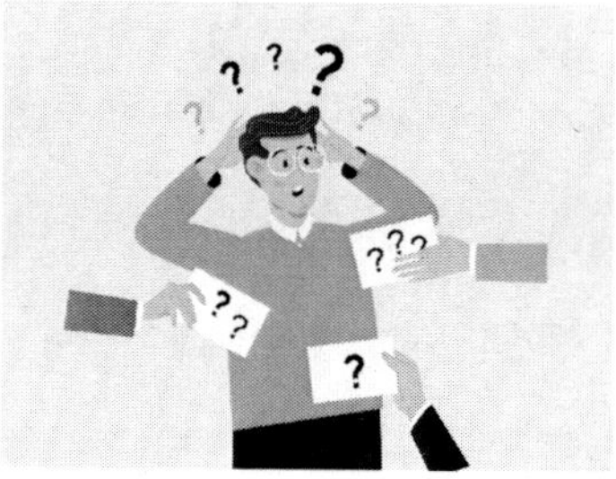

Be sure to eat a substantial breakfast the morning of the exam. If you are taking the exam in the afternoon, be sure to have a good lunch as well. Being hungry is distracting and can make it difficult to focus. You have hopefully spent lots of time preparing for the exam. Don't let an empty stomach get in the way of success!

When travelling to the testing center, leave earlier than needed. That way, you have a buffer in case you experience any delays. This will help you remain calm and will keep you from missing your appointment time at the testing center.

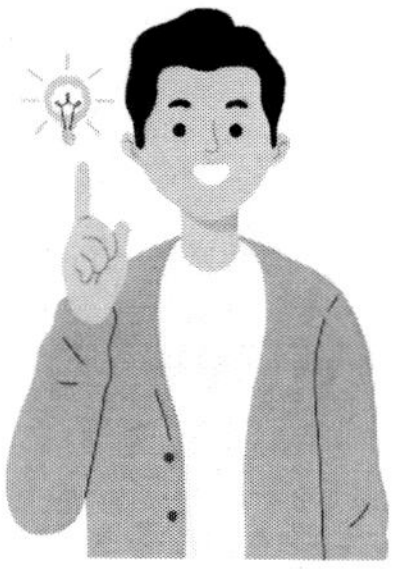

Be sure to pace yourself during the exam. Don't try to rush through the exam. There is no need to risk performing poorly on the exam just so you can leave the testing center early. Allow yourself to use all of the allotted time if needed.

Remain positive while taking the exam even if you feel like you are performing poorly. Thinking about the content you should have mastered will not help you perform better on the exam.

Once the exam is complete, take some time to relax. Even if you feel that you need to take the exam again, you will be well served by some down time before you begin studying again. It's often easier to convince yourself to study if you know that it will come with a reward!

Test-Taking Strategies

1. Predicting the Answer

When you feel confident in your preparation for a multiple-choice test, try predicting the answer before reading the answer choices. This is especially useful on questions that test objective factual knowledge. By predicting the answer before reading the available choices, you eliminate the possibility that you will be distracted or led astray by an incorrect answer choice. You will feel more confident in your selection if you read the question, predict the answer, and then find your prediction among the answer choices. After using this strategy, be sure to still read all of the answer choices carefully and completely. If you feel unprepared, you should not attempt to predict the answers. This would be a waste of time and an opportunity for your mind to wander in the wrong direction.

2. Reading the Whole Question

Too often, test takers scan a multiple-choice question, recognize a few familiar words, and immediately jump to the answer choices. Test authors are aware of this common impatience, and they will sometimes prey upon it. For instance, a test author might subtly turn the question into a negative, or he or she might redirect the focus of the question right at the end. The only way to avoid falling into these traps is to read the entirety of the question carefully before reading the answer choices.

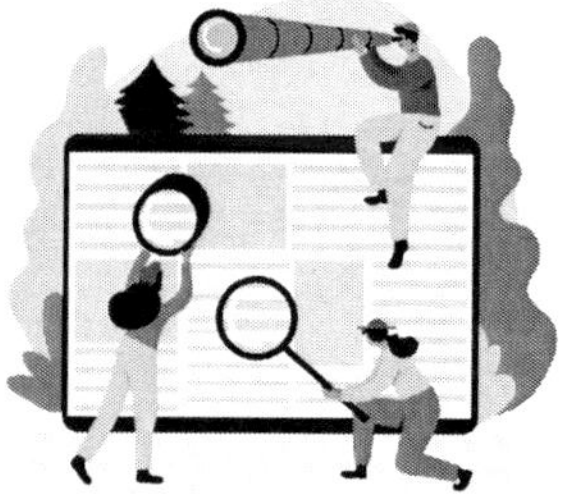

3. Looking for Wrong Answers

Long and complicated multiple-choice questions can be intimidating. One way to simplify a difficult multiple-choice question is to eliminate all of the answer choices that are clearly wrong. In most sets of answers, there will be at least one selection that can be dismissed right away. If the test is administered on paper, the test taker could draw a line through it to indicate that it may be ignored; otherwise, the test taker will have to perform this operation mentally or on scratch paper. In either case, once the obviously incorrect answers have been eliminated, the remaining choices may be considered. Sometimes identifying the clearly wrong answers will give the test taker some information about the correct answer. For instance, if one of the remaining answer choices is a direct opposite of one of the eliminated answer choices, it may well be the correct answer. The opposite of obviously wrong is obviously right! Of course, this is not always the case. Some answers are obviously incorrect simply because they are irrelevant to the question being asked. Still, identifying and eliminating some incorrect answer choices is a good way to simplify a multiple-choice question.

4. Don't Overanalyze

Anxious test takers often overanalyze questions. When you are nervous, your brain will often run wild, causing you to make associations and discover clues that don't actually exist. If you feel that this may be a problem for you, do whatever you can to slow down during the test. Try taking a deep breath or counting to ten. As you read and consider the question, restrict yourself to the particular words used by the author. Avoid thought tangents about what the author *really* meant, or what he or she was *trying* to say. The only things that matter on a multiple choice test are the words that are actually in the question. You must avoid reading too much into a multiple-choice question, or supposing that the writer meant something other than what he or she wrote.

5. No Need for Panic

It is wise to learn as many strategies as possible before taking a multiple-choice test, but it is likely that you will come across a few questions for which you simply don't know the answer. In this situation, avoid panicking. Because most multiple-choice tests include dozens of questions, the relative value of a single wrong answer is small. As much as possible, you should compartmentalize each question on a multiple-choice test. In other words, you should not allow your feelings about one question to affect your success on the others. When you find a question that you either don't understand or don't know how to answer, just take a deep breath and do your best. Read the entire question slowly and carefully. Try rephrasing the question a couple of different ways. Then, read all of the answer choices carefully. After eliminating obviously wrong answers, make a selection and move on to the next question.

6. Confusing Answer Choices

When working on a difficult multiple-choice question, there may be a tendency to focus on the answer choices that are the easiest to understand. Many people, whether consciously or not, gravitate to the answer choices that require the least concentration, knowledge, and memory. This is a mistake. When you come across an answer choice that is confusing, you should give it extra attention. A question might be confusing because you do not know the subject matter to which it refers. If this is the case, don't eliminate the answer before you have affirmatively settled on another. When you come across an answer choice of this type, set it aside as you look at the remaining choices. If you can confidently assert that one of the other choices is correct, you can leave the confusing answer aside. Otherwise, you will need to take a moment to try to better understand the confusing answer choice. Rephrasing is one way to tease out the sense of a confusing answer choice.

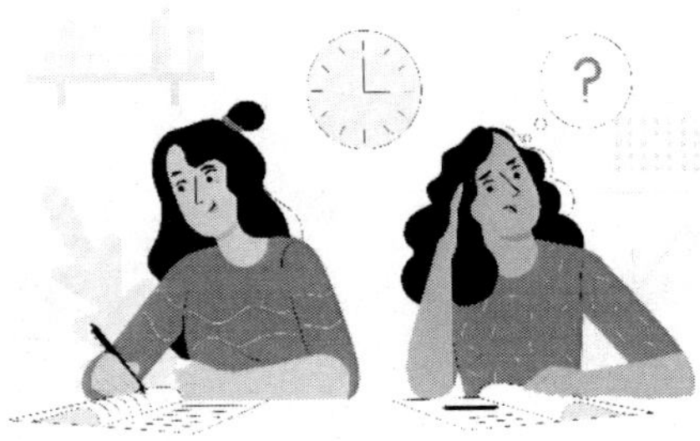

7. Your First Instinct

Many people struggle with multiple-choice tests because they overthink the questions. If you have studied sufficiently for the test, you should be prepared to trust your first instinct once you have carefully and completely read the question and all of the answer choices. There is a great deal of research suggesting that the mind can come to the correct conclusion very quickly once it has obtained all of the relevant information. At times, it may seem to you as if your intuition is working faster even than your reasoning mind. This may in fact be true. The knowledge you obtain while studying may be retrieved from your subconscious before you have a chance to work out the associations that support it. Verify your instinct by working out the reasons that it should be trusted.

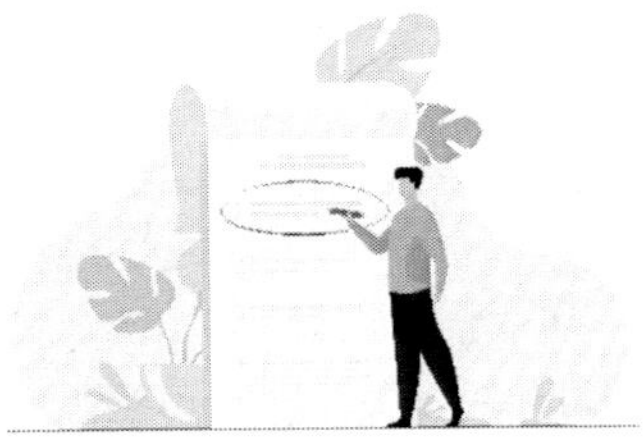

8. Key Words

Many test takers struggle with multiple-choice questions because they have poor reading comprehension skills. Quickly reading and understanding a multiple-choice question requires a mixture of skill and experience. To help with this, try jotting down a few key words and phrases on a piece of scrap paper. Doing this concentrates the process of reading and forces the mind to weigh the relative importance of the question's parts. In selecting words and phrases to write down, the test taker thinks about the question more deeply and carefully. This is especially true for multiple-choice questions that are preceded by a long prompt.

9. Subtle Negatives

One of the oldest tricks in the multiple-choice test writer's book is to subtly reverse the meaning of a question with a word like *not* or *except*. If you are not paying attention to each word in the question, you can easily be led astray by this trick. For instance, a common question format is, "Which of the following is…?" Obviously, if the question instead is, "Which of the following is not…?," then the answer will be quite different. Even worse, the test makers are aware of the potential for this mistake and will include one answer choice that would be correct if the question were not negated or reversed. A test taker who misses the reversal will find what he or she believes to be a correct answer and will be so confident that he or she will fail to reread the question and discover the original error. The only way to avoid this is to practice a wide variety of multiple-choice questions and to pay close attention to each and every word.

10. Reading Every Answer Choice

It may seem obvious, but you should always read every one of the answer choices! Too many test takers fall into the habit of scanning the question and assuming that they understand the question because they recognize a few key words. From there, they pick the first answer choice that answers the question they believe they have read. Test takers who read all of the answer choices might discover that one of the latter answer choices is actually *more* correct. Moreover, reading all of the answer choices can remind you of facts related to the question that can help you arrive at the correct answer. Sometimes, a misstatement or incorrect detail in one of the latter answer choices will trigger your memory of the subject and will enable you to find the right answer. Failing to read all of the answer choices is like not reading all of the items on a restaurant menu: you might miss out on the perfect choice.

11. Spot the Hedges

One of the keys to success on multiple-choice tests is paying close attention to every word. This is never truer than with words like *almost*, *most*, *some*, and *sometimes*. These words are called "hedges" because they indicate that a statement is not totally true or not true in every place and time. An absolute statement will contain no hedges, but in many subjects, the answers are not always straightforward or absolute. There are always exceptions to the rules in these subjects. For this reason, you should favor those multiple-choice questions that contain hedging language. The presence of qualifying words indicates that the author is taking special care with his or her words, which is certainly important when composing the right answer. After all, there are many ways to be wrong, but there is only one way to be right! For this reason, it is wise to avoid answers that are absolute when taking a multiple-choice test. An absolute answer is one that says things are either all one way or all another. They often include words like *every*, *always*, *best*, and *never*. If you are taking a multiple-choice test in a subject that doesn't lend itself to absolute answers, be on your guard if you see any of these words.

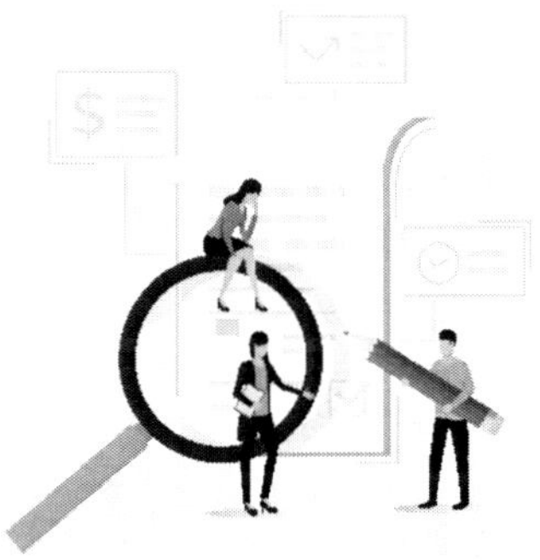

12. Long Answers

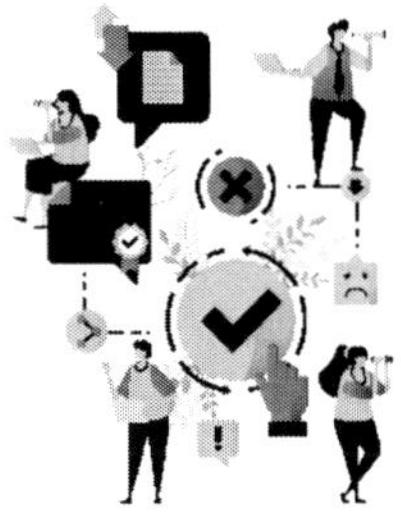

In many subject areas, the answers are not simple. As already mentioned, the right answer often requires hedges. Another common feature of the answers to a complex or subjective question are qualifying clauses, which are groups of words that subtly modify the meaning of the sentence. If the question or answer choice describes a rule to which there are exceptions or the subject matter is complicated, ambiguous, or confusing, the correct answer will require many words in order to be expressed clearly and accurately. In essence, you should not be deterred by answer choices that seem excessively long. Oftentimes, the author of the text will not be able to write the correct answer without offering some qualifications and modifications. Your job is to read the answer choices thoroughly and completely and to select the one that most accurately and precisely answers the question.

13. Restating to Understand

Sometimes, a question on a multiple-choice test is difficult not because of what it asks but because of how it is written. If this is the case, restate the question or answer choice in different words. This process serves a couple of important purposes. First, it forces you to concentrate on the core of the question. In order to rephrase the question accurately, you have to understand it well. Rephrasing the question will concentrate your mind on the key words and ideas. Second, it will present the information to your mind in a fresh way. This process may trigger your memory and render some useful scrap of information picked up while studying.

14. True Statements

Sometimes an answer choice will be true in itself, but it does not answer the question. This is one of the main reasons why it is essential to read the question carefully and completely before proceeding to the answer choices. Too often, test takers skip ahead to the answer choices and look for true statements. Having found one of these, they are content to select it without reference to the question above. The savvy test taker will always read the entire question before turning to the answer choices. Then, having settled on a correct answer choice, he or she will refer to the original question and ensure that the selected answer is relevant. The mistake of choosing a correct-but-irrelevant answer choice is especially common on questions related to specific pieces of objective knowledge.

15. No Patterns

One of the more dangerous ideas that circulates about multiple-choice tests is that the correct answers tend to fall into patterns. These erroneous ideas range from a belief that B and C are the most common right answers, to the idea that an unprepared test-taker should answer "A-B-A-C-A-D-A-B-A." It cannot be emphasized enough that pattern-seeking of this type is exactly the WRONG way to approach a multiple-choice test. To begin with, it is highly unlikely that the test maker will plot the correct answers according to some predetermined pattern. The questions are scrambled and delivered in a random order. Furthermore, even if the test maker was following a pattern in the assignation of correct answers, there is no reason why the test taker would know which pattern he or she was using. Any attempt to discern a pattern in the answer choices is a waste of time and a distraction from the real work of taking the test. A test taker would be much better served by extra preparation before the test than by reliance on a pattern in the answers.

Introduction to the MCAT

Function of the Test

All medical schools in the United States, as well as many Canadian schools, require candidates to submit Medical College Admission Test (MCAT) scores as part of the admissions process. Most schools require that an applicant's scores were obtained within the prior three years. The MCAT is a standardized test that assesses several different areas such as critical thinking and problem solving; knowledge of natural, behavioral, and social science concepts; and other principles related to the medical field. The AAMC develops and writes the MCAT. Candidates are eligible to take the MCAT if they are applying to a professional school of medicine in the following areas: allopathic, osteopathic, podiatric, or veterinary medicine. Candidates should apply and take the MCAT about a year before entering medical school. Although there are no prerequisites required to take the MCAT, the exam covers topics on introductory biology, general and organic chemistry, physics, and first-semester psychology, sociology and biochemistry; college-level science labs and statistics concepts and skills are also assessed on the MCAT.

Test Administration

The MCAT is given at hundreds of testing sites throughout the country at multiple times throughout the year between January and September. Registration for the following year typically starts in the fall prior to the year of administration. International students may apply for the MCAT if they hold a MBBS degree or are in a program to obtain an MBBS. Since the MCAT is for candidates wishing to apply to a professional medical school, there are "special permissions" granted to individuals who are not planning on attending such a school. These special requests can be granted via email to mcat@aamc.org and will typically be reviewed within five business days. Details for special requests can be viewed on the official MCAT website: https://students-residents.aamc.org/applying-medical-school/faq/mcat-faqs/

Candidates should attempt to take the exam early in the year, in case a retest is necessary. This gives a student sufficient time to study and find a second available seat. The MCAT can be taken three times in a year and four times in two consecutive years. The MCAT can be taken up to seven times in a lifetime. No shows and voids count as attempts against the candidate's test limits.

Test Format

The MCAT is a standardized, multiple-choice test. There are 230 questions and the test takes about 6 hours and 15 minutes to complete, with additional time for breaks. There are four sections on the MCAT: biological and biochemical foundations of living systems; chemical and physical foundations of biological systems; psychological, social, and biological foundations of behavior; and critical analysis and reasoning. The first three sections include scientific inquiry and reasoning skills. The following table displays the categories, number of questions, and allotted time:

Category	Number of Questions	Time Limit (min)
Biological and Biochemical Foundations of Living Systems	59	95
Chemical and Physical Foundations of Biological Systems	59	95
Psychological, Social, and Biological Foundations of Behavior	59	95
Critical Analysis and Reasoning Skills	53	90

Scoring

Scores for the MCAT are released approximately a month after the date the exam was taken. If the MCAT was taken in April or May, the scores take longer to reach the candidate, but a percentile ranking will be sent about three weeks after taking the exam. This will help a candidate decide if a retest is necessary. There are five scores for the MCAT exam: a score will be given for each of the four sections and one combined score will be given for the total test. The four individual sections range from 118-132 and the total score ranges from 472-528. Scores are scaled and are not curved. However, since some forms of the test are more difficult than others, raw scores are converted to scaled score, which consider test difficulty.

Recent/Future Developments

The current version of the MCAT discussed above is reflective of the latest updates from April of 2015. Periodic updates are necessary because the field of medicine continues to change and the MCAT needs to reflect these changes. The required knowledge, skills, and training that a new physician needs has changed since the MCAT's previous 1991 version, and will likely dictate future revisions.

Study Prep Plan for the MCAT

1. **Schedule** - Use one of our study schedules below or come up with one of your own.

2. **Relax** - Test anxiety can hurt even the best students. There are many ways to reduce stress. Find the one that works best for you.

3. **Execute** - Once you have a good plan in place, be sure to stick to it.

One Week Study Schedule

Day 1	Biological and Biochemical Foundations of...
Day 2	Chemical and Physical Foundations of...
Day 3	Nature of Molecules and Intermolecular...
Day 4	Psychological, Social, and Biological...
Day 5	Critical Analysis and Reasoning Skills
Day 6	Practice Test #1
Day 7	Take Your Exam!

Two Week Study Schedule

Day 1	Biological and Biochemical...	Day 8	Making Sense of the Environment
Day 2	Principles of Bioenergetics and Fuel...	Day 9	Attitude and Behavior Change
Day 3	Structure and Integrative Functions...	Day 10	Demographic Characteristics and...
Day 4	Chemical and Physical Foundations of...	Day 11	Critical Analysis and Reasoning Skills
Day 5	Importance of Fluids for the Circulation of...	Day 12	Practice Test #1
Day 6	Nature of Molecules and Intermolecular...	Day 13	Practice Test #2
Day 7	Psychological, Social, and Biological...	Day 14	Take Your Exam!

One Month Study Schedule

Day 1	Biological and Biochemical...	Day 11	Translational Motion, Forces, Work, Energy...	Day 21	Self-identity
Day 2	Structure and Function of Proteins and Their...	Day 12	Importance of Fluids for the Circulation of...	Day 22	Social Interactions
Day 3	Transmission of Genetic Information...	Day 13	Atoms, Nuclear Decay, Electronic Structure...	Day 23	Understanding Social Structure
Day 4	Transmission of Heritable...	Day 14	Nature of Molecules and Intermolecular...	Day 24	Demographic Characteristics and...
Day 5	Principles of Bioenergetics and...	Day 15	Structure, Function, and Reactivity of...	Day 25	Social Inequality
Day 6	Assemblies of Molecules, Cells, and...	Day 16	Principles of Chemical Thermodynamics and...	Day 26	Critical Analysis and Reasoning Skills
Day 7	The Structure, Growth, Physiology, and...	Day 17	Psychological, Social, and Biological...	Day 27	Practice Test #1
Day 8	Processes of Cell Division...	Day 18	Making Sense of the Environment	Day 28	Practice Test #2
Day 9	Structure and Integrative Functions...	Day 19	Responding to the World	Day 29	Practice Test #3
Day 10	Chemical and Physical Foundations of...	Day 20	Individual Influences on Behavior	Day 30	Take Your Exam!

Build your own prep plan by visiting the Online Resources page.

Instructions and a QR code can be found on the last page of this guide.

As you study for your test, we'd like to take the opportunity to remind you that you are capable of great things! With the right tools and dedication, you truly can do anything you set your mind to. The fact that you are holding this book right now shows how committed you are. In case no one has told you lately, you've got this! Our intention behind including this coloring page is to give you the chance to take some time to engage your creative side when you need a little brain-break from studying. As a company, we want to encourage people like you to achieve their dreams by providing good quality study materials for the tests and certifications that improve careers and change lives. As individuals, many of us have taken such tests in our careers, and we know how challenging this process can be. While we can't come alongside you and cheer you on personally, we can offer you the space to recall your purpose, reconnect with your passion, and refresh your brain through an artistic practice. We wish you every success, and happy studying!

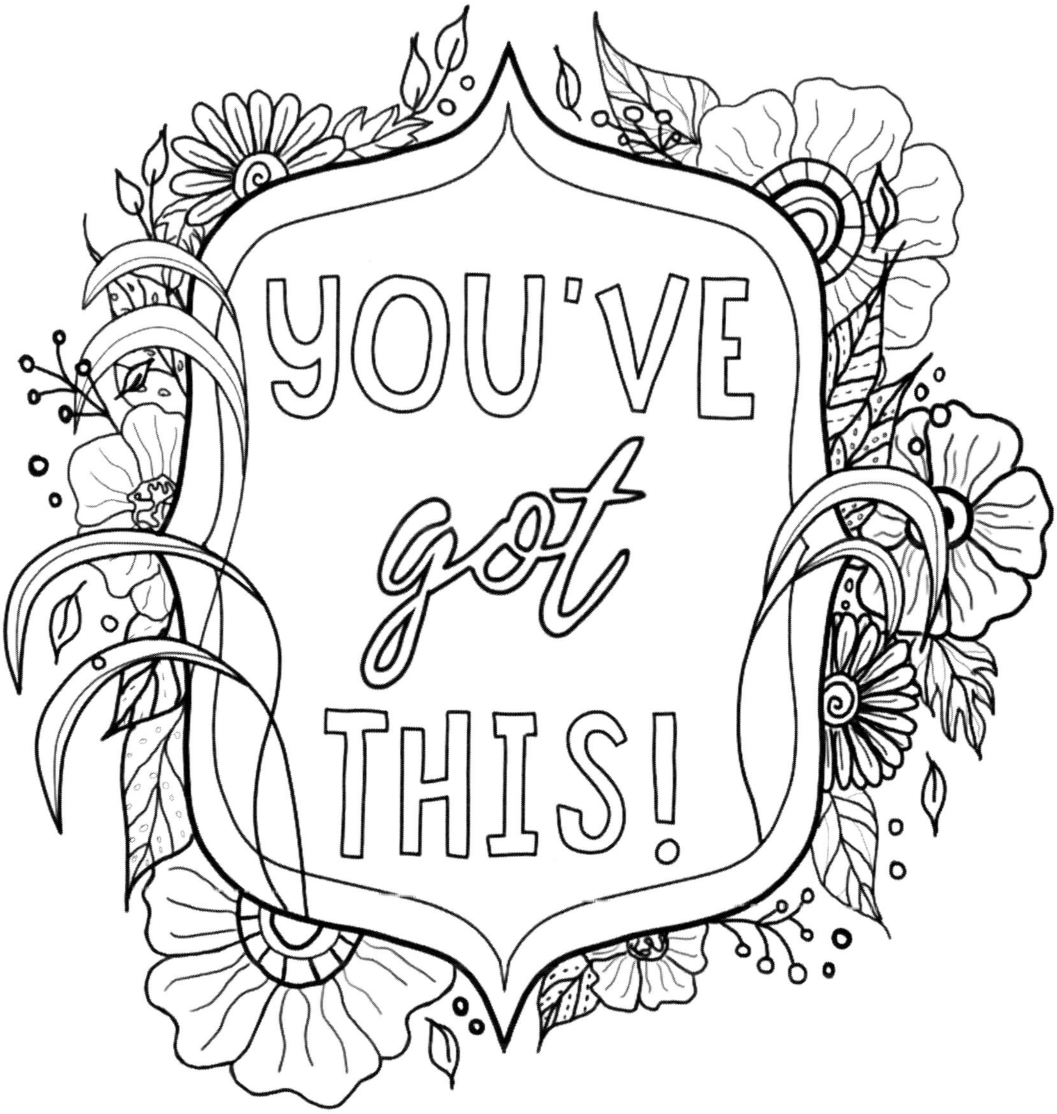

Biological and Biochemical Foundations of Living Systems

Foundational Concept 1: Biomolecules have unique properties that determine how they contribute to the structure and function of cells and how they participate in the processes necessary to maintain life.

Structure and Function of Proteins and Their Constituent Amino Acids

Amino Acids

Proteins are molecules that consist of carbon, hydrogen, oxygen, nitrogen, and other atoms, and they have a wide variety of functions. The monomers that make up proteins are amino acids. All amino acids have the same basic structure. They contain an **amine group** (-NH), a **carboxylic acid group** (-COOH), and an **R group**. The R group, also called the **functional group**, is different in each amino acid.

The functional groups give the different amino acids their unique chemical properties. There are twenty naturally-occurring amino acids that can be divided into groups based on their chemical properties. Glycine, alanine, valine, leucine, isoleucine, methionine, phenylalanine, tryptophan, and proline have non-polar, hydrophobic functional groups. Serine, threonine, cysteine, tyrosine, asparagine, and glutamine have polar functional groups. Arginine, lysine, and histidine have charged functional groups that are basic, and aspartic acid and glutamic acid have charged functional groups that are acidic.

A **peptide bond** can form between the carboxylic-acid group of one amino acid and the amine group of another amino acid, joining the two amino acids. A long chain of amino acids is called a polypeptide or a protein. Because there are so many different amino acids and because they can be arranged in an infinite number of combinations, proteins can have very complex structures.

There are four levels of protein structure, which will be discussed in more depth in another section. Briefly, **primary structure** is the linear sequence of the amino acids; it determines the overall structure of the protein and how the functional groups are positioned in relation to each other, as well as how they interact.

Secondary structure is the interaction between different atoms in the backbone chain of the protein. The two main types of secondary structure are the **alpha helix** and the **beta sheet**. Alpha helices are formed when the N-H of one amino acid forms a hydrogen bond with the C=O of an amino acid positioned three or four residues earlier in the chain.

The functional groups of certain amino acids—including methionine, alanine, uncharged leucine, glutamate, and lysine—make the formation of alpha helices more likely. The functional groups of other amino acids, such as proline and glycine, make the formation of alpha helices less likely. Alpha helices are right-handed and have 3.6 residues per turn. Proteins with alpha helices can span the cell membrane and are often involved in DNA, or deoxyribonucleic acid, binding.

Beta sheets are formed when a protein strand is stretched out, allowing for hydrogen bonding with a neighboring strand. Similar to alpha helices, certain amino acids have an increased propensity to form beta sheets.

Tertiary protein structure forms from the interactions between the different functional groups and gives the protein its overall geometric shape. Interactions that are important for tertiary structure include hydrophobic interactions between non-polar side groups, hydrogen bonds, salt bridges, and disulfide bonds.

Quaternary structure is the interaction that occurs between two different polypeptide chains and involves the same properties as tertiary structure. Only proteins that have more than one chain have quaternary structure.

Protein Structure

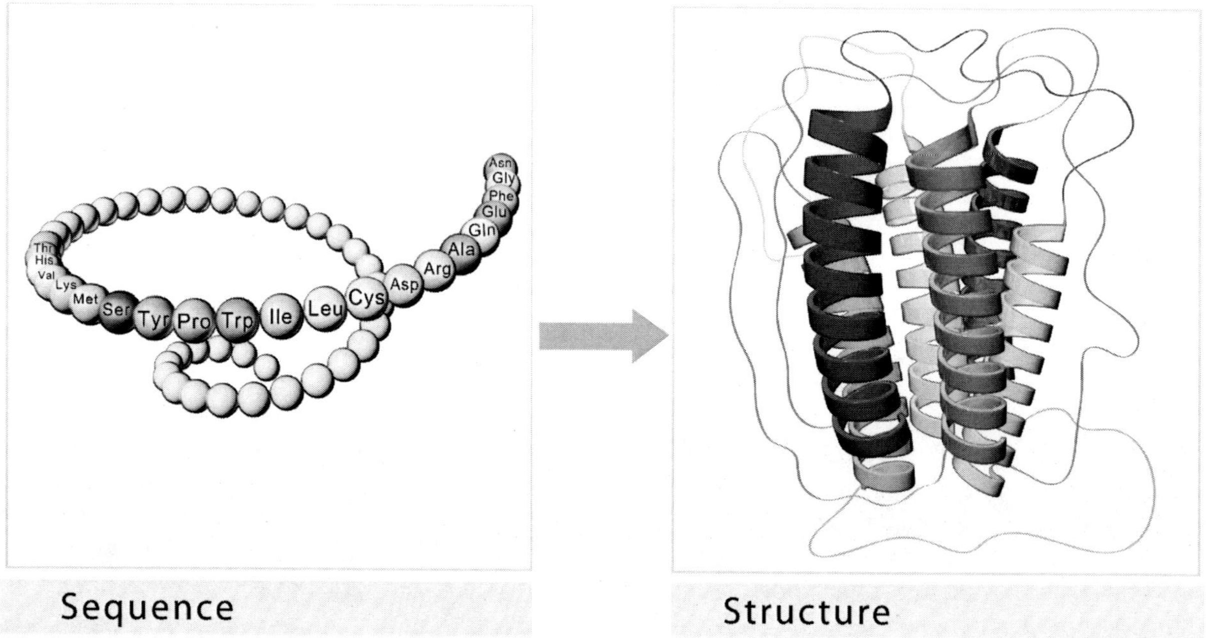

As mentioned, the primary protein structure refers to the chain of amino acids. In living organisms, this structure is oriented in a left to right linear chain with the terminal amino group on the left, and the terminal carboxyl group on the right. Amino acids are classified as chiral or achiral, where **chiral** refers to the presence of the central carbon atom adjacent to the carboxyl group, which results in isomerism. All chiral amino acids are designated as L (**levorotary**), and the achiral molecules are designated as D (**dexter**) because the amine groups are positioned to the right of the central carbon. Examination of the primary structure can be used to predict the secondary and tertiary structures.

Depending on the hydrogen bonds, the secondary structure of proteins takes one of three forms: the α-helix, the β-sheet, and the β-turns. The **α-helix** is a right-handed coiled strand. The side-chain structures of the amino acid groups extend to the outside of the helix. The oxygen molecules of the C=O of the peptide bonds form hydrogen bonds with the hydrogen of the N-H structure located four amino acids below in the helical structure. The side chains are positioned beside the N-H groups.

The **β-sheets** are characterized by strands of amino acids lying side by side, which are joined by hydrogen bonds between the carbonyl oxygen molecules in one strand and the amino hydrogen molecules in an adjacent strand. Depending on the orientation of the N-terminus to the C-terminus, the two strands in the β-sheet are identified as parallel or anti-parallel.

β -Turns result when two anti-parallel β strands change direction, forming loops or "hairpin" turns as opposed to a helix or sheet. Hydrogen bonds between the carbonyl oxygen and the amine hydrogen secure the structure of the loop. Loops are most often located on the surface of the protein, and therefore they can interact with other proteins and molecules.

The development of the three-dimensional tertiary protein structure is the result of the bending and folding of the protein that results in the most stable configuration, which is also at the lowest possible energy state. The bonds that form between the side chains of the amino acids provide additional support to the tertiary structure.

Large proteins may have protein subunits that consist of numerous polypeptide chains. The quaternary structure is determined by the interaction between these subunits. Hydrogen bonds, disulfide-bridges, and salt bridges reflecting the interaction among these subunits define the final structure of the protein.

The **Ramachandran plot** is used to theorize possible configurations for the residue in a protein or to validate the structure of a protein by recording data points that occur in theorized areas of the plot.

Chemical Reactions

Types of Chemical Reactions

Chemical reactions are characterized by a chemical change in which the starting substances, or reactants, differ from the substances formed, or products. Chemical reactions may involve a change in color, the production of gas, the formation of a precipitate, or changes in heat content. The following table lists the five basic types of chemical reactions:

Reaction Type	Definition	Example
Decomposition	A compound is broken down into two or more smaller elements or compounds	$2H_2O \rightarrow 2H_2 + O_2$
Synthesis	Two or more elements or compounds are joined together to form a new compound	$2H_2 + O_2 \rightarrow 2H_2O$
Single Displacement (Substitution Reaction)	A single element or ion takes the place of another in a compound	$Zn + 2HCl \rightarrow ZnCl_2 + H_2$
Double Displacement (Metathesis Reaction)	Two elements or ions each exchange a single atom to form two different compounds, resulting in different combinations of cations and anions in the final compounds	$H_2SO_4 + 2NaOH \rightarrow Na_2SO_4 + 2H_2O$
Oxidation-Reduction (Redox Reaction)	Elements undergo a change in oxidation number	$2S_2O_3{}^2(aq) + I_2(aq) \rightarrow S_4O_6{}^2(aq) + 2I(aq)$
Acid-Base	Involves a reaction between an acid and a base, which usually produces a salt and water	$HBr + NaOH \rightarrow NaBr + H_2O$
Combustion	A hydrocarbon (a compound composed of only hydrogen and carbon) reacts with oxygen to form carbon dioxide and water	$CH_4 + 2O_2 \rightarrow CO_2 + 2H_2O$

Balancing Chemical Reactions

Chemical reactions are expressed using **chemical equations**. Chemical equations must be balanced with equivalent numbers of atoms for each type of element on each side of the equation. Antoine Lavoisier, a French chemist, was the first to propose the **Law of Conservation of Mass** for the purpose of balancing a chemical equation. The law states, "Matter is neither created nor destroyed during a chemical reaction."

The **reactants** are located on the left side of the arrow, while the **products** are located on the right side of the arrow. **Coefficients** are the numbers in front of the chemical formulas. **Subscripts** are the numbers to the lower right of chemical symbols in a formula. To tally atoms, one should multiply the formula's coefficient by the subscript of each chemical symbol. For example, the chemical equation $2 H_2 + O_2 \rightarrow 2H_2O$ is balanced. For H, the coefficient of 2 multiplied by the subscript 2 = 4 hydrogen atoms. For O, the coefficient of 1 multiplied by the subscript 2 = 2 oxygen atoms. Coefficients and subscripts of 1 are understood and never written. When known, the form of the substance is noted with (g)=gas, (s)=solid, (l)=liquid, or (aq)=aqueous.

Catalysts

Catalysts are substances that accelerate the speed of a chemical reaction. A catalyst remains unchanged throughout the course of a chemical reaction. In most cases, only small amounts of a catalyst are needed. Catalysts increase the rate of a chemical reaction by providing an alternate pathway, requiring less **activation energy**. Activation energy refers to the amount of energy required for the initiation of a chemical reaction.

Catalysts can be homogeneous or heterogeneous. Catalysts in the same phase of matter as the reaction's reactants are **homogeneous**, while catalysts in a different phase than the reactants are **heterogeneous**. It is important to remember that catalysts are selective. They don't accelerate the speed of any and all chemical reactions, but they do accelerate specific chemical reactions.

Enzymes

Enzymes are a class of catalysts instrumental in biochemical reactions. They are always, or nearly always, proteins. Like all catalysts, enzymes increase the rate of a chemical reaction by providing an alternate path, which lowers the activation energy. Enzymes catalyze thousands of chemical reactions in the human body. The protein structure of the enzyme contains an active site, which is the part of the molecule that binds the reacting molecule, or **substrate**. The "lock and key" analogy is used to describe the substrate "key" fitting precisely into the active site of the enzyme "lock" to form an enzyme-substrate complex.

Many enzymes work in tandem with cofactors or coenzymes to catalyze chemical reactions. **Cofactors** can be either **inorganic** (not containing carbon) or **organic** (containing carbon). Organic cofactors can be either coenzymes or prosthetic groups tightly bound to an enzyme. **Coenzymes** transport chemical groups from one enzyme to another. Within a cell, coenzymes are continuously regenerating and their concentrations are held at a steady state.

Several factors, including temperature, pH, and concentrations of the enzyme and substrate, can affect the catalytic activity of an enzyme. For humans, the optimal temperature for peak enzyme activity is approximately that of body temperature, at 98.6 °F, while the optimal pH for peak enzyme activity is approximately 7 to 8. Increasing the concentrations of either the enzyme or substrate will also increase the rate of reaction, up to a certain point.

The activity of enzymes can be regulated. A common form of metabolic control is **feedback inhibition**, where the pathway is controlled by inhibitory binding of the product to an enzyme earlier in the pathway.

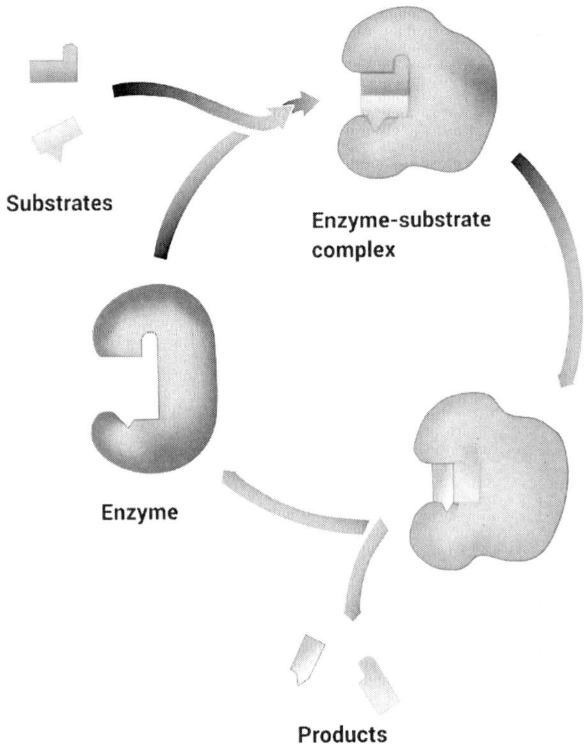

Transmission of Genetic Information from Gene to Protein

Nucleic Acids

Nucleic acids are made of nucleotides. Nucleotides consist of a five-carbon sugar, a nitrogen-containing base, and a phosphate group. **Deoxyribonucleic acid (DNA)** exists as two nucleotide chains arranged in a double helix. Each deoxyribose sugar is connected to a nitrogen base and an electrically-negative phosphate group. The nitrogen bases are adenine and guanine (the two-ringed purines), and cytosine and thymine (the one-ringed pyrimidines). The double helix is held together by weak hydrogen bonds that connect adenine to thymine and cytosine to guanine.

Ribonucleic acid (RNA) has a slightly different structure. It is usually single-stranded, has a ribose sugar as opposed to deoxyribose, and contains uracil instead of thymine.

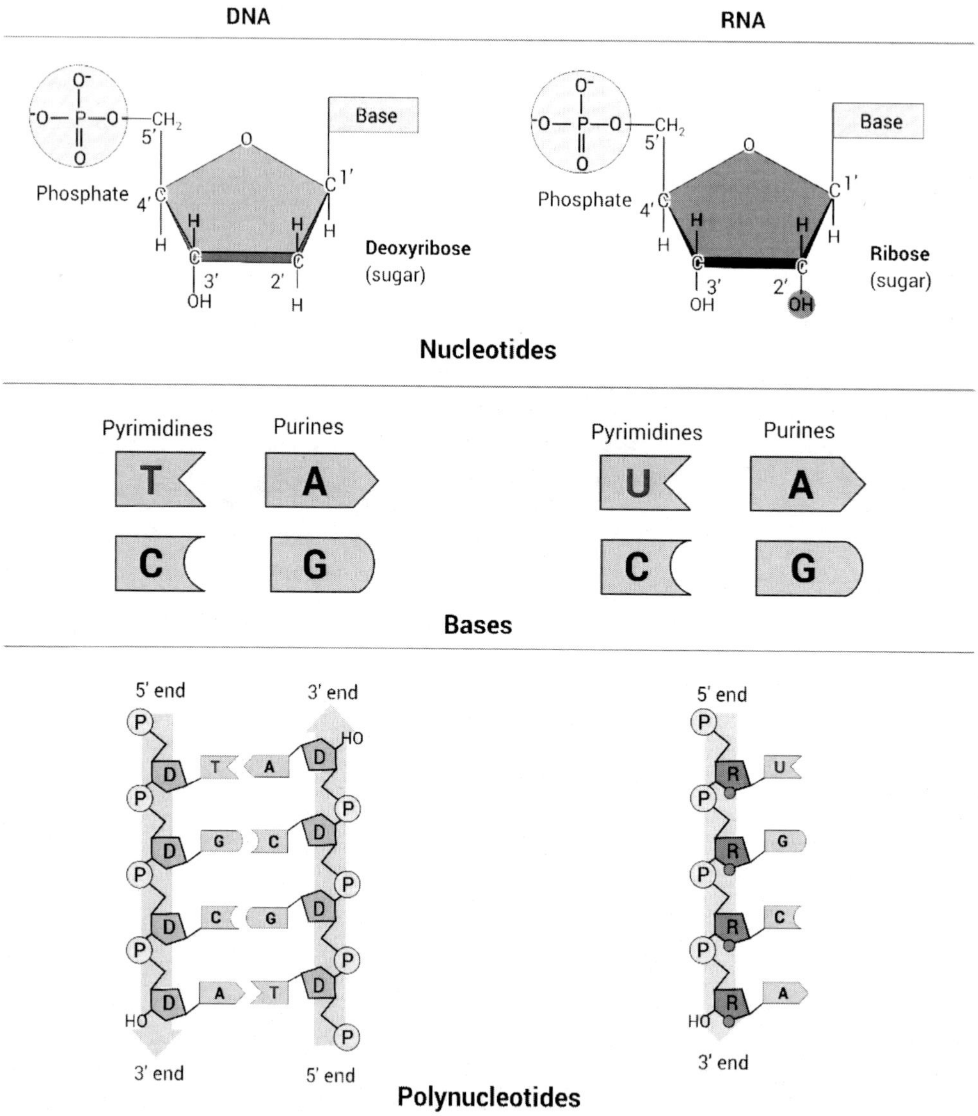

DNA forms the genetic code in the nucleus of eukaryotes, and RNA is the interpreter of that code. RNA exists in the following subtypes:

- **Messenger RNA** (mRNA) copies the DNA into a complementary transcript. This process is called **transcription**.
- **Ribosomal RNA** (rRNA) makes up the protein-manufacturing structure, called a ribosome, which reads the transcript in a process called **translation.**
- **Transfer RNA** (tRNA) carries amino acids and delivers them to the ribosomes. Each three letters of the mRNA transcript, or codon, recruits the anti-codon of a tRNA molecule, which carries the corresponding amino acid.

Genes and Heredity

Genes are the basis of heredity. The German scientist Gregor Mendel first suggested the existence of genes in 1866. A gene can be pinpointed to a locus, or a particular position, on DNA. It is estimated that humans have approximately 20,000 to 25,000 genes. For any particular gene, a human inherits one copy from each parent for a total of two.

Chromosomes, Genes, Proteins, RNA, and DNA

Chromosomes are composed of hundreds to thousands of genes. Human cells contain 23 pairs of chromosomes for a total of 46 chromosomes. As explained above, genes are inherited in pairs, one from each parent.

Proteins are made of long chains of amino acids. In total, there are 20 amino acids, 11 of which humans can synthesize on their own and the remaining 9 of which are procured through diet. DNA contains the information for the synthesis of proteins, but that information on DNA has to undergo transcription and translation by RNA in order to produce proteins.

Codons

A **codon** represents a sequence of three nucleotides that codes for either one specific amino acid or a stop signal during protein synthesis. Codons are found on messenger RNA (mRNA).

Twenty essential amino acids are utilized in the process of protein synthesis. The full set of codons encompasses 64 possible combinations and is termed the **genetic code**. In the genetic code, 61 codons represent amino acids and three codons are stop signals. The genetic code is **redundant**, since a single amino acid may be produced by multiple codons. For example, the codons AAA and AAG both produce the amino acid lysine. The codons UAA, UAG, and UGA are stop signals. The codon AUG codes for both the amino acid methionine and the start signal. As a result, AUG, when found in mRNA, marks the initiation point of protein translation.

RNA

Ribonucleic acid (RNA) plays crucial roles in protein synthesis and gene regulation. RNA is made of nucleotides consisting of ribose (a sugar), a phosphate group, and one of four possible nitrogen bases—adenine (A), cytosine (C), guanine (G), and uracil (U). RNA utilizes the nitrogen base uracil in place of the base thymine found in DNA. Another difference between RNA and DNA is that RNA is typically found as a single-stranded structure, while DNA typically exists in a double-stranded structure.

As mentioned, RNA can be categorized into three major groups—messenger RNA (mRNA), ribosomal RNA (rRNA), and transfer RNA (tRNA). Messenger RNA (mRNA) transports instructions from DNA in the nucleus of a cell to the areas responsible for protein synthesis in the cytoplasm of a cell. This process is known as transcription. Transfer RNA (tRNA) deciphers the amino acid sequence for the construction of proteins found in mRNA. Both tRNA and ribosomal RNA (rRNA) are found in the ribosomes of cells. Ribosomes are responsible for protein synthesis. The process is also known as translation and both tRNA and rRNA play crucial roles. Both translation and transcription are further described below.

DNA

Deoxyribonucleic acid, or DNA, contains the genetic material that is passed from parent to offspring. It contains specific instructions for the development and function of a unique eukaryotic organism. The great majority of cells in a eukaryotic organism contain the same DNA.

The majority of DNA can be found in the cell's nucleus and is referred to as **nuclear DNA**. A small amount of DNA can be located in the mitochondria and is referred to as **mitochondrial DNA**. Mitochondria are the site of aerobic energy production for the cell. All offspring inherit mitochondrial DNA from their mother. James Watson, an American geneticist, and Frances Crick, a British molecular biologist, first outlined the structure of DNA in 1953.

The structure of DNA visually approximates a twisting ladder and is described as a double helix. DNA is made of nucleotides consisting of deoxyribose (a sugar), a phosphate group, and one of four possible nitrogen bases—thymine (T), adenine (A), cytosine (C), and guanine (G). It is estimated that human DNA contains three billion bases. The sequence of these bases dictates the instructions contained in the DNA, making each species singular or unique. The bases in DNA pair in a particular manner—thymine (T) with adenine (A) and guanine (G) with cytosine (C). Weak hydrogen bonds amongst the nitrogen bases ensure easy uncoiling of DNA's double helical structure in preparation for replication.

Transcription

Transcription refers to a portion of DNA being copied into RNA, specifically mRNA. It represents the first crucial step in gene expression. The process begins with the enzyme **RNA polymerase** binding to the **promoter region** of DNA, which initiates transcription of a specific gene. RNA polymerase then untwists the double helix of DNA by breaking weak hydrogen bonds between its nucleotides. Once DNA is untwisted, RNA polymerase travels down the strand reading the DNA sequence and adding complementary nitrogen bases. With the assistance of RNA polymerase, the pentose sugar and phosphate functional group are added to the nitrogen base to form a nucleotide. Lastly, the weak hydrogen bonds uniting the DNA-RNA complex are broken to free the newly formed mRNA. The mRNA travels from the nucleus of the cell out to the cytoplasm of the cell where translation occurs.

Translation

Translation refers to the process of ribosomes synthesizing proteins. It represents the second crucial step in gene expression. The instructions encoding specific proteins to be made are contained in codons on mRNA, which have previously been transcribed from DNA. Each codon represents a specific amino acid or stop signal in the genetic code.

Amino acids are the building blocks of proteins. Ribosomes contain transfer RNA (tRNA) and ribosomal RNA (rRNA). Translation occurs in ribosomes located in the cytoplasm of cells and consists of the following three phases:

1. **Initiation**: The ribosome gathers at a target point on the mRNA, and tRNA attaches at the start codon (AUG), which is also the codon for the amino acid methionine.

2. **Elongation**: A new tRNA reads the next codon on the mRNA and links the two amino acids together with a peptide bond. The process is repeated until a polypeptide, or long chain of amino acids, is formed.

3. **Termination**: The ribosome disengages from the mRNA when it encounters a stop codon (UAA, UAG, or UGA). This event releases the polypeptide molecule. Proteins are made of one or more polypeptide molecules.

Genotypes and Phenotypes

Genotype refers to the genetic makeup of an individual within a species. **Phenotype** refers to the visible characteristics and observable behavior of an individual within a species.

Genotypes are written with pairs of letters that represent alleles. **Alleles** are different versions of the same gene, and, in simple systems, each gene has one dominant allele and one recessive allele. The letter of the **dominant** trait is capitalized, while the letter of the **recessive** trait is not capitalized. An individual can be homozygous dominant, homozygous recessive, or heterozygous for a particular gene. **Homozygous** means that the individual inherits two alleles of the same type while **heterozygous** means that the organism inherited one dominant allele and one recessive allele.

If an individual has homozygous dominant alleles or heterozygous alleles, the dominant allele is expressed. If an individual has homozygous recessive alleles, the recessive allele is expressed. For example, imagine a species of bird can develop either white or black feathers. The white feathers are the dominant allele, or trait (*A*), while the black feathers are the recessive allele (*a*). Homozygous dominant (*AA*) and heterozygous (*Aa*) birds will develop white feathers. Homozygous recessive (aa) birds will develop black feathers.

Genotype (genetic makeup)	Phenotype (observable traits)
AA	white feathers
Aa	white feathers
aa	black feathers

Influence of Phenotype on Genotype

The genetic material (DNA) inherited from an individual's parents determines genotype. Natural selection leads to adaptations within a species, which affects the phenotype. Over time, individuals within a species with the most advantageous phenotypes will survive and reproduce. As result of reproduction, the subsequent generation of phenotypes receives the fittest genotype. Eventually, the individuals within a species with genetic fitness flourish and those without it are erased from the environment. This is also referred to as the concept of "survival of the fittest." When this process is duplicated over numerous generations, the outcome is offspring with a level of genetic fitness that meets or exceeds that of their parents.

Mendel's Laws of Genetics and Punnett Squares

Mendel's first law of genetics is the principle of **segregation** and states that alleles will segregate into different cells during the formation of gametes in meiosis. Mendel's second law of genetics is the principle of **independent assortment** and states that genes for different traits will be assigned to different gametes independent of the others. Together, these two laws state the assumptions on which genetic probabilities are based.

Punnett squares are simple graphic representations of all the possible genotypes of offspring, given the genotypes of the parent organisms. For instance, in the above example with the species of bird with black or white feathers, *A* represents a dominant allele and determines white colored feathers on a bird. The recessive allele *a* determines black colored feathers on a bird. If both parents are heterozygous (*Aa*, the x- and y-axis of the square) the offspring will have the possible genotypes *AA*, *Aa*, *Aa*, and *aa*. Phenotypically, three offspring would have white feathers and one would have black feathers, as shown in the below Punnett square.

	A	a
A	White	White
a	White	Black

Monohybrid and Dihybrid Genetic Crosses

Genetic crosses represent all possible permutations of gene combinations, or alleles. A **monohybrid cross** investigates the inheritance pattern of a single gene such as in the above example of the birds with black or white feathers. Both parents must have heterozygous gene pairs in a monohybrid cross.

The phenotypic ratio for a monohybrid cross is 3:1 (*AA*, *Aa*, *Aa*, *aa*), in favor of the dominant gene. A **dihybrid cross** investigates the inheritance patterns of two genes that are related, for example *A* and *B*. A dihybrid cross has a phenotypic ratio of 9:3:3:1, with nine offspring inheriting both dominant genes, six offspring inheriting a single dominant and a single recessive gene, and one offspring inheriting both recessive genes.

Transmission of Heritable Information from Generation to Generation

Natural Selection and Adaptation

The **theory of natural selection** is one of the fundamental tenets of evolution. It affects the phenotype, or visible characteristics, of individuals in a species, which ultimately affects the genotype, or genetic makeup, of those same individuals. Charles Darwin was the first to explain the theory of natural selection, and it was described by Herbert Spencer as favoring **survival of the fittest.** Natural selection encompasses three assumptions:

1. A species has **heritable** traits: All traits have some likelihood of being propagated to offspring.
2. The traits of a species vary: Some traits are more advantageous than others.
3. Individuals of a species are subject to differing rates of reproduction: Some individuals of a species may not get the opportunity to reproduce while others reproduce frequently.

Over time, certain variations in traits may increase both the survival and reproduction of certain individuals within a species. The desirable heritable traits are passed on from generation to generation. Eventually, the desirable traits will become more common and permeate the entire species. **Natural selection** is one of the processes leading to the theory of evolutionary change and is the primary determinant of how a species adapts to its environment.

Adaptation

The theory of **adaptation** is defined as an alteration in a species that causes it to become more well-suited to its environment. It increases the probability of survival, thus increasing the rate of successful reproduction. As a result, an adaptation becomes more common within the population of that species.

For examples, bats use reflected sound waves (echolocation) to prey on insects, and chameleons change colors to blend in with their surroundings to evade detection by its prey and predators. Adaptations are brought about by natural selection.

Adaptive radiation refers to rapid diversification within a species into an array of unique forms. It may occur as a result of changes in a habitat, which creates new challenges, ecological niches, or natural resources.

A classic example of the theory of adaptive radiation is that of Darwin's finches. Charles Darwin documented 13 varieties of finches on the Galapagos Islands. Each island in the chain presented a unique and changing environment, which caused rapid adaptive radiation among the finches. There was also diversity among finches inhabiting the same island. Because of natural selection, each variety of finch developed adaptations to fit into its native environment.

A major adaptation of Darwin's finches had to do with the size and shapes of their beaks. The variation in beaks allowed the finches to access different foods and natural resources, which decreased competition and preserved resources. As a result, various finches of the same species could coexist, thrive, and diversify. Finches had:

- Short beaks, which were better adapted to foraging for seeds
- Thin, sharp beaks, which were better adapted to preying on insects
- Long beaks, which were better suited for probing for food inside plants

The adaptive radiation among Darwin's finches on the Galapagos Islands resulted from chance mutations in genes transmitted from generation to generation.

Principles of Bioenergetics and Fuel Molecule Metabolism

Bioenergetics

Bioenergetics refers to the flow of energy within a biological system and is primarily focused on how chemical energy in the macronutrients from food (i.e., carbohydrates, proteins, fats) is converted into biologically-usable forms of energy (i.e., substrates) that organisms can use to perform work.

Catabolism

Catabolism is the process of breaking large molecules into smaller molecules to make energy available to the organism. For example, carbohydrates are catabolized to provide fuel for exercise and daily living. Catabolism also can involve the breakdown of muscle tissue during periods of heavy training volumes, low caloric intake, or high stress.

Anabolism

Anabolism is the process of restructuring or building larger compounds from catabolized materials, such as assembling amino acids into structural proteins, which are needed to maintain homeostasis and to generate new muscle tissue.

Metabolism is the sum total of the chemical processes that occur within a cell for the maintenance of life. It includes both the synthesizing and breaking down of substances. A **metabolic pathway** begins with a molecule and ends with a specific product after going through a series of reactions, often involving an enzyme at each step. **Catabolic pathways** are metabolic pathways in which energy is released, as complex molecules are broken down into simpler molecules. In contrast, **anabolic pathways** use energy to build complex molecules out of simpler molecules. With cell metabolism, it is important to remember the first law of thermodynamics: Energy can be transformed, but it cannot be created or destroyed. Therefore, the energy released in a cell by catabolic pathways is used up in anabolic pathways.

The reactions that occur within metabolic pathways are classified as either exergonic reactions or endergonic reactions. **Exergonic reactions** end in a release of free energy, while endergonic reactions absorb free energy from the surroundings. **Free energy** is the portion of energy in a system, such as a living cell, that can be used to perform work, such as a chemical reaction. It is denoted as the capital letter G, and the change in free energy from a reaction or set of reactions is denoted as delta G (ΔG). When reactions do not require an input of energy, they are said to occur spontaneously. Exergonic reactions are considered **spontaneous** because they result in a negative delta G ($-\Delta G$), where the products of the reaction have less free energy within them than the reactants. **Endergonic reactions** require an input of energy and result in a positive delta G ($+\Delta G$), with the products of the reaction containing more free energy than the individual reactants. When a system no longer has free energy to do work, it has reached **equilibrium**. Since cells always need to do work, they are no longer alive if they reach true equilibrium.

Cells balance their energy resources by using the energy from exergonic reactions to drive endergonic reactions forward, a process called **energy coupling**. **Adenosine triphosphate**, or ATP, is a molecule that is an immediate source of energy for cellular work. When it is broken down, it releases energy used in endergonic reactions and anabolic pathways. ATP breaks down into **adenosine diphosphate**, or ADP, and a separate phosphate group, releasing energy in an exergonic reaction. As ATP is used up by reactions, it is also regenerated by having a new phosphate group added onto the ADP products within the cell in an endergonic reaction.

As mentioned, **enzymes** are special proteins that help speed up metabolic reactions and pathways. They do not change the overall free energy release or consumption of reactions; they just make the reactions occur more quickly by lowering the required activation energy. Enzymes are designed to act only on specific substrates. Their physical shape fits snugly onto their matched substrates, so enzymes only speed up reactions that contain the substrates to which they are matched.

Adenosine Triphosphate (ATP)

ATP is a high-energy molecule used for muscle contractions, endergonic reactions, movement, and other life-sustaining metabolic processes. ATP is an **intermediate molecule** (consisting of three primary parts—an adenine, a ribose, and three phosphates in a chain) that allows energy to transfer from exergonic to endergonic and catabolic to anabolic reactions. ATP is generated and replenished in skeletal muscles by three energy systems: phosphagen, glycolytic, and oxidative.

ATP Hydrolysis

Hydrolysis is a general term for any chemical reaction that breaks a chemical body via the addition of water. ATP hydrolysis splits the ATP molecule into adenosine diphosphate (ADP) and usable energy. The enzyme **adenosine triphosphatase** (ATPase) is the catalyst for the hydrolysis of ATP. The following equation shows the **reactants** (left of arrow), enzyme (middle), and **products** (right of arrow) for ATP hydrolysis:

$$\text{ATP} + \text{H}_2\text{O} \leftarrow \text{ATPase} \rightarrow \text{ADP} + \text{P}_\text{i} + \text{H}^+ + \text{Energy}$$

When ATP undergoes hydrolysis, ADP (containing two phosphate groups), an inorganic phosphate molecule, a hydrogen ion, and free energy are produced.

ATPase is the enzyme responsible for catalyzing the breakdown of ATP to ADP. The dephosphorylation reaction results in the release of energy, which is then used to carry out other chemical reactions.

Myosin ATPase catalyzes ATP hydrolysis, providing the energy for cross-bridge recycling.

Calcium ATPase provides the energy used to regulate calcium movement, by pumping it into the sarcoplasmic reticulum.

The ATP - ADP Cycle

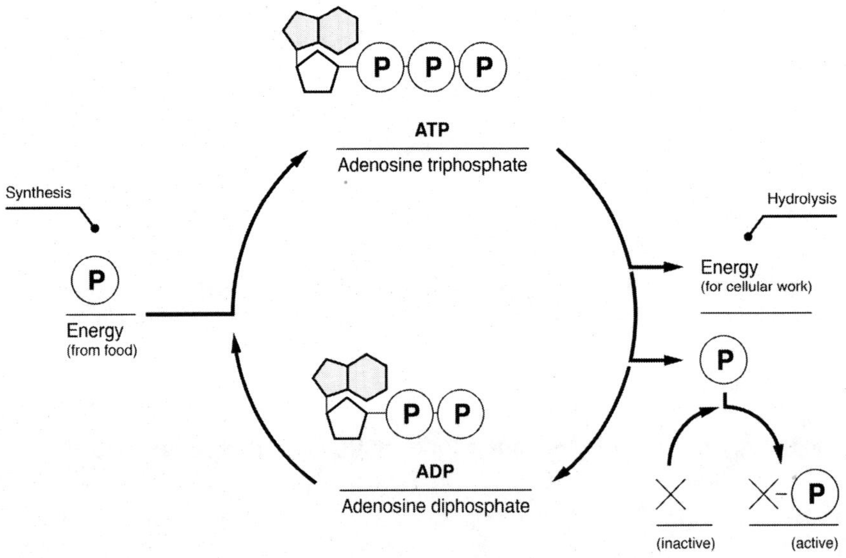

Sodium-Potassium ATPase controls the sodium potassium concentration gradient in the sarcolemma after depolarization to maintain the cellular resting potential. For every two K^+ ions pumped in, there are three NA^+ ions pumped out of the cell.

Adenosine Monophosphate (AMP)

Adenosine Monophosphate (AMP) results from ADP hydrolysis, which cleaves the second phosphate group, leaving one.

Biological Energy Systems

There are several basic biological energy systems in muscle cells that replace ATP. The **phosphagen** and **glycolytic** systems are **anaerobic** mechanisms, operating in the sarcoplasm, and do not require oxygen. The **electron transport chain** (ETC) and **Krebs cycle** are **aerobic** mechanisms that require oxygen and occur in the mitochondria. The cellular respiration systems act in concert, rather than individually, to provide all of the required energy during exercise or rest.

Phosphagen System (ATP-phosphocreatine [PC])

The **phosphagen** system utilizes ATP hydrolysis for high-intensity, short duration activities (e.g., resistance training; short, intense sprints; other vigorous bouts up to about 10 seconds in duration) and this system is also active at the start of all types of exercise of varying intensities until the other systems have time to produce energy. This system relies on the breakdown of **creatine phosphate** (CP) for energy. Because ATP stores are quickly depleted and ATP is required for cellular functions other than muscle contractions, the phosphagen system uses CP stores to maintain ATP concentrations. This system is rapidly depleted after about 10 seconds of maximal intensity work, so the glycolytic system starts to engage and contribute energy after this point. It takes longer for glycolysis, and especially oxidative energy systems, to generate energy, which is why the phosphagen system is the initial source.

Creatine Phosphate (CP)

CP, also called **phosphocreatine** (PC), concentrations in muscles are four to six times greater than ATP muscle stores, with higher CP concentrations in Type II muscle fibers. The phosphagen system uses creatine kinase in the chemical reaction that combines a phosphate group from CP with ADP to replenish ATP. CP is stored in small amounts, limiting the phosphagen system to only supplying energy for intense, short bouts of exercise.

$$\text{ADP} + \text{CP} \leftarrow \text{creatine kinase} \rightarrow \text{ATP} + \text{Creatine}$$

Creatine Kinase

Creatine kinase is the enzyme required to catalyze the reaction that combines ADP and CP to form ATP and creatine. Elevated levels of creatine kinase in blood serum tests are indicative of muscle damage (e.g., kidney failure, heart attack). In athletes, too much work performed in a training session (single or aggregate sessions) can cause **rhabdomyolysis**, the rapid breakdown of muscle tissue, which elevates circulating levels of creatine kinase.

Adenylate Kinase

Also called **myokinase**, this enzyme catalyzes a reaction that replenishes ATP:

$$2\text{ADP} \leftarrow \text{adenylate kinase} \rightarrow \text{ATP} + \text{AMP}$$

Law of Mass Action/Mass Action Effect

This law states that the concentration of reactants, products, or both in a solution will influence the direction of the reactions. These are often referred to as near-equilibrium reactions because they continue in the direction based on the concentration of available reactants. This equilibrium is specific to the amount of ATP needed for the particular physical work being completed by the individual. The reactions will continue until the physical activity intensity is low enough for another energy system to take over or the exercise ends.

Glycolytic System

Glycolysis

Glycolysis is the breakdown of carbohydrates, either stored in the muscles or liver as glycogen or circulating in blood as glucose, to replenish ATP. ATP replenished during glycolysis is slower than the replenishment provided by the single-step phosphagen system because glycolysis has several steps and actually requires an investment of energy to drive some of the early steps in the energy pathway. The glycolytic system has an advantage, as it can produce significantly more ATP because of the relatively large supply of glucose and glycogen in the body versus the limited supply of CP.

Anaerobic Glycolysis

ATP is produced by breaking down glucose without oxygen available during glycolysis. This process relies on converting pyruvate to lactate to replace ATP during short, high-intensity activity lasting two minutes or less. Once the lactate threshold is reached, pyruvate is shuttled to the mitochondria for the Krebs cycle.

Pyruvate

Pyruvate is the result of anaerobic glycolysis; one glucose molecule produces two pyruvate molecules. Pyruvate can either be converted to lactate in the sarcoplasm or it can be transported to the mitochondria for the **Krebs cycle**. Compared to pyruvate's conversion to lactate, the Krebs cycle takes longer to replenish ATP because more reactions are required. However, the Krebs cycle can continue for a longer duration when exercise intensity is low. This process is **aerobic glycolysis** (also called **slow glycolysis**).

Pyruvate conversion to lactate: The enzyme lactate dehydrogenase catalyzes lactate from pyruvate. The reaction converting pyruvate to lactate is provided below. **Lactate** produced by anaerobic glycolysis can be cleared by oxidation within the muscle fiber, or it can be moved to the liver via the blood, where it is converted into glucose. The process of the liver turning lactate to glucose is referred to as the **Cori cycle**.

The net reaction of glycolysis when pyruvate is converted to lactate:

$$\text{Glucose} + 2\text{P}_\text{i} + 2\text{ADP} \rightarrow 2\text{Lactate} + 2\text{ATP} + \text{H}_2\text{O}$$

Pyruvate transported to mitochondria for Krebs cycle: If oxygen is available, pyruvate will be transported to the mitochondria along with two molecules of **nicotinamide adenine dinucleotide** (NADH). Pyruvate is converted to acetyl-coenzyme A (acetyl-CoA) by pyruvate dehydrogenase, resulting in the loss of carbon dioxide (CO_2), and enters the Krebs cycle to resynthesize ATP. The **Krebs cycle**, a continuation of the substrate oxidation from glycolysis, is a series of reactions that results in the production of two ATP molecules.

The net reaction for glycolysis when pyruvate is transported to the mitochondria:

$$\text{Glucose} + 2\text{P}_\text{i} + 2\text{ADP} + 2\text{NAD} \rightarrow 2\text{Pyruvate} + 2\text{ATP} + 2\text{NADH} + 2\text{H}_2\text{O}$$

Phosphorylation

Phosphorylation is the addition of an inorganic phosphate to a molecule. Phosphorylation of ADP to ATP occurs by adding a phosphoryl (PO_3) group to ADP.

Substrate-Level Phosphorylation

Substrate-level phosphorylation refers to a single enzyme-generated reaction that uses ADP to directly resynthesize ATP. Substrate-level phosphorylation occurs during **anaerobic glycolysis** (fast phosphorylation) and can occur during both anaerobic and aerobic activities.

Oxidative Phosphorylation

This is the process of ATP being resynthesized via the actions of the electron transport chain (ETC). The oxidative system produces approximately thirty-eight ATP molecules when a molecule of glucose is processed through glycolysis, the Krebs cycle, and the ETC. The oxidative system produces approximately 90 percent of ATP, while substrate-level phosphorylation accounts for approximately 10 percent of ATP production.

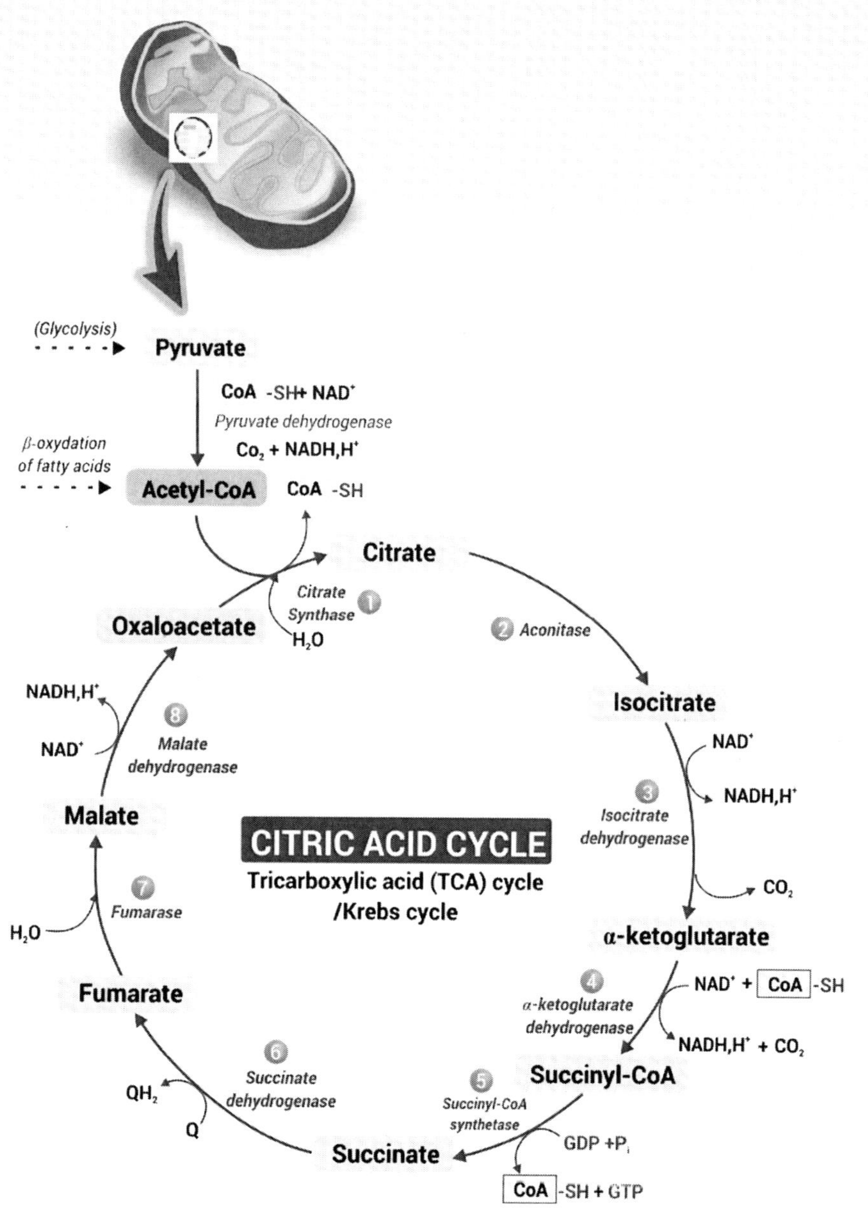

Electron Transport Chain (ETC)

In addition to two pyruvate molecules produced by glycolysis, six molecules of NADH and two molecules of flavin adenine dinucleotide ($FADH_2$) are produced and used by the ETC. Hydrogen atoms, transported by NADH and $FADH_2$ to the ETC, are used to produce ATP from ADP. The hydrogen atoms form a proton concentration gradient down the

ETC, which produces energy required to form ATP. NADH and $FADH_2$ molecules re-phosphorylate ADP to ATP via the ETC, with each NADH producing three ATP molecules and each $FADH_2$ producing two ATP molecules.

Oxidative System

During low-intensity activity and while the body is at rest, the primary source of ATP is the oxidative system, which utilizes carbohydrates and fats as substrates. Fats, compared to carbohydrates and proteins, have the greatest capacity for ATP production through their metabolism. Protein is not a primary substrate and is only used for energy during long-duration exercise (more than 90 minutes) or times of starvation. During rest, the majority of ATP (approximately 70 percent) is produced from fat, with approximately 30 percent coming from carbohydrates. With the initiation of high-intensity activity, nearly 100 percent of ATP comes from carbohydrates. During long bouts of submaximal exercise, carbohydrates are used initially (due to their faster metabolism), but there is a slow shift back to using fats, as glycogen stores deplete.

Net ATP Production

The **net ATP production** from the oxidation of one glucose molecule can be determined by adding the number of ATP molecules produced during each process. During glycolysis, substrate-level phosphorylation and oxidative phosphorylation produce four and six ATP molecules, respectively. During the Krebs cycle, substrate-level phosphorylation produces two ATP molecules, oxidative phosphorylation of eight NADH produces twenty-four ATP molecules, and two $FADH_2$ molecules produce four ATP. These processes combined yield a total of forty ATP molecules. Two ATP molecules are used by glycolysis, so the net ATP production from one molecule of glucose is thirty-eight ATP molecules.

Substrates

Carbohydrates

Carbohydrates are usually sweet, ring-like sugar molecules that are built from carbon (carbo-), oxygen, and hydrogen (-hydrates, meaning water). They can exist as one-ring **monosaccharides**, like glucose, fructose, and galactose, or as two-ring **disaccharides**, like lactose, maltose, and sucrose. These simple sugars can be easily broken down and used via glycolysis to provide a source of quick energy. **Polysaccharides** are repeating chains of monosaccharide rings. They are more complex carbohydrates, and there are several types. For example:

- Plants store energy in the form of **starch**.
- Animals store energy in the form of **glycogen**. Vertebrates store glycogen in the liver and in muscle cells.
- **Cellulose** is the chief structural component of plant cell walls.
- **Chitin** is the chief structural component of fungi cell walls and the exoskeletons of arthropods.

Lipids

Lipids are mostly non-polar, hydrophobic molecules that are insoluble in water. **Triglycerides** are a type of lipid with a glycerol backbone attached to three long fatty acid chains. These energy-storage molecules can exist as any of the following types:

- **Saturated fats** have no double bonds within their fatty acid tails. These are solid at room temperature and are mostly animal fats like bacon fat.
- **Unsaturated fats** have double bonds within any of their fatty acid tails. Due to the kinks caused by the double bonds, these fats are liquid at room temperature and are mostly plant fats like olive oil.

Phospholipids are also composed of glycerol, except they only have two fatty acid tails. The third tail is replaced with a hydrophilic phosphate group. The **amphipathic** nature of this molecule results in a lipid bilayer where the "water-loving" **hydrophilic** heads face the extracellular matrix and cytoplasm, and the "water-fearing" **hydrophobic** tails face each other on the inside.

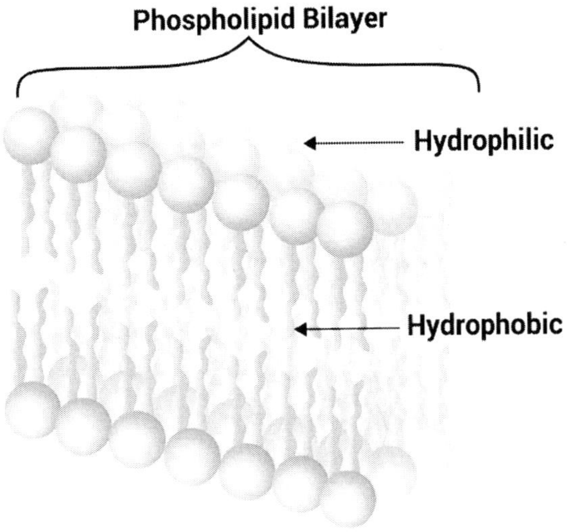

Steroids are another type of lipid. **Cholesterol** is a steroid that is embedded in the cell membranes of animal cells and acts as a fluidity buffer. Steroid hormones, such as testosterone and estrogen, are responsible for transcriptional regulation in certain cells.

Foundational Concept 2: Highly-organized assemblies of molecules, cells, and organs interact to carry out the functions of living organisms.

Assemblies of Molecules, Cells, and Groups of Cells Within Unicellular and Multicellular Organisms

Cell Structure and Function

The **cell** is the main functional and structural component of all living organisms. Robert Hooke, an English scientist, coined the term "cell" in 1665. Hooke's discovery laid the groundwork for the **cell theory**, which is composed of three principles:

1. All organisms are composed of cells.
2. All existing cells are created from other living cells.
3. The cell is the most fundamental unit of life.

Organisms can be **unicellular** (composed of one cell) or **multicellular** (composed of many cells). All cells are bounded by a cell membrane, filled with cytoplasm of some sort, and are coded for by a genetic sequence.

The cell membrane separates a cell's internal and external environments. It is a **selectively permeable** membrane, which usually only allows the passage of certain molecules by diffusion. Phospholipids and proteins are crucial components of all cell membranes. The **cytoplasm** is the cell's internal environment and is **aqueous**, or water-based. The **genome** represents the genetic material inside the cell that is passed on from generation to generation.

Prokaryotes and Eukaryotes

Prokaryotic cells are much smaller than eukaryotic cells. The vast majority of prokaryotes are unicellular, while the majority of eukaryotes are multicellular. Prokaryotic cells have no nucleus, and their genome is found in an area known as the **nucleoid**. They also do not have membrane-bound **organelles**, which are "little organs" that perform specific functions within a cell.

Eukaryotic cells have a proper **nucleus**, which contains the genome. They also have numerous membrane-bound organelles such as lysosomes, endoplasmic reticula (rough and smooth), Golgi complexes, and mitochondria.

The majority of prokaryotic cells have cell walls, while most eukaryotic cells do not have cell walls. The DNA of prokaryotic cells is contained in a single circular chromosome, while the DNA of eukaryotic cells is contained in multiple linear chromosomes. Prokaryotic cells divide using binary fission, while eukaryotic cells divide using mitosis. Examples of prokaryotes are bacteria and archaea, while examples of eukaryotes are animals and plants.

Nuclear Parts of a Cell

Nucleus (plural nuclei): Houses a cell's genetic material, deoxyribonucleic acid (DNA), which is used to form chromosomes. A single nucleus is the defining characteristic of eukaryotic cells. The nucleus of a cell controls gene expression. It ensures genetic material is transmitted from one generation to the next.

Chromosomes: Complex thread-like arrangements composed of DNA that is found in a cell's nucleus. Humans have 23 pairs of chromosomes, for a total of 46.

Chromatin: An aggregate of genetic material, consisting of DNA and proteins, that forms chromosomes during cell division.

Nucleolus (plural nucleoli): The largest component of the nucleus of a eukaryotic cell. With no membrane, the primary function of the nucleolus is the production of ribosomes, which are crucial to the synthesis of proteins.

Cell Membranes

Cell membranes enclose the cell's cytoplasm, separating the intracellular environment from the extracellular environment. They are selectively permeable, which enables them to control molecular traffic entering and exiting cells. Cell membranes are made of a double layer of phospholipids studded with proteins. Cholesterol is also dispersed in the phospholipid bilayer of cell membranes to provide stability. The proteins in the phospholipid bilayer aid the transport of molecules across cell membranes.

Scientists use the term "fluid mosaic model" to refer to the arrangement of phospholipids and proteins in cell membranes. In this model, phospholipids have a head region and a tail region. The head region of the phospholipids is attracted to water (hydrophilic), while the tail region is repelled by it (hydrophobic). Because they are hydrophilic, the heads of the phospholipids are facing the water, on the outside of the cell and lining the inside. Because they are hydrophobic, the tails of the phospholipids are oriented inward between both head regions. This orientation constructs the phospholipid bilayer.

As mentioned, cell membranes have the distinct trait of selective permeability. The fact that cell membranes are **amphiphilic** (having hydrophilic and hydrophobic zones) contributes to this trait. As a result, cell membranes can regulate the flow of molecules into and out of the cell.

Factors relating to molecules, such as size, polarity, and solubility, determine their likelihood of passage across cell membranes. Small molecules can diffuse easily across cell membranes compared to large molecules. **Polarity** refers to the charge present in a molecule. **Polar** molecules have regions, or poles, of positive and negative charge and are water-soluble, while **non-polar** molecules have no charge and are fat-soluble. **Solubility** refers to the ability of a substance, called a **solute**, to dissolve in a solvent. A **soluble** substance can be dissolved in a solvent, while an

insoluble substance cannot be dissolved in a solvent. Non-polar, fat-soluble substances have a much easier time passing through cell membranes compared to polar, water-soluble substances.

Passive Transport Mechanisms

Passive transport refers to the migration of molecules across a cell membrane that does not require energy. The three types of passive transport are simple diffusion, facilitated diffusion, and osmosis.

Simple diffusion relies on a **concentration gradient**, or differing quantities of molecules inside or outside of a cell. During simple diffusion, molecules move from an area of high concentration to an area of low concentration. **Facilitated diffusion** utilizes carrier proteins to transport molecules across a cell membrane. **Osmosis** refers to the transport of water across a selectively-permeable membrane. During osmosis, water moves from a region of low solute concentration to a region of high solute concentration.

Active Transport Mechanisms

Active transport refers to the energy-requiring migration of molecules across a cell membrane. It's a useful way to move molecules from an area of low concentration to an area of high concentration. Adenosine triphosphate (ATP), the currency of cellular energy, is needed to work against the concentration gradient.

Active transport can involve carrier proteins that cross the cell membrane to pump molecules and ions across the membrane, like in facilitated diffusion. The difference is that active transport uses the energy from ATP to drive this transport, as typically the ions or molecules are going against their concentration gradients. For example, glucose pumps in the kidney pump all of the glucose into the cells from the lumen of the nephron even though there is a higher concentration of glucose inside the cell than in the lumen. This is because glucose is a precious food source and the body wants to conserve as much as possible. Pumps can either send a molecule in one direction, multiple molecules in the same direction (**symports**), or multiple molecules in different directions (**antiports**).

Active transport can also involve the movement of membrane-bound particles, either into a cell (**endocytosis**) or out of a cell (**exocytosis**). The three major forms of endocytosis are: **pinocytosis**, where the cell is drinking and intakes only small molecules; **phagocytosis**, where the cell is eating and intakes large particles or small organisms; and **receptor-mediated endocytosis**, where the cell's membrane splits off to form an internal vesicle in response to molecules activating receptors on its surface. Exocytosis is the inverse of endocytosis, and the membranes of the vesicle join to that of the cell's surface while the molecules inside the vesicle are released outside. This is common in nervous and muscle tissue for the release of neurotransmitters, and in endocrine cells for the release of hormones. The two major categories of exocytosis are excretion and secretion. **Excretion** is defined as the removal of waste from a cell. **Secretion** is defined as the transport of molecules, such as hormones or enzymes, from a cell.

Structure and Function of Cellular Organelles

Organelles are specialized structures that perform specific tasks in a cell. The term literally means "little organs." Most organelles are membrane bound and serve as sites for the production or degradation of chemicals. The following are organelles found in eukaryotic cells:

Nucleus

A cell's **nucleus** contains genetic information in the form of DNA. The nucleus is surrounded by the **nuclear envelope**. A single nucleus is the defining characteristic of eukaryotic cells. The nucleus is also the most important organelle of the cell. It contains the nucleolus, which manufactures ribosomes (another organelle) that are crucial in **protein synthesis** (also called **gene expression**).

Mitochondria

The **mitochondrion** is the primary site of respiration and adenosine triphosphate (ATP) synthesis inside the cell. Mitochondria have two lipid bilayers that create the **intermembrane space**, which is the space between the two membranes, and the **matrix**, which is the space inside the inner membrane. While the outer membrane is smooth, the inner membrane is folded and forms **cristae**. The outer membrane is permeable to small molecules. The cristae contain many proteins involved in ATP synthesis. In the mitochondria, the products of glycolysis are further oxidized during the citric-acid cycle and the electron-transport chain. The two-layer structure of the mitochondria allows for the buildup of H+ ions produced during the electron-transport chain in the intermembrane space, which creates a proton gradient and an energy potential. This gradient drives the formation of ATP. Mitochondria have their own DNA and are capable of replication.

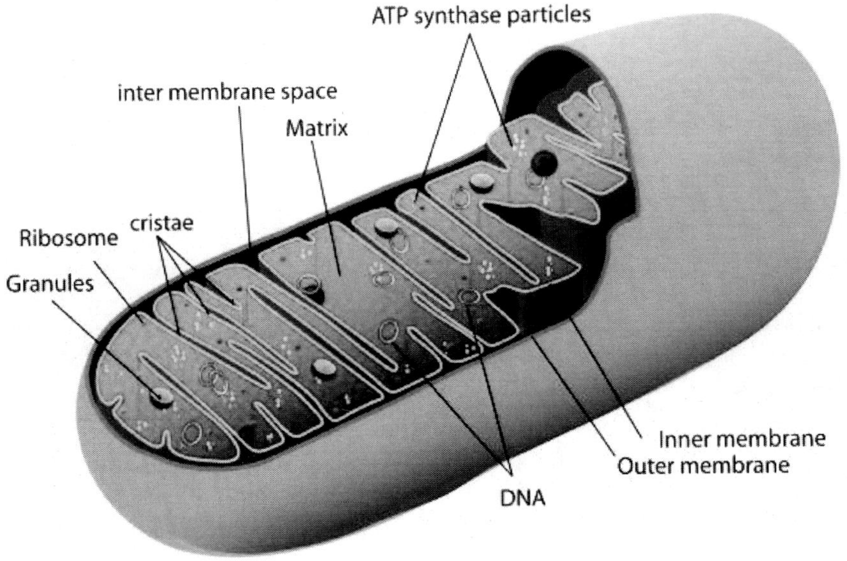

Rough Endoplasmic Reticulum

The **rough endoplasmic reticulum** (RER) is composed of linked membranous sacs called *cisternae* with ribosomes attached to their external surfaces. The RER is responsible for the production of proteins that will eventually get shipped out of the cell.

Smooth Endoplasmic Reticulum

The **smooth endoplasmic reticulum** (SER) is composed of linked membranous sacs called cisternae without ribosomes, which distinguishes it from the RER. The SER's main function is the production of carbohydrates and lipids, which can be created expressly for the cell, or to modify the proteins from the RER that will eventually get shipped out of the cell.

Golgi Apparatus

The **Golgi apparatus** is the site where proteins are modified; it is involved in the transport of proteins, lipids, and carbohydrates within the cell. The Golgi apparatus is made up of flat layers of membranes called **cisternae**. Material is transported in transfer vesicles from the ER to the **cis region** of the Golgi apparatus. From there, the material moves through the medial region, where it is sometimes modified, and then leaves through the **trans region** of the ER in a secretory vesicle.

Lysosomes

Lysosomes are specialized vesicles that contain enzymes capable of digesting food, surplus organelles, and foreign invaders such as bacteria and viruses. They often destroy dead cells in order to recycle cellular components. Lysosomes are found only in animal cells.

Secretory Vesicles

Secretory vesicles transport and deliver molecules into or out of the cell via the cell membrane. **Endocytosis** refers to the movement of molecules into a cell via secretory vesicles. **Exocytosis** refers to the movement of molecules out of a cell via secretory vesicles.

Ribosomes

Ribosomes are made up of ribosomal RNA molecules and a variety of proteins, and they are the structures that synthesize proteins. They consist of two subunits: small and large. The ribosomes use mRNA as a template for the protein and they use tRNA to bring amino acids to the ribosomes, where they are synthesized into peptide strands using the genetic code provided by the messenger RNA. Most ribosomes are attached to the ER membrane.

Cilia and Flagella

Cilia are specialized hair-like projections on some eukaryotic cells that aid in movement, while **flagella** are long, whip-like projections that are used in the same capacity.

The following organelles are *not* found in animal cells:

Cell Walls

Cell walls can be found in plants, bacteria, and fungi, and are made of cellulose, peptidoglycan, and lignin in these organisms, respectively. Each of these materials is a type of sugar recognized as a structural carbohydrate. The carbohydrates form rigid structures located outside of the cell membrane. Cell walls protect the cell, help maintain a cell's shape, and provide structural support.

Chloroplasts

Chloroplasts are organelles found primarily in plants and are the site of photosynthesis. They have a double membrane and also contain membrane-bound **thylakoids**, or discs, that are organized into **grana**, or stacks. Chlorophyll is present in the thylakoids, and the light stage of photosynthesis—which includes the production of ATP and $NADPH_2$—occurs there. Chlorophyll is green and traps the light energy necessary for photosynthesis. Chloroplasts also contain **stroma**—which are the site of the dark reaction stage of photosynthesis—during which sugar is made. The membrane structure of chloroplasts allows for the compartmentalization of the light and dark stages of photosynthesis.

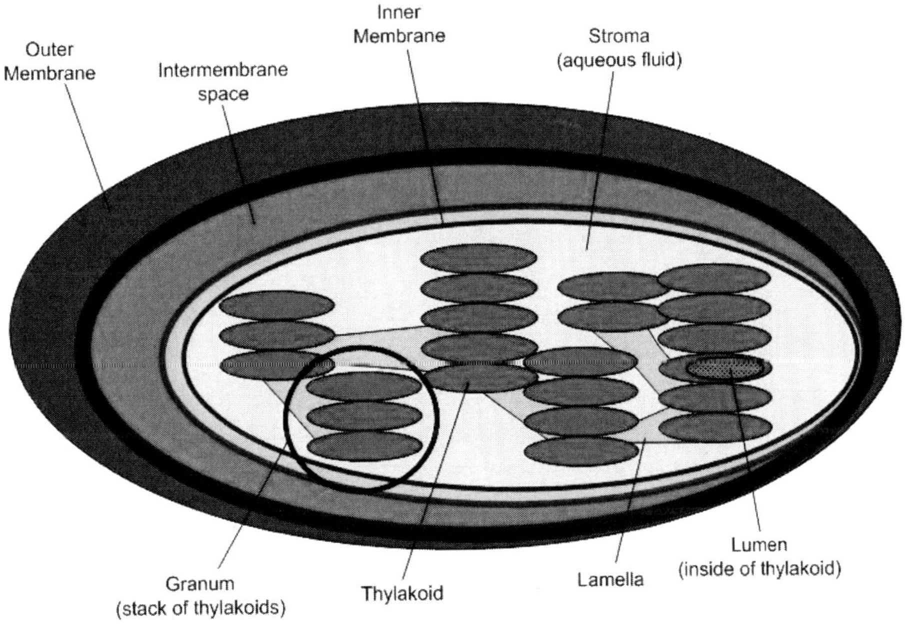

Vacuoles

Vacuoles are membrane-bound organelles primarily found in plant and fungi cells, but also in some animal cells. Vacuoles are filled with water and some enzymes and are important for intracellular digestion and waste removal. The membrane-bound nature of the vacuole allows for the storage of harmful material and poisonous substances. The pressure from the water inside the vacuole also contributes to the structure of plant cells.

Here is an illustration of the cell:

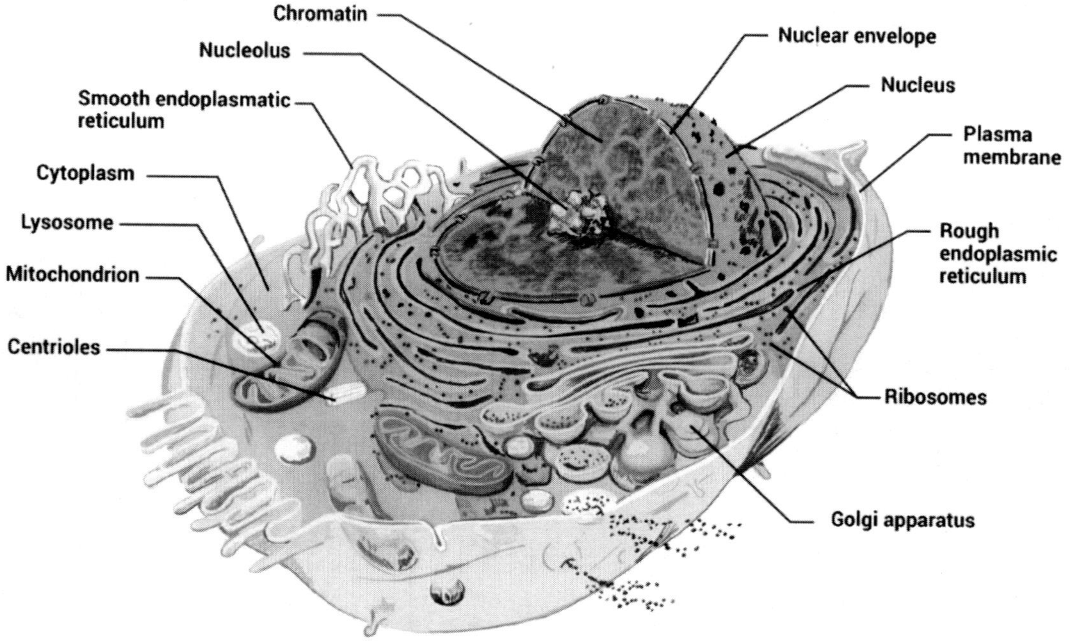

The Structure, Growth, Physiology, and Genetics of Prokaryotes and Viruses

Prokaryotic Organelles

Prokaryotic cells are usually structurally less complex than eukaryotic cells because they lack membrane-bound organelles. While they do contain some of the same structures as eukaryotic cells—including ribosomes, cytoplasm, and plasma membranes—they have several unique structures as well including the following:

- **Chromosome:** Located in the nucleotide region of the cell, the bacterial chromosome is a single loop of DNA that carries the genes for the cell's protein synthesis.
- **Plasmids:** Some bacterial cells have plasmids, which are small extra-chromosomal rings of DNA that contain genes that code for resistance to various antibiotics. Through **transposons**, genetic information can be moved between the chromosome and plasmids.
- **Cell wall:** Like plant cells, most bacteria have a cell wall on the outer surface of their cell membrane. It usually contains peptidoglycan in either a single or double layer. **Gram-positive** bacteria have a single layer of peptidoglycan in their cell walls, while **gram-negative** bacteria have a double layer.

- **Flagella:** Flagella provide motility to the cell but differ in structure from those of eukaryotic cells because they have a hollow helical confirmation anchored into the cell membrane. The power for their rotation is provided by a proton pump in the cell membrane. Prokaryotic cells may have one, multiple, or no flagella; of course, those that contain more are more mobile.
- **Spores:** There are a few species of prokaryotes that can create spores during unfavorable environmental conditions, which enables them to survive for several years in spore form and then germinate into the vegetative cell form when conditions improve.
- **Capsule** and **slime layers:** Some bacterial cells have a sticky layer of sugars and proteins on their outer surface, which enables the cell to attach to various surfaces.
- **Pili:** Some prokaryotes have pili, which are tiny proteins covering the cell's surface. Like slime layers, pili assist in the attachment of the cell to other surfaces.

Bacterial Morphology

Most bacterial cells are one of three general shapes. **Cocci** are circular and may exist singly or in pairs, clusters, or chains. **Spirilli** are spiral-shaped and **bacilli** are rod-shaped and may also occur in chains.

Bacterial Reproduction

Bacterial cells only contain a single chromosome so their division is much less complex than eukaryotic mitosis. Genetic material can be passed down through binary fission, conjugation, or transformation.

1. **Binary fission:** Binary fission is a type of asexual reproduction in which bacteria replicate their single chromosome of DNA, pass a copy to each of two daughter cells, and divide. Because prokaryotes are unicellular, binary fission creates an entirely new organism. Because each division produces offspring that are genetically identical to the parent cell, genetic variation is only introduced is through mutation, conjugation, or transformation.

Transformation	Transduction	Conjugation
Exogenous snippets of DNA enter bacterial cells.	Bacteriophages (viruses that infect bacteria) introduce foreign DNA into a bacterial cell	One bacterial cell extends a pili into another and releases DNA.

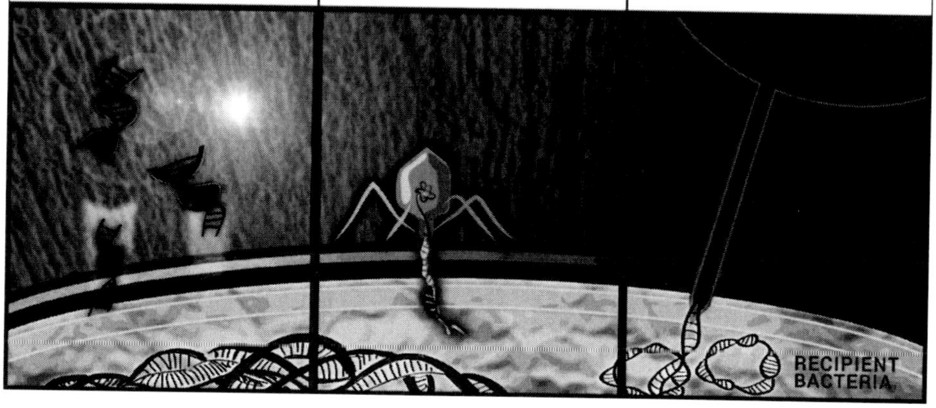

2. **Conjugation:** Some bacterial cells are capable of conjugation, which is the rapid process by which the cell copies its plasmid and passes it to another cell through a direct physical connection, termed a **sex pilus**. The cell that contains the plasmid is referred to as **male** or **F+**, while the cell that the male bridges to is called **female**, or **F-**. After conjugation, both cells contain the plasmid and are both considered male. Sometimes during conjugation, plasmids can become integrated into the chromosome and some of the bacterial chromosome may be transferred along with the plasmid. Through conjugation, antibiotic resistance can rapidly spread through a bacterial population, as plasmids encode for resistance to antibiotics.

3. **Transformation:** Transformation is the process by which some prokaryotes, called **competent bacteria**, can absorb and incorporate foreign DNA from their environment into their own chromosomal DNA.

Bacterial Growth Cycle

The typical growth cycle of bacterial cells consists of four stages and is governed by environmental factors and nutrient availability. In the first stage, the **lag**, growth is initially, albeit briefly, slow as the new population of bacteria begins to reproduce. In the next stage, **logarithmic growth**, growth increases quickly because the bacteria start to rapidly undergo binary fission. The third stage, the **stationary stage**, is the slowing and ultimate plateau of growth, caused by the increased number of bacteria competing for limited resources. Essentially, the rate of division and cell death are equivalent, and this is the point that the maximum population is reached. In the last stage, **decline** or death, the lack of nutrients and resources causes a greater number of cells in the population to die than those that are being produced. This is the phase in which those bacteria capable of spore production would do so.

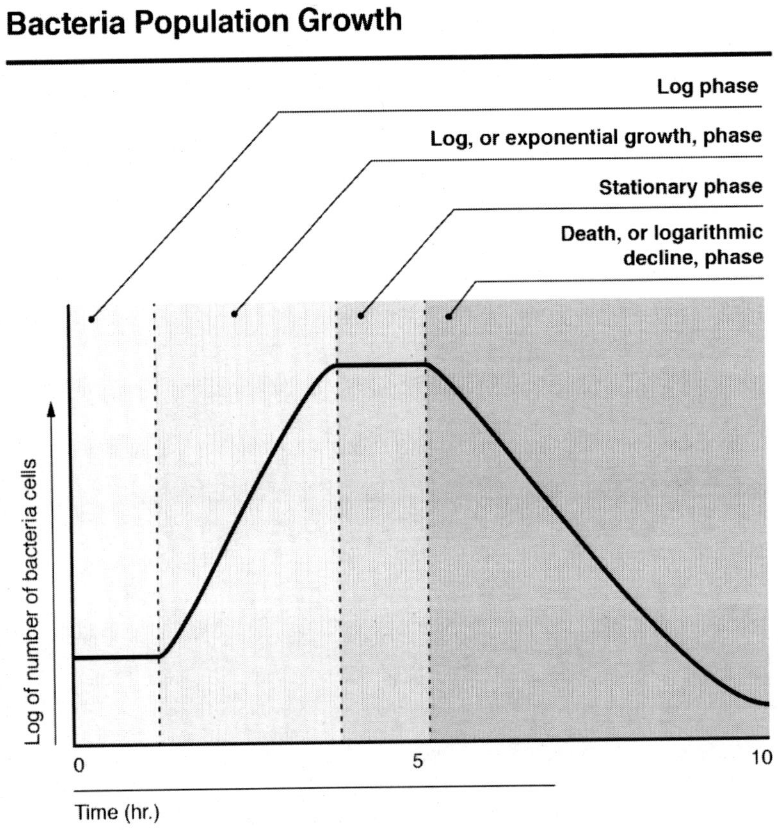

Viruses

Viruses do not resemble any of the classes of typical cells and are sometimes not even considered living things because without a host cell, they cannot reproduce or perform a variety of other functions of living organisms.

Viruses are quite small because they do not contain organelles and usually just have a piece of genetic material—which can be either DNA or RNA—protected by a protein coating, and which codes for just a few to a few hundred genes. They are categorized as animal or plant viruses or bacteriophages, depending on the type of host cell they infect. They can be more specifically categorized by the type of nucleic acid they contain.

For a host cell to be infected by a virus, it must have a receptor for that specific virus, and viruses are specific to the host cell they infect. Typically, viruses mimic a needed substance for which the host cell has the required receptor. That way, the virus can bind to the receptor on the host cell's membrane in place of the needed substance. After binding, the genetic material contained in the virus is injected or transferred via endocytosis through the cell membrane of the host cell. The host cell begins to transcribe and translate the viral genes and nucleic acids, producing new viruses and releasing them.

The host cells for animal viruses (various animal cells), can release the new viruses they assemble by either lysis or budding. In lysis, the host cell immediately dies because its cell membrane is lost through the process, but in budding, the new viruses leave the host cell via exocytosis, so the host cell does not immediately die. The released viruses seek out their own host cells to subsequently infect. Some host cells can harbor the virus for some time in their chromosome in a latent phase and then produce and release new viruses at a later time. Mutations are the only way that variation is introduced into the viral population because each virus is genetically identical and contains a copy of the original genetic material.

Retroviruses, such as HIV, are a type of RNA virus that must enter the host cell in RNA form that then has to be converted to DNA form. This process, which takes place in the opposite direction of the typical information flow in a cell, is called **reverse transcription** and is carried out by an enzyme coded for by the viral genome called **reverse transcriptase**. As soon as the retrovirus enters the host cell, the RNA is transcribed, which produces reverse transcriptase, which, in turn, produces a copy of the viral genome's DNA. At some point, depending on the specific retrovirus, the host chromosome excises the viral DNA, and the DNA becomes active and produces new viruses.

Bacteriophages exclusively infect bacteria. They are DNA viruses that inject into the host bacterial cell. Once inside the cell, they can undergo a lytic cycle or a lysogenic cycle. In the **lytic cycle**, they immediately activate, and new viruses are created and leave the cell via lysis, killing their host. The first step of this cycle is **attachment**, in which the capsid combines with the receptor. Then **penetration** occurs, and the viral DNA enters the bacterial host cell. In the third step, **biosynthesis**, the viral components are synthesized in the host cell for step four, **maturation**, or the assembly of the viral components. The final stage, the **release**, is when the new viruses leave the host cell and are free to infect other hosts. Some viruses can undergo the **lysogenic cycle**, wherein they inject their DNA into the host cell, where it is incorporated into the bacterial chromosome for some time. When the host bacterial cell undergoes binary fission to divide, the daughter cells receive a copy of the viral genome. The viral DNA that has integrated into the host cell's chromosome is excised at some point and then the new viruses begin infecting other bacterial hosts.

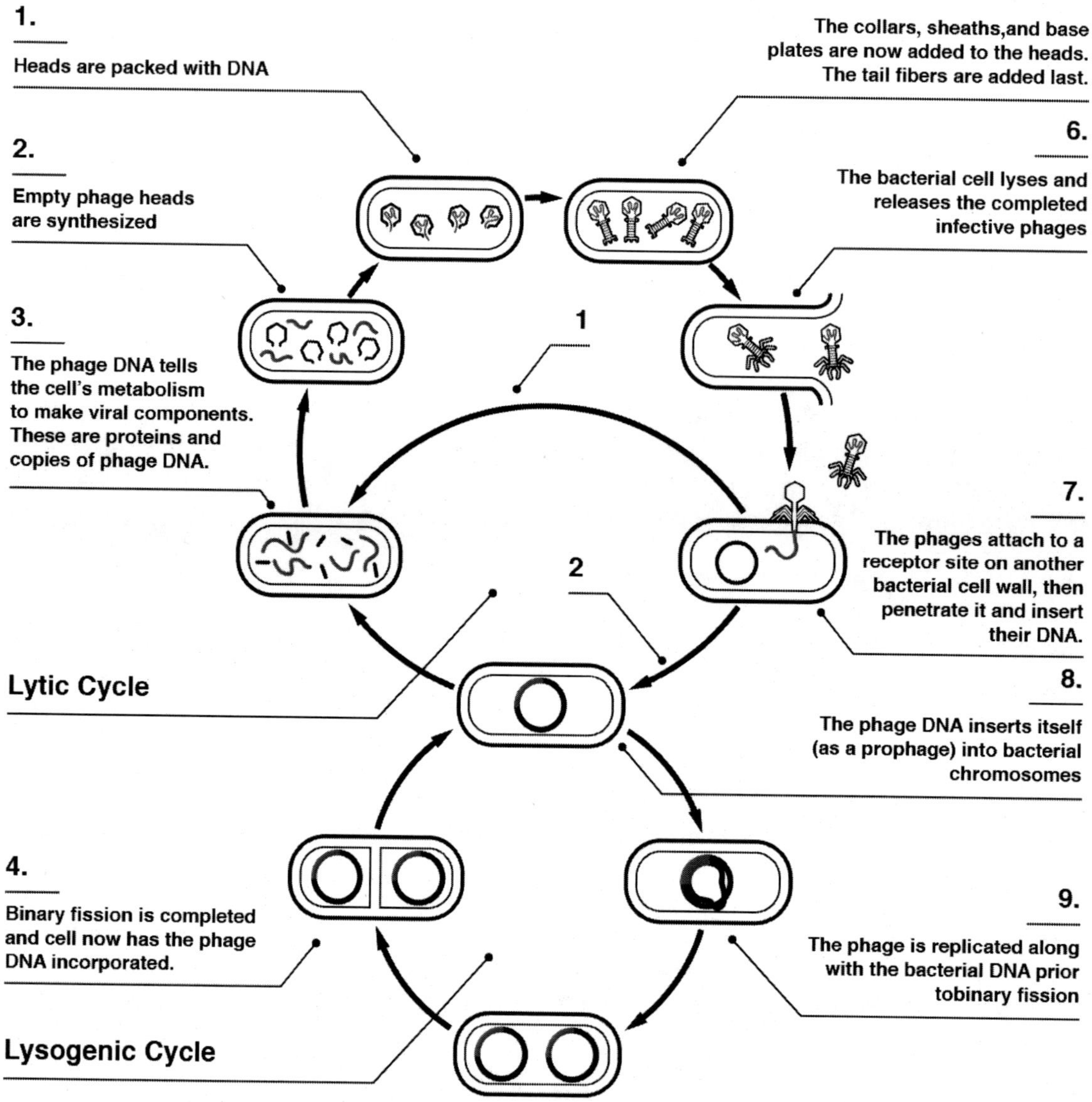

Transduction

Transduction is the process by which some portion of the host cell's chromosome gets packaged and transferred out of the cell in the new copy of the virus, and then gets incorporated into the subsequent host cell when the virus delivers its viral DNA during infection.

Processes of Cell Division, Differentiation, and Specialization

Cell Differentiation

Cell differentiation refers to the process of a cell transforming into another type of cell. It most commonly involves a less specialized cell transforming into a more specialized cell.

The human body contains a vast array of cells which undergo division and differentiation to compose each unique human being. The trillions of cells composing the human body are derived from one cell, a fertilized egg called a **zygote**. The zygote not only divides, but also differentiates into cells that perform specific tasks.

Genes control the process of cell differentiation during human development. The zygote divides through mitosis into a **blastula** and then into a **gastrula**. At this stage, the three embryonic germ layers (endoderm, mesoderm, and ectoderm) are formed. Most of the human body systems develop from one or more of the embryonic germ layers. For example, the digestive system develops from the **endoderm**, or innermost germ layer; the cardiovascular system develops from the **mesoderm**, or middle germ layer; and the nervous system develops from the **ectoderm**, or outer germ layer.

Mitosis and Meiosis

Mitosis

Mitosis, or asexual reproduction, produces two new cells that are genetically identical to the parent cell. It can happen in virtually every healthy adult cell, although some cells like red blood cells and neurons do not typically divide. When a cell is not undergoing cell division, it is in a stage called **interphase** which is characterized by growth, typical maintenance, and DNA synthesis in the nucleus. Each healthy human cell nucleus typically has 46 chromosomes and is said to be **diploid** (2n), as this count comes from 23 pairs of **homologous chromosomes**. Homologous chromosomes are pairs of chromatids with similar sections that correspond to similar genes, as in pairs of chromosome 1 or pairs of chromosome 21.

Mitosis is divided into the following events:

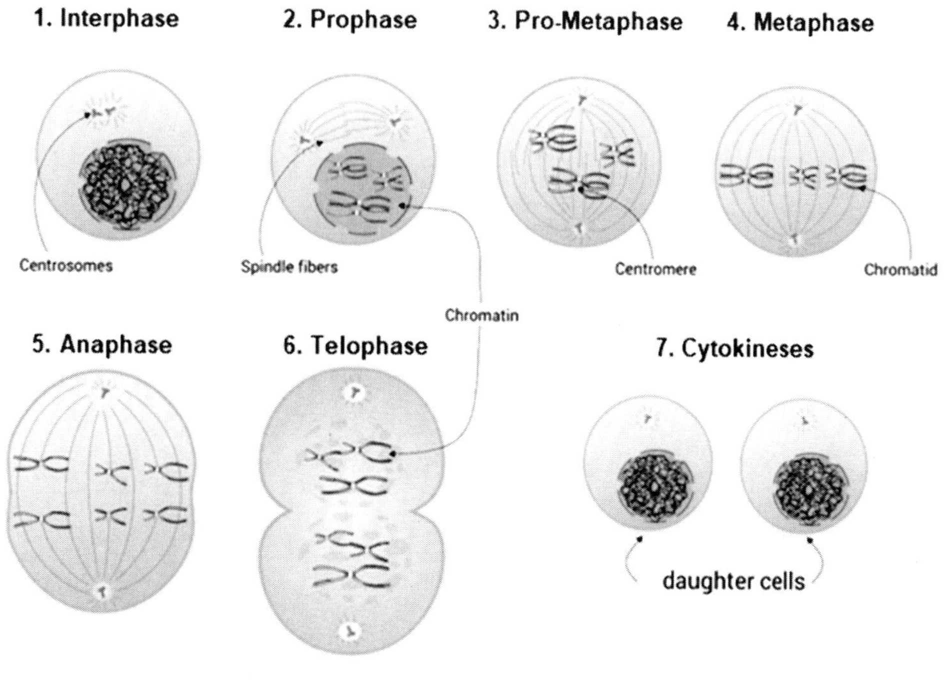

Prophase: The already-duplicated chromatin condenses to form chromosomes. Each new chromosome is made up of two identical sister chromatids joined by a structure called a **centromere**. The nuclear envelope is degraded and spindle fibers form and attach to structures called **centrioles**. The centrioles separate and proceed to opposite poles of the cell.

Pro-metaphase: The centrioles build spindle fibers and attach them to the chromosomes.

Metaphase: Using tension from spindle fibers, the chromosomes align in the middle of the cell.

Anaphase: The spindle fibers contract and separate the chromosomes at their centromere. The single chromatids, pulled by the spindle fibers, begin migrating to opposite poles of the cell.

Telophase: The chromatids arrive at opposite poles of the cell. The spindle fibers disappear, the nuclear envelope reforms, and the chromosomes uncoil back into chromatin.

Cytokinesis: The process refers to the cleaving of the cytoplasm to form two daughter cells that are genetically identical to the parent cell. In animal cells, this happens via a **cleavage furrow**. A cleavage furrow is a pinching of the cell membrane near the center that deepens until it reaches the point that the cell membrane can recombine and split the entity into two separate cells.

Meiosis

Meiosis, or sexual division, happens only in specialized sex cells and produces four cells called gametes. In humans, sex cells are found in the ovaries and in the testes, and contrast with somatic cells, which constitute the rest of the body of the organism. Each gamete contains half the number of chromosomes of a normal cell, and each is said to be **haploid** (n), rather than **diploid** (2n). In humans, a gamete has 23 chromosomes instead of the 46 that are typically found in somatic cells. The female gamete is called an **egg,** and the male gamete is called a **sperm**.

Preceding meiosis, the DNA is synthesized, and the chromatin coalesces into chromosomes, as in mitosis. However, the pairs of sister chromatids that are homologous combine, joining their centromeres into a single **chiasma** and forming a **tetrad**. At this point, sections of the different chromatids may break off and rejoin, possibly in another place. Half of a leg of one chromatid may swap with that of another chromatid; the chromatids essentially exchange some of their genes with one another. This process, called **crossing over** or **genetic recombination**, happens in prophase I and increases genetic diversity.

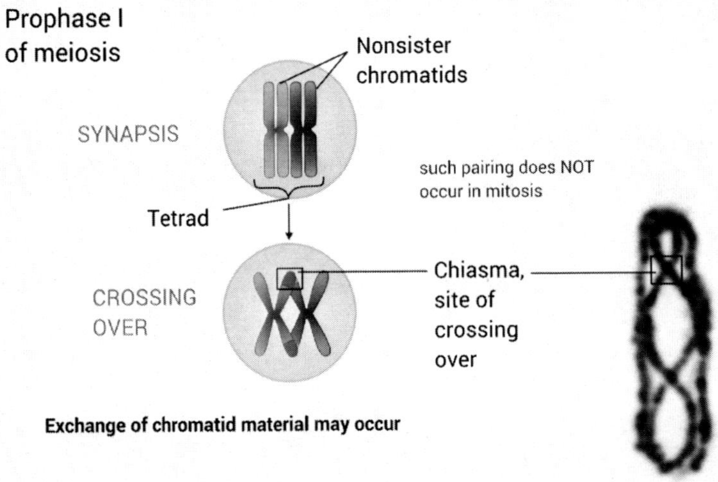

Like mitosis, meiosis is divided into stages of prophase, metaphase, anaphase, telophase, and cytokinesis. However, as the end products have half the genetic material as do the end products of mitosis, another round of division is necessary, so meiosis is first partitioned into meiosis I and meiosis II, with each round similar in scope to mitosis. During meiosis I, homologous chromosome pairs are separated into two daughter cells. Each daughter cell is haploid

(n) because, although each cell at the end of meiosis I has 46 chromatids, half of them are duplicates of the others and not considered unique genetic material.

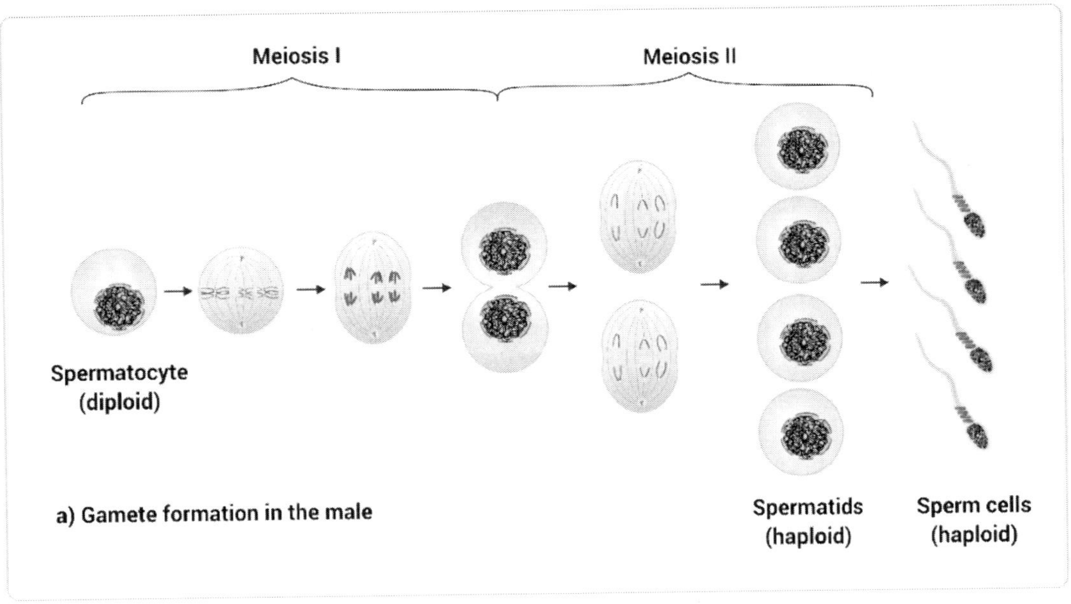

After cytokinesis I, the daughter cells immediately enter prophase II, rather than duplicating DNA or entering interphase. The nucleus disintegrates, the centrioles migrate to the ends of the cell, and the next round of divisions begins. This results in four haploid (n) daughter cells—the gametes of egg and sperm referenced earlier.

A common problem that arises in both meiosis and mitosis (but that is especially noticeable in meiosis) is that of **nondisjunction**. Nondisjunction is the failure of homologous chromosomes or sister chromatids to separate during anaphase. This causes the daughter cells to have one more or one fewer chromosomes than usual and can ultimately result in genetic conditions like Down's syndrome, wherein a meiotic egg with nondisjunction is fertilized.

Cell Replication

Cell replication in eukaryotes involves duplicating the genetic material (DNA) and then dividing to yield two daughter cells that are clones of the parent cell. The cell cycle is a series of stages leading to the growth and division of a cell. The cell cycle helps to replenish damaged or depleted cells. On average, eukaryotic cells go through a complete cell cycle every 24 hours. Some cells such as epithelial, or skin, cells are constantly dividing, while other cells, such as mature nerve cells, do not divide. Prior to mitosis, cells exist in a non-divisional stage of the cell cycle called interphase. During interphase, the cell begins to prepare for division by duplicating DNA and its cytoplasmic contents. Interphase is divided into three phases: gap 1 (G_1), synthesis (S), and gap 2 (G_2).

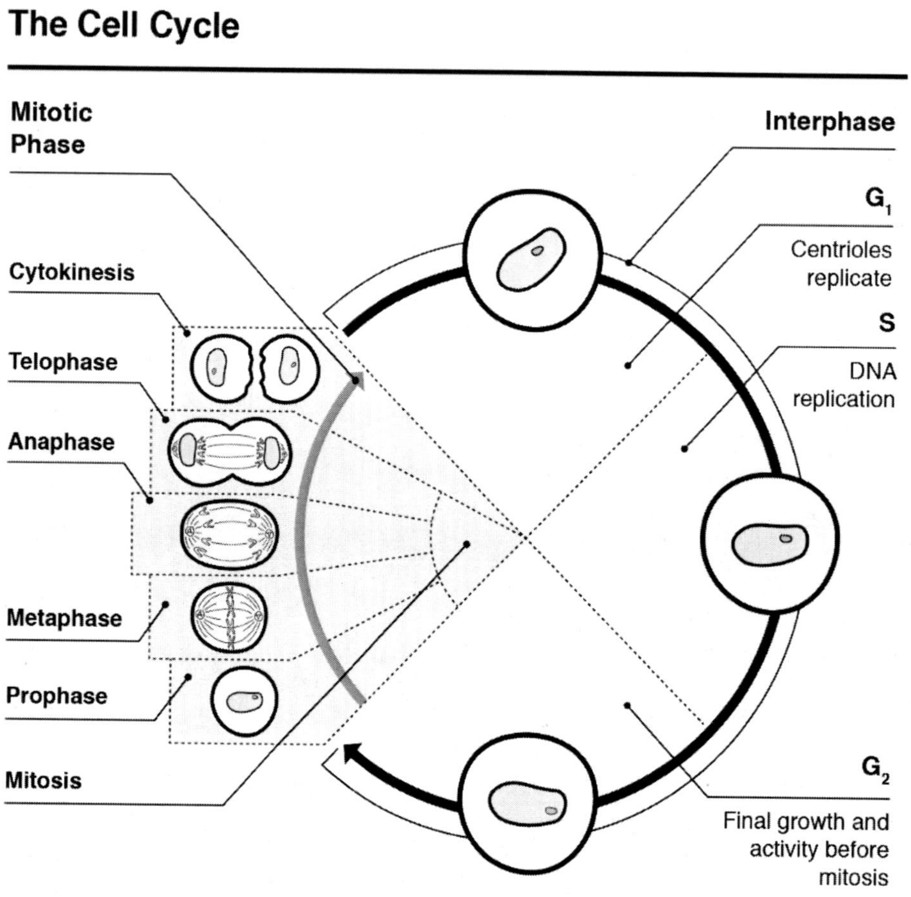

DNA Replication

Replication refers to the process during which DNA makes copies of itself. Enzymes govern the major steps of DNA replication.

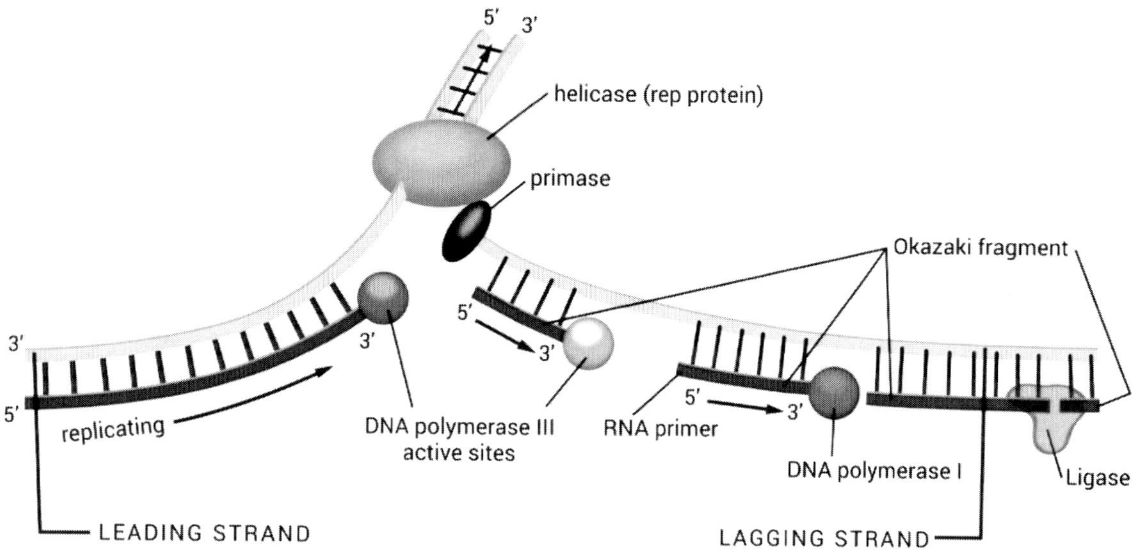

The process begins with the uncoiling of the double helix of DNA. **Helicase**, an enzyme, accomplishes this task by breaking the weak hydrogen bonds uniting base pairs. The uncoiling of DNA gives rise to the **replication fork**, which has a Y-shape. Each separated strand of DNA will act as a template to produce a new molecule of DNA. The strand of DNA oriented toward the replication fork is called the **leading strand** and the strand oriented away from the replication fork is named the **lagging strand.**

Replication of the leading strand is continuous. **DNA polymerase**, an enzyme, binds to the leading strand and adds complementary bases. Replication of the lagging strand of DNA on the other hand is discontinuous. DNA polymerase produces discontinuous segments, called **Okazaki fragments**, which are later joined together by another enzyme, **DNA ligase**. To start the DNA synthesis on the lagging strand, the protein **primase** lays down a strip of RNA, called an **RNA primer**, to which the DNA polymerase can bind. As a result, two clones of the original DNA emerge from this process. DNA replication is considered **semiconservative**, since half of the new molecule is old and the other half is new.

Foundational Concept 3: Complex systems of tissues and organs sense the internal and external environments of multicellular organisms, and through integrated functioning, maintain a stable internal environment within an ever-changing external environment.

Structure and Functions of the Nervous and Endocrine Systems and Ways in Which These Systems Coordinate the Organ Systems

Endocrine System

The **endocrine system** is made of the ductless tissues and glands that secrete hormones into the interstitial fluids of the body. Interstitial fluid is the solution that surrounds tissue cells within the body. This system works closely with the nervous system to regulate the physiological activities of the other systems of the body to maintain homeostasis. While the nervous system provides quick, short-term responses to stimuli, the endocrine system acts by releasing hormones into the bloodstream that get distributed to the whole body. The response is slow but long-lasting, ranging from a few hours to a few weeks.

Hormones are chemical substances that change the metabolic activity of tissues and organs. While regular metabolic reactions are controlled by enzymes, hormones can change the type, activity, or quantity of the enzymes involved in the reaction. They bind to specific cells and start a biochemical chain of events that changes the enzymatic activity. Hormones can regulate development and growth, digestive metabolism, mood, and body temperature, among other things. Often small amounts of a hormone will lead to significant changes in the body.

Major Endocrine Glands

Hypothalamus: A part of the brain, the hypothalamus connects the nervous system to the endocrine system via the pituitary gland. Although it is considered part of the nervous system, the hypothalamus plays a dual role in regulating endocrine organs.

Pituitary Gland: A pea-sized gland found at the bottom of the hypothalamus with two lobes, called the anterior and posterior lobes. The pituitary gland plays an important role in regulating the function of other endocrine glands. The hormones it releases control growth, blood pressure, certain functions of the sex organs, salt concentration of the kidneys, internal temperature regulation, and pain responses.

Thyroid Gland: This gland releases hormones, such as thyroxine, which are important for metabolism, growth and development, temperature regulation, and brain development during infancy and childhood. Thyroid hormones also monitor the amount of circulating calcium in the body.

Parathyroid Glands: These are four pea-sized glands located on the posterior surface of the thyroid. The main hormone secreted is called **parathyroid hormone** (PTH), which helps with the thyroid's regulation of calcium in the body.

Thymus Gland: The thymus is in the chest cavity, embedded in connective tissue. It produces several hormones important for development and maintenance of normal immunological defenses. One hormone promotes the development and maturation of **lymphocytes**, which strengthens the immune system.

Adrenal Gland: One adrenal gland is attached to the top of each kidney. Each adrenal gland produces **epinephrine**, which is responsible for the "fight or flight" reactions in the face of danger or stress. The hormones epinephrine and **norepinephrine** cooperate to regulate states of arousal.

Pancreas: The pancreas is an organ that has both endocrine and exocrine functions. The endocrine functions are controlled by the pancreatic **islets of Langerhans**, which are groups of beta cells scattered throughout the gland that secrete insulin to lower blood sugar levels in the body. Neighboring alpha cells secrete glucagon to raise blood sugar.

Pineal Gland: The pineal gland secretes melatonin, a hormone derived from the neurotransmitter **serotonin**. **Melatonin** can slow the maturation of sperm, oocytes, and reproductive organs. It also regulates the body's circadian rhythm, which is the natural awake/asleep cycle. It also serves an important role in protecting the CNS tissues from neural toxins.

Testes and **Ovaries:** These glands secrete testosterone and estrogen, respectively, and are responsible for secondary sex characteristics, as well as reproduction.

Nervous System

The human **nervous system** coordinates the body's response to stimuli from inside and outside the body. There are two major types of nervous system cells: neurons and neuroglia. **Neurons** are the workhorses of the nervous system and form a complex communication network that transmits electrical impulses termed action potentials, while **neuroglia** connect and support the neurons.

Although some neurons monitor the senses, some control muscles, and some connect the brain to other neurons, all neurons have four common characteristics:

- **Dendrites:** These receive electrical signals from other neurons across small gaps called **synapses**.
- **Nerve cell body:** This is the hub of processing and protein manufacturing for the neuron.
- **Axon:** This transmits the signal from the cell body to other neurons.
- **Terminals:** These bridge the neuron's axon to dendrites of other neurons and are involved with delivering the nervous signal via chemical messengers called neurotransmitters.

Here is an illustration of a typical nerve cell:

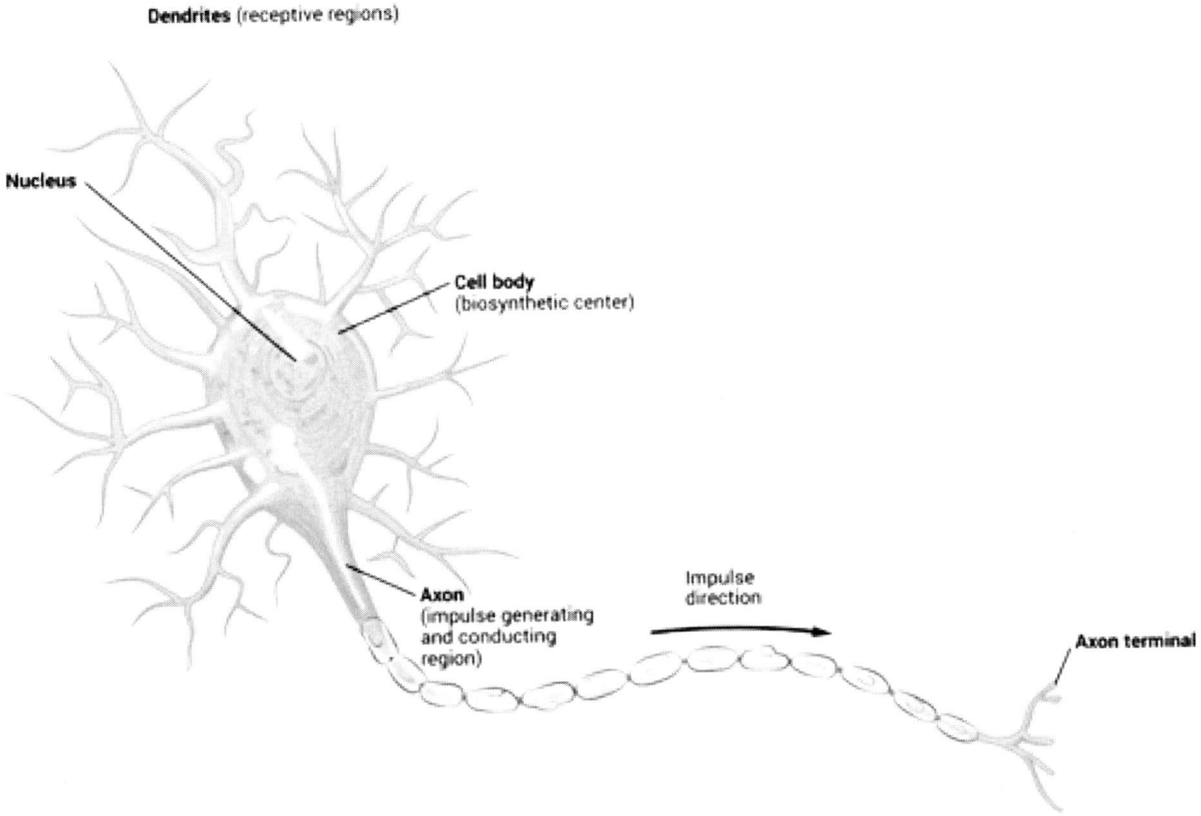

There are two major divisions of the nervous system: central and peripheral.

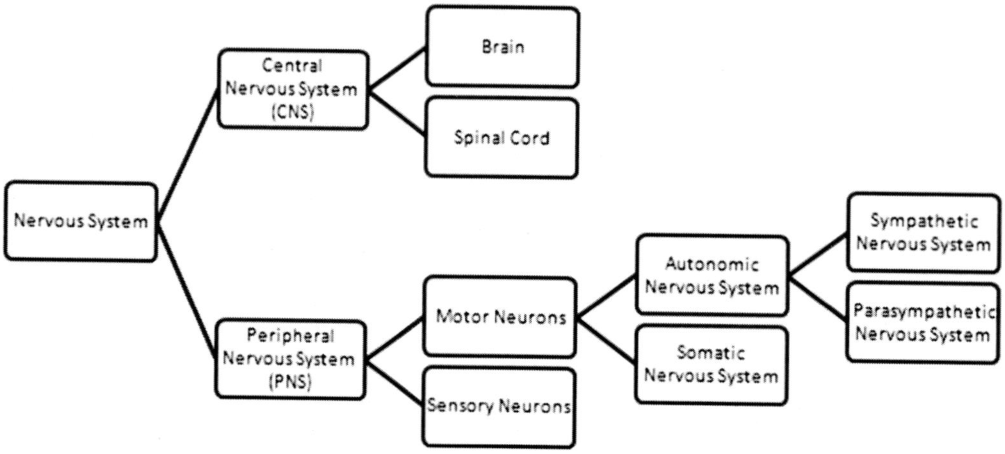

Central Nervous System

The **central nervous system** (CNS) consists of the brain and spinal cord. Three layers of membranes, called the **meninges,** cover and separate the CNS from the rest of the body.

The major divisions of the brain are the forebrain, the midbrain, and the hindbrain.

The **forebrain** consists of the cerebrum, the thalamus and hypothalamus, and the rest of the limbic system. The **cerebrum** is the largest part of the brain, and its most well-researched part is the outer cerebral cortex. The cerebrum is divided into right and left hemispheres, and each cerebral cortex hemisphere has four discrete areas, or **lobes**: frontal, temporal, parietal, and occipital. The **frontal lobe** governs duties such as voluntary movement, judgment, problem solving, and planning, while the other lobes have more sensory involvement. The **temporal lobe** integrates hearing and language comprehension, the **parietal lobe** processes sensory input from the skin, and the **occipital lobe** processes visual input from the eyes. For completeness, the other two senses, smell and taste, are processed via the olfactory bulbs. The **thalamus** helps organize and coordinate all of this sensory input in a meaningful way for the brain to interpret.

The **hypothalamus** controls the endocrine system and all of the hormones that govern long-term effects on the body. Each hemisphere of the **limbic system** includes a **hippocampus** (which plays a vital role in memory), an

amygdala (which is involved with emotional responses like fear and anger), and other small bodies and nuclei associated with memory and pleasure.

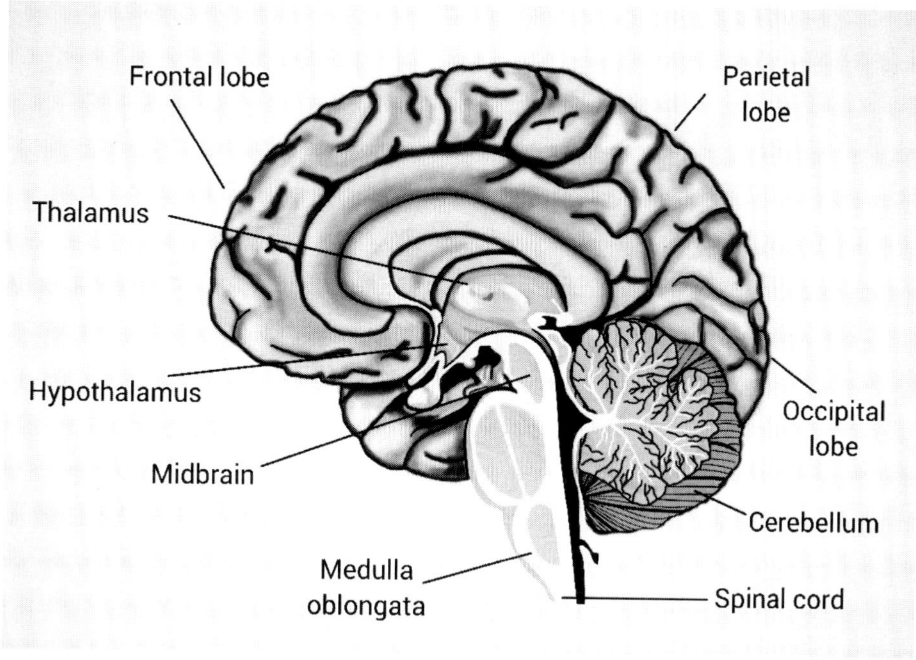

The **midbrain** oversees alertness, sleep/wake cycles, and temperature regulation, and it includes the **substantia nigra**, which produces **melatonin** to regulate sleep patterns. The notable components of the **hindbrain** include the medulla oblongata and cerebellum. The **medulla oblongata** is located just above the spinal cord and is responsible for crucial involuntary functions such as breathing, swallowing, and the regulation of heart rate and blood pressure. Together with other parts of the hindbrain, the midbrain and medulla oblongata form the **brain stem**. The brain stem connects the spinal cord to the rest of the brain. To the rear of the brain stem sits the **cerebellum**, which plays key roles in posture, balance, and muscular coordination. The spinal cord itself carries sensory information to the brain and motor information to the body. It is encapsulated by its protective bony spinal column.

Peripheral Nervous System

The **peripheral nervous system** (PNS) includes all nervous tissue besides the brain and spinal cord. The PNS consists of the sets of **cranial** and **spinal nerves** and relays information between the CNS and the rest of the body. The PNS has two divisions: the autonomic nervous system and the somatic nervous system.

Autonomic Nervous System

The **autonomic nervous system** (ANS) governs involuntary, or reflexive, body functions. Ultimately, the autonomic nervous system controls functions such as breathing, heart rate, digestion, body temperature, and blood pressure.

The ANS is split between **parasympathetic** nerves and **sympathetic** nerves. These two nerve types are antagonistic, so they have opposite effects on the body. Parasympathetic nerves typically are useful when resting or during "safe" conditions; they decrease heart rate, decrease inhalation speed, prepare digestion, and allow urination and excretion. Sympathetic nerves, on the other hand, become active when a person is under stress or excited, and they increase heart rate, increase breathing rates, and inhibit digestion, urination, and excretion.

Somatic Nervous System and the Reflex Arc

The **somatic** nervous system (SNS) governs the conscious, or voluntary, control of skeletal muscles and their corresponding body movements. The SNS contains afferent and efferent neurons. Afferent neurons carry sensory messages from the skeletal muscles, skin, or sensory organs to the CNS. Efferent neurons relay motor messages from the CNS to skeletal muscles, skin, or sensory organs.

The SNS also has a role in involuntary movements called **reflexes**. A reflex is defined as an involuntary response to a stimulus. Reflexes are transmitted via what is termed a **reflex arc**, where a stimulus is sensed by a receptor and its afferent neuron, interpreted and rerouted by an **interneuron**, and delivered to effector muscles by an efferent neuron to respond to the initial stimulus. A reflex can bypass the brain by being rerouted through the spinal cord; the interneuron decides the proper course of action, rather than the brain. The reflex arc results in an instantaneous, involuntary response. For example, a physician tapping on the knee produces an involuntary knee jerk referred to as the **patellar tendon reflex.**

Structure and Integrative Functions of the Main Organ Systems

Anatomy and Physiology of Various Systems of the Body

Circulatory System

The **circulatory** system is a network of organs and tubes that transport blood, hormones, nutrients, oxygen, and other gases to cells and tissues throughout the body. It is also known as the **cardiovascular** system. The major components of the circulatory system are the blood vessels, blood, and heart.

Blood Vessels

In the circulatory system, blood vessels are responsible for transporting blood throughout the body. The three major types of blood vessels in the circulatory system are arteries, veins, and capillaries. **Arteries** carry blood from the heart to the rest of the body. Veins carry blood from the body back to the heart. **Capillaries** connect arteries to veins and form networks that exchange materials between the blood and the cells.

In general, arteries are stronger and thicker than veins, as they need to withstand the high pressures exerted by the blood as the heart pumps it through the body. Arteries control blood flow through either **vasoconstriction** (narrowing of the blood vessel's diameter) or **vasodilation** (widening of the blood vessel's diameter). The blood in veins is under much lower pressures than that in arteries, so veins have **valves** to prevent the backflow of blood.

Most of the exchange between the blood and tissues takes place through the capillaries. There are three types of capillaries: continuous, fenestrated, and sinusoidal.

1. **Continuous capillaries** are made up of epithelial cells tightly connected together. As a result, they limit the types of materials that pass into and out of the blood. Continuous capillaries are the most common type of capillary.

2. **Fenestrated capillaries** have openings that allow materials to be freely exchanged between the blood and tissues. They are commonly found in the digestive, endocrine, and urinary systems.

3. **Sinusoidal capillaries** have larger openings to allow proteins and blood cells through. They are found primarily in the liver, bone marrow, and spleen.

Blood

Blood is vital to the human body. It is a liquid connective tissue that serves as a transport system to supply cells with nutrients and to carry away their wastes. The average adult human has five to six quarts of blood circulating through their body. Approximately 55% of blood is **plasma** (the fluid portion), and the remaining 45% is composed of whole cells and cell parts.

There are three major types of blood cells:

- **Red blood cells** transport oxygen throughout the body. They contain a protein called **hemoglobin** that allows them to carry oxygen. The iron in the hemoglobin gives the cells and the blood their red colors.
- **White blood cells** are responsible for fighting infectious diseases and maintaining the immune system. There are five types of white blood cells: neutrophils, lymphocytes, eosinophils, monocytes, and basophils.
- **Platelets** are cell fragments that play a central role in the blood-clotting process.

All blood cells in adults are produced in the bone marrow—red blood cells from red marrow and white blood cells from yellow marrow.

Heart

The **heart** is a two-part, muscular pump that forcefully pushes blood throughout the human body. The human heart has four chambers—two upper **atria** and two lower ventricles separated by a partition called the septum. There is a pair on the left and a pair on the right. Anatomically, *left* and *right* correspond to the sides of the body that the patient themselves would refer to as left and right.

Four valves help to section off the chambers from one another. Between the right atrium and ventricle, the three flaps of the **tricuspid valve** keep blood from flowing backwards from the ventricle to the atrium, similar to how the two flaps of the **mitral valve** work between the left atrium and ventricle. As these two valves lie between an atrium and a ventricle, they are referred to as **atrioventricular** (AV) valves. The other two valves are called **semilunar** (SL); they control blood flow into the two great arteries that leave the ventricles. The **pulmonary valve** connects the right ventricle to the pulmonary artery, while the **aortic valve** connects the left ventricle to the aorta.

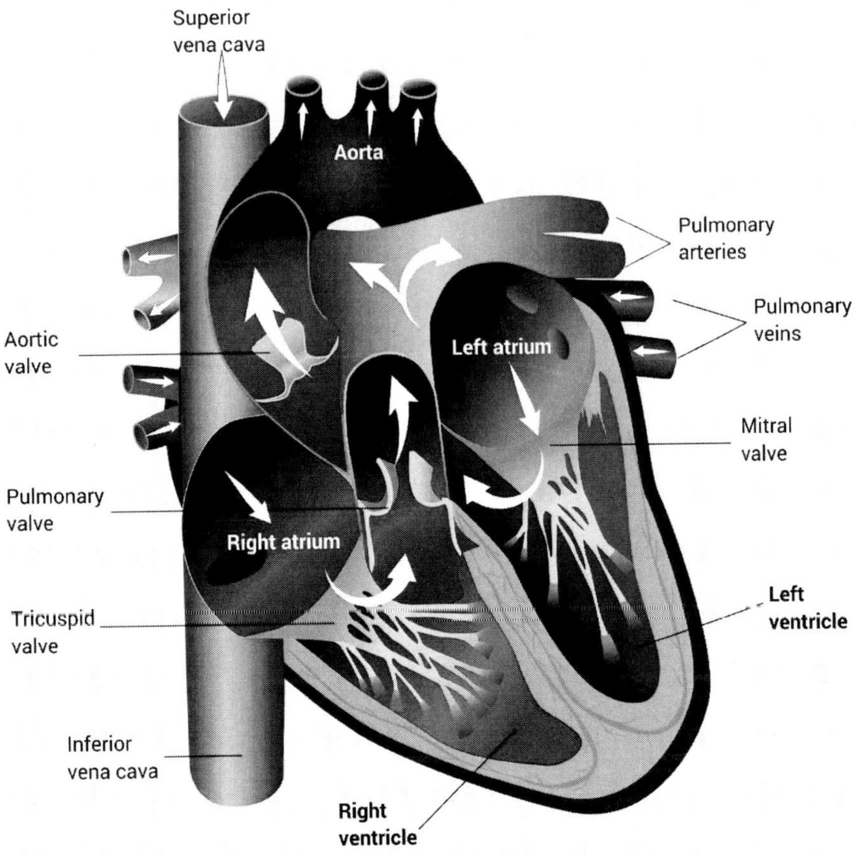

Cardiac Cycle

A **cardiac cycle** is one complete sequence of cardiac activity. The cardiac cycle represents the relaxation and contraction of the heart and can be divided into two phases: diastole and systole.

Diastole is the phase during which the heart relaxes and fills with blood. It gives rise to the **diastolic blood pressure** (DBP), which is the bottom number of a blood pressure reading. **Systole** is the phase during which the heart contracts and discharges blood. It gives rise to the **systolic blood pressure** (SBP), which is the top number of a blood pressure reading. The heart's electrical conduction system coordinates the cardiac cycle.

Types of Circulation

Five major blood vessels manage blood flow to and from the heart: the superior and inferior venae cavae, the aorta, the pulmonary artery, and the pulmonary vein.

The **superior vena cava** is a large vein that drains blood from the head and upper body. The **inferior vena cava** is a large vein that drains blood from the lower body. The **aorta** is the largest artery in the human body; it carries blood from the heart to body tissues. The **pulmonary arteries** carry blood from the heart to the lungs. The **pulmonary veins** transport blood from the lungs to the heart.

In the human body, there are two types of circulation: pulmonary circulation and systemic circulation. **Pulmonary circulation** supplies blood to the lungs. Deoxygenated blood enters the right atrium of the heart and is routed through the tricuspid valve into the right ventricle. Deoxygenated blood then travels from the right ventricle of the heart through the pulmonary valve and into the pulmonary arteries. The pulmonary arteries carry the deoxygenated blood to the lungs. In the lungs, oxygen is absorbed, and carbon dioxide is released. The pulmonary veins carry oxygenated blood to the left atrium of the heart.

Systemic circulation supplies blood to all other parts of the body, except the lungs. Oxygenated blood flows from the left atrium of the heart through the mitral, or bicuspid, valve into the left ventricle of the heart. Oxygenated blood is then routed from the left ventricle of the heart through the aortic valve and into the aorta. The aorta delivers blood to the systemic arteries, which supply the body tissues. In the tissues, oxygen and nutrients are exchanged for carbon dioxide and other wastes. The deoxygenated blood, carrying carbon dioxide and waste, enters the systemic veins, where it is returned to the right atrium of the heart via the superior and inferior venae cavae.

Digestive System

The human body relies entirely on the **digestive system** to meet its nutritional needs. After food and drink are ingested, the digestive system breaks them down into their component nutrients and absorbs them so that the circulatory system can transport the nutrients to other cells to use for growth, energy, and cell repair. These nutrients may be classified as proteins, lipids, carbohydrates, vitamins, and minerals.

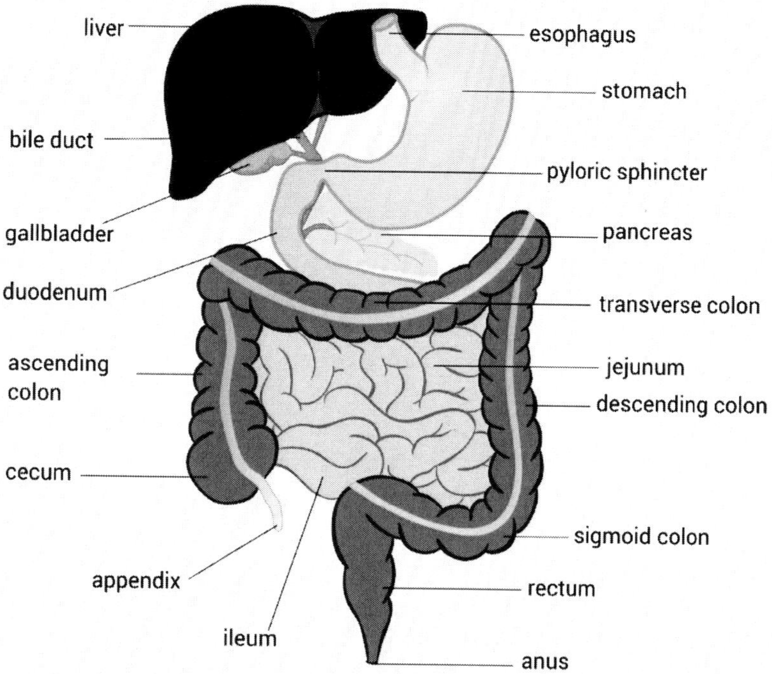

The digestive system is thought of chiefly in two parts: the **digestive tract** (also called **the alimentary tract** or **gastrointestinal tract**) and the **accessory digestive organs**. The digestive tract is the pathway in which food is ingested, digested, absorbed, and excreted. It is composed of the mouth, pharynx, esophagus, stomach, small and large intestines, rectum, and anus. **Peristalsis**, or wave-like contractions of smooth muscle, moves food and wastes through the digestive tract. The accessory digestive organs are the salivary glands, liver, gallbladder, and pancreas.

Mouth and Stomach

The **mouth** is the entrance to the digestive system. Here, the mechanical and chemical digestion of the food begins. The food is chewed mechanically by the teeth and shaped into a **bolus** by the tongue so that it can be more easily swallowed by the esophagus. The food also becomes more watery and pliable with the addition of saliva secreted from the salivary glands, the largest of which are the **parotid glands**. The glands also secrete **amylase** in the saliva, an enzyme which begins chemical digestion and the breakdown of the carbohydrates and sugars in the food.

The food then moves through the pharynx and down the muscular esophagus to the stomach.

The **stomach** is a large, muscular sac-like organ at the distal end of the esophagus. Here, the bolus is subjected to more mechanical and chemical digestion. As it passes through the stomach, it is physically squeezed and crushed while additional secretions turn it into a watery nutrient-filled liquid that exits into the small intestine as **chyme.**

The stomach secretes many substances into the **lumen** of the digestive tract. Some cells produce **gastrin**, a hormone that prompts other cells in the stomach to secrete a gastric acid composed mostly of **hydrochloric acid** (HCl). The HCl is at such a high concentration and low pH that it denatures most proteins and degrades a lot of organic matter. The stomach also secretes mucous to form a protective film that keeps the corrosive acid from dissolving its own cells; gaps in this mucous layer can lead to peptic ulcers. Finally, the stomach also uses digestive enzymes like **proteases** and **lipases** to break down proteins and fats; although there are some gastric lipases here, the stomach mostly breaks down proteins.

Small Intestine

The chyme from the stomach enters the first part of the small intestine, the **duodenum**, through the **pyloric sphincter**, and its extreme acidity is partly neutralized by sodium bicarbonate secreted along with mucous. The presence of chyme in the duodenum triggers the secretion of the hormones **secretin** and **cholecystokinin** (CCK). Secretin acts on the pancreas to dump more sodium bicarbonate into the small intestine so that the pH is kept at a reasonable level, while CCK acts on the gallbladder to release the **bile** that it has been storing. Bile, a substance produced by the liver and stored in the gallbladder, helps to emulsify or dissolve fats and lipids.

Because of the bile, which aids in lipid absorption, and the secreted lipases, which break down fats, the duodenum is the chief site of fat digestion in the body. The duodenum also represents the last major site of chemical digestion in the digestive tract, as the other two sections of the small intestine (the **jejunum** and **ileum**) are, instead, heavily involved in absorption of nutrients.

The small intestine reaches 40 feet in length, and its cells are arranged in small finger-like projections called **villi.** This is arrangement is necessary for the small intestine's key role in the absorption of nearly all nutrients from the ingested and digested food, effectively transferring them from the lumen of the GI tract to the bloodstream, where they travel to the cells which need them. These nutrients include simple sugars like glucose from carbohydrates, amino acids from proteins, emulsified fats, electrolytes like sodium and potassium, minerals like iron and zinc, and vitamins like D and B12. Although the absorption of vitamin B12 takes place in the intestines, it is actually aided by **intrinsic factor**, which was released into the chyme back in the stomach.

Large Intestine

The leftover parts of food that remain unabsorbed or undigested in the lumen of the small intestine next travel through the **large intestine**, which may also be referred to as the **large bowel** or **colon**. The large intestine is mainly responsible for water absorption. As the chyme at this stage no longer has any useful nutrients that can be absorbed by the body, it is now referred to as **waste**, and it is stored in the large intestine until it can be excreted from the body. Removing the liquid from the waste transforms it from liquid to solid stool, or **feces**.

This waste first passes from the small intestine to the cecum, a pouch that forms the first part of the large intestine. In herbivores, it provides a place for bacteria to digest cellulose, but in humans, most of it is vestigial and is known as the **appendix**. The appendix has no known function other than arbitrarily becoming inflamed. From the cecum, waste next travels up the ascending colon, across the transverse colon, down the descending colon, and through the sigmoid colon to the **rectum**. The rectum is responsible for the final storage of waste before it is expelled through the anus. The **anal canal** is a small portion of the rectum leading through to the anus and the outside of the body.

Pancreas

The **pancreas** has endocrine and exocrine functions. The endocrine function involves releasing the hormone insulin, which decreases blood sugar (glucose) levels, and **glucagon**, which increases blood sugar (glucose) levels, directly into the bloodstream. Both hormones are produced in the **islets of Langerhans**—insulin in the beta cells and glucagon in the alpha cells.

The major part of the gland has an exocrine function, which consists of acinar cells secreting inactive digestive enzymes (**zymogens**) into the main pancreatic duct. The main pancreatic duct joins the common bile duct, which empties into the small intestine (specifically the duodenum). The digestive enzymes are then activated and take part in the digestion of carbohydrates, proteins, and fats within chyme (the mixture of partially digested food and digestive juices).

Immune System

The **immune system** is the body's defense against invading microorganisms (bacteria, viruses, fungi, and parasites) and other harmful, foreign substances. It is capable of limiting or preventing infection.

There are two general types of immunity: innate immunity and acquired immunity. **Innate immunity** uses physical and chemical barriers to block the entry of microorganisms into the body. The skin forms a physical barrier that blocks microorganisms from entering underlying tissues. Mucous membranes in the digestive, respiratory, and urinary systems secrete mucus to block and remove invading microorganisms. Saliva, tears, and stomach acids are examples of chemical barriers intended to block infection with microorganisms. In addition, macrophages and other white blood cells can recognize and eliminate foreign objects through phagocytosis or direct lysis.

Acquired immunity refers to a specific set of events used by the body to fight a particular infection. Essentially, the body accumulates and stores information about the nature of an invading microorganism. As a result, the body can mount a specific attack that is much more effective than innate immunity. It also provides a way for the body to prevent future infections by the same microorganism.

Acquired immunity is divided into a primary response and a secondary response. The **primary immune response** occurs the first time that a particular microorganism enters the body, where macrophages engulf the microorganism and travel to the lymph nodes. In the lymph nodes, macrophages present the invader to helper T lymphocytes, which then activate humoral and cellular immunity. **Humoral immunity** refers to immunity resulting from antibody production by B lymphocytes. After being activated by helper T lymphocytes, B lymphocytes multiply and divide into plasma cells and memory cells. Plasma cells are B lymphocytes that produce immune proteins called **antibodies**, or **immunoglobulins**. Antibodies then bind to the microorganism to flag it for destruction by other white blood cells. **Cellular immunity** refers to the immune response coordinated by T lymphocytes. After being activated by helper T lymphocytes, other T lymphocytes attack and kill cells that cause infection or disease.

The **secondary immune response** takes place during subsequent encounters with a known microorganism. Memory cells respond to the previously encountered microorganism by immediately producing antibodies. Memory cells are B lymphocytes that store information to produce antibodies. The secondary immune response is swift and powerful because it eliminates the need for the time-consuming macrophage activation of the primary immune response. Suppressor T lymphocytes also take part to inhibit the immune response, as an overactive immune response could cause damage to healthy cells.

Active and Passive Immunity

Immunization is the process of inducing immunity. **Active immunization** refers to immunity gained by exposure to infectious microorganisms or viruses and can be **natural** or **artificial.** Natural immunization refers to an individual being exposed to an infectious organism as a part of daily life. For example, it was once common for parents to expose their children to childhood diseases such as measles or chicken pox. Artificial immunization refers to therapeutic exposure to an infectious organism as a way of protecting an individual from disease. Today, the medical community relies on artificial immunization as a way to induce immunity.

Vaccines are used for the development of active immunity. A vaccine contains a killed, weakened, or inactivated microorganism or virus that is administered through injection, by mouth, or by aerosol. Vaccinations are administered to prevent an infectious disease, but they do not always guarantee immunity.

Passive immunity refers to immunity gained by the introduction of antibodies. This introduction can be natural or artificial. The process occurs when antibodies from the mother's bloodstream are passed on to the bloodstream of the developing fetus. Breast milk can also transmit antibodies to a baby. Babies are born with passive immunity, which provides protection against general infection for approximately the first six months of life.

Integumentary System (Skin)

Skin consists of three layers: epidermis, dermis, and the hypodermis. There are four types of cells that make up the keratinized stratified squamous epithelium in the epidermis. They are keratinocytes, melanocytes, Merkel cells, and Langerhans cells. Skin is composed of many layers, starting with a basement membrane. On top of that sits the stratum germinativum, the stratum spinosum, the stratum granulosum, the stratum lucidum, and then the stratum corneum at the outer surface. Skin can be classified as thick or thin. These descriptions refer to the epidermal layer. Most of the body is covered with thin skin, but areas such as the palms of the hands are covered with thick skin. The **dermis** consists of a superficial papillary layer and a deeper reticular layer. The **papillary layer** is made of loose connective tissue, containing capillaries and the axons of sensory neurons. The **reticular layer** is a meshwork of tightly packed irregular connective tissue, containing blood vessels, hair follicles, nerves, sweat glands, and sebaceous glands. The **hypodermis** is a loose layer of fat and connective tissue. Since it is the third layer, if a burn reaches this tissue, it can cause serious damage.

Sweat glands and sebaceous glands are important exocrine glands found in the skin. **Sweat glands** regulate temperature, and remove bodily waste by secreting water, nitrogenous waste, and sodium salts to the surface of the body. Some sweat glands, such as those in the armpits and genitalia, are classified as **apocrine glands**. **Sebaceous glands** are holocrine glands that secrete sebum, which is an oily mixture of lipids and proteins. **Sebum** protects the skin from water loss, as well as bacterial and fungal infections.

The three major functions of skin are protection, regulation, and sensation. Skin acts as a barrier and protects the body from mechanical impacts, variations in temperature, microorganisms, and chemicals. It regulates body temperature, peripheral circulation, and fluid balance by secreting sweat. It also contains a large network of nerve cells that relay changes in the external environment to the body.

Lymphatic System

The **lymphatic** system, like the circulatory system, is a network of vessels and organs that move fluid—in this case, lymph—throughout the body. The lymphatic system works in concert with the immune system to help the body process toxins and waste. **Lymph** has a high concentration of white blood cells, which help attack viruses and bacteria throughout body cells and tissues. Lymph is filtered in nodes along the vessels; the body has 600 to 700 lymph nodes, which may be superficial (like those in the armpit and groin) or deep (such as those around the heart and lungs). The spleen is the largest organ of the lymphatic system and it helps produce the lymphocytes (white blood cells) to control infections. It also controls the number of red blood cells in the body. Other lymphatic organs include the tonsils, adenoids, and thymus.

Muscular System

The **muscular system** of the human body is responsible for all movements that the body produces. There are approximately 700 muscles in the body that are attached to the bones of the skeletal system and they make up half of the body's weight. Muscles are attached to the bones through **tendons**. Tendons are made up of dense bands of connective tissue and have collagen fibers that firmly attach to the bone on one side and to the muscle on the other. Their fibers are actually woven into the coverings of the bone and muscle so they can withstand the large forces that are put on them when the body is moving. There are three types of muscle tissue in the body: **skeletal muscle** tissue pulls on the bones of the skeleton and causes body movement, **cardiac muscle** tissue helps pump blood through veins and arteries, and **smooth muscle** tissue helps move fluids and solids along the digestive tract and contributes to movement in other body systems. All of these muscle tissues have four important properties in common:

1. They are **excitable**, meaning they respond to stimuli.
2. They are **contractile**, meaning they can shorten and pull on connective tissue.
3. They are **extensible**, meaning they can be stretched repeatedly but still maintain the ability to contract.
4. They are **elastic**, meaning they rebound to their original length after a contraction.

Muscles begin at an **origin** and end at an **insertion**. Generally, the origin is proximal to the insertion and the origin remains stationary while the insertion moves. For example, when bending the elbow and moving the hand up toward the head, the part of the forearm that is closest to the wrist moves and the part closer to the elbow is stationary. Therefore, a muscle in the forearm has an origin at the elbow and an insertion at the wrist.

Body movements occur by muscle **contraction**. Each contraction causes a specific action. Muscles can be classified into one of four muscle groups based on the action they perform. **Primary movers**, or **agonists**, produce a specific movement, such as flexion of the elbow. **Synergists** oversee helping the primary movers complete their specific movements. They can help stabilize the point of origin or provide extra pull near the insertion. Some synergists can aid an agonist in preventing movement at a joint. **Antagonists** are muscles whose actions are the opposite of that of the agonist. If an agonist is contracting during a specific movement, the antagonist is stretched. During flexion of the elbow, the biceps brachii muscle contracts and acts as an agonist, while the triceps brachii muscle on the opposite side of the upper arm acts as an antagonist and stretches.

Skeletal muscle tissue has several important functions. It causes movement of the skeleton by pulling on tendons, which moves the bones. It maintains body posture through the contraction of specific muscles responsible for the stability of the skeleton. Skeletal muscles help support the weight of internal organs and protect these organs from external injury. They also help to regulate body temperature within a normal range; muscle contractions require energy and produce heat, which heats the body when cold.

Reproductive System

The **reproductive system** is responsible for producing, storing, nourishing, and transporting functional reproductive cells, or gametes, in the human body. It includes the reproductive organs (also known as **gonads**), the reproductive tract, the accessory glands and organs that secrete fluids into the reproductive tract, and the **perineal** structures, which are the external genitalia.

The Male System

The male gonads are called **testes**. The testes secrete **androgens**—mainly testosterone—and produce and store 500 million **spermatocytes**, which are the male gametes, each day. An androgen is a steroid hormone that controls the development and maintenance of male characteristics. Once the sperm are mature, they move through a duct system, where they mix with additional fluids secreted by accessory glands, forming a mixture called **semen**.

The Female System

The female gonads are the **ovaries**. Ovaries generally produce one immature gamete, an egg or **oocyte**, per month. They are also responsible for secreting the hormones estrogen and progesterone. When the oocyte is released from the ovary, it travels along the uterine tubes, or **Fallopian tubes**, and then into the uterus. The uterus opens into the vagina. When sperm cells enter the vagina, they swim through the uterus and may fertilize the oocyte in the Fallopian tubes. The resulting zygote travels down the tube and implants into the uterine wall. The uterus protects and nourishes the developing embryo for nine months until it is ready for the outside environment. If the oocyte is not fertilized, it is released in the uterine, or menstrual, cycle. The **menstrual cycle** occurs monthly and involves the shedding of the functional part of the uterine lining.

Human Reproduction

Humans procreate through sexual reproduction. Sexual reproduction involves the fusion of gametes, one from each parent. A **gamete** is a reproductive cell that contains half the chromosomes of a normal cell. Chromosomes are found in the nucleus of cells and contain DNA. The female gamete is called an **ovum**, or **egg**, and the male gamete is called a **sperm**. In sexual reproduction, the gametes fuse through a process called fertilization. Thus, sexual reproduction often produces offspring with varying characteristics.

Gametes are created by the human reproductive systems. In women, the ovaries produce eggs, the female gamete. On average, the ovaries produce one mature egg per month, which is referred to as the menstrual cycle. The release of an egg from the ovaries is termed **ovulation**. The female menstrual cycle is under the control of hormones such as luteinizing hormone (LH), follicle stimulating hormone (FSH), estrogen, and progesterone. In men, the testes produce sperm, the male gamete, and they produce millions of sperm at a time. The hormones LH and testosterone regulate the production of sperm in the testes. **Leydig cells** in the testes produce testosterone, while sperm is manufactured in the seminiferous tubules of the testes.

As mentioned previously, the fusion of the gametes (egg and sperm) is termed **fertilization**, and the resulting fusion creates a **zygote**. The zygote takes approximately seven days to travel through the fallopian tube and implant itself into the uterus. Upon implantation, it has developed into a **blastocyst** and will next grow into a **gastrula**. It is during this stage that the embryological **germ layers** are formed. The three germ layers are the **ectoderm** (outer layer), **mesoderm** (middle layer), and **endoderm** (inner layer). All of the human body systems develop from one or more of the germ layers. The gastrula further develops into an **embryo** which then matures into a **fetus**. The entire process takes approximately nine months and culminates in labor and birth.

Respiratory System

The **respiratory system** mediates the exchange of gas between the air and the blood, mainly through the act of breathing. This system is divided into the upper respiratory system and the lower respiratory system. The **upper respiratory system** comprises the nose, the nasal cavity and sinuses, and the pharynx. The **lower respiratory system** comprises the larynx (voice box), the trachea (windpipe), the small passageways leading to the lungs, and the lungs. The upper respiratory system is responsible for filtering, warming, and humidifying the air that gets passed to the lower respiratory system, protecting the lower respiratory system's more delicate tissue surfaces. The process of breathing in is referred to as **inspiration**, while the process of breathing out is referred to as **expiration**.

The Lungs

Bronchi are tubes that lead from the trachea to each lung. They are lined with cilia and mucus that collect dust and germs along the way. The bronchi, which carry air into the lungs, branch into **bronchioles** and continue to divide into smaller and smaller passageways, until they become **alveoli**, which are the smallest structures. Most of the gas exchange in the lungs occurs between the blood-filled pulmonary capillaries and the air-filled alveoli. Within the lungs, oxygen and carbon dioxide are exchanged between the air in the alveoli and the blood in the pulmonary capillaries. Oxygen-rich blood returns to the heart and is pumped through the systemic circuit. Carbon dioxide-rich air is exhaled from the body. Together, due to all the branching, the lungs contain approximately 1,500 miles of airway passages.

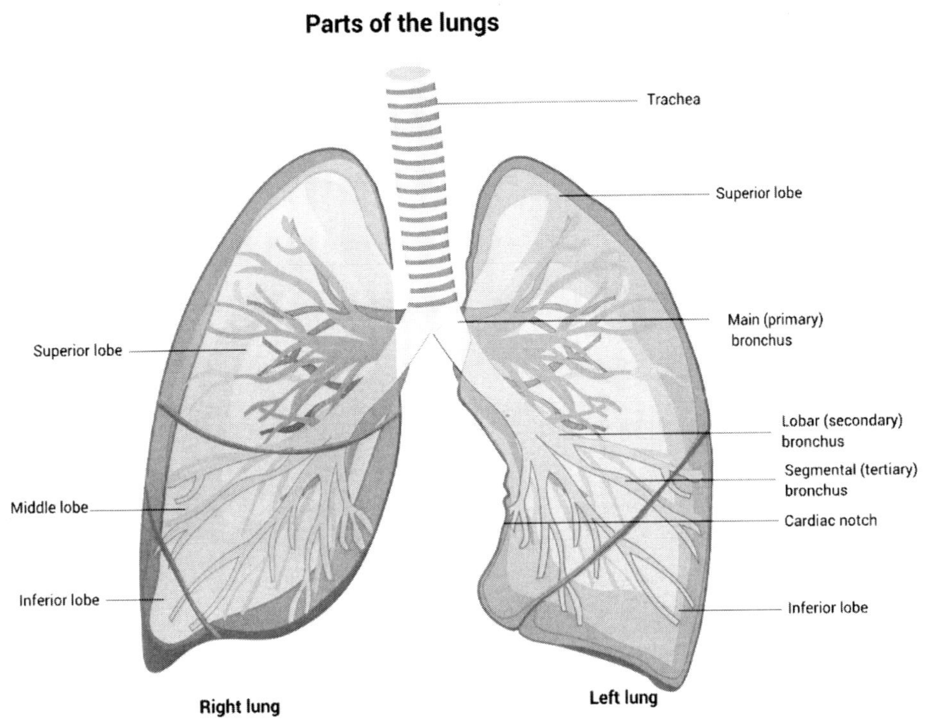

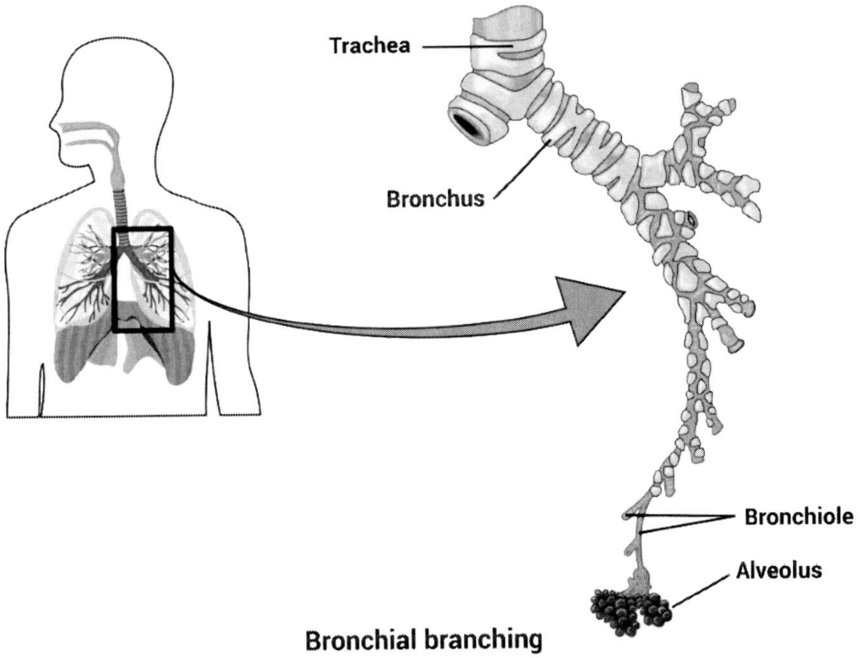

Breathing is possible due to the muscular diaphragm pulling on the lungs, increasing lung volume and decreasing pulmonary pressure. Air flows from the external high-pressure system to the low-pressure system inside the lungs. When breathing out, the diaphragm releases its pressure difference, decreases the lung volume, and forces the stale air back out.

Functions of the Respiratory System

The respiratory system has many functions. Most importantly, it provides a large area for gas exchange between the air and the circulating blood. It protects the delicate respiratory surfaces from environmental variations and defends them against pathogens. It is responsible for producing the sounds that the body makes for speaking and singing, as well as for non-verbal communication. It also helps regulate blood volume and blood pressure by releasing **vasopressin**, and it is a regulator of blood pH due to its control over carbon dioxide release, as the aqueous form of carbon dioxide is the chief buffering agent in blood.

Skeletal System

The **skeletal system** consists of the 206 bones that make up the adult skeleton, as well as the cartilage, ligaments, and other connective tissues that stabilize them.

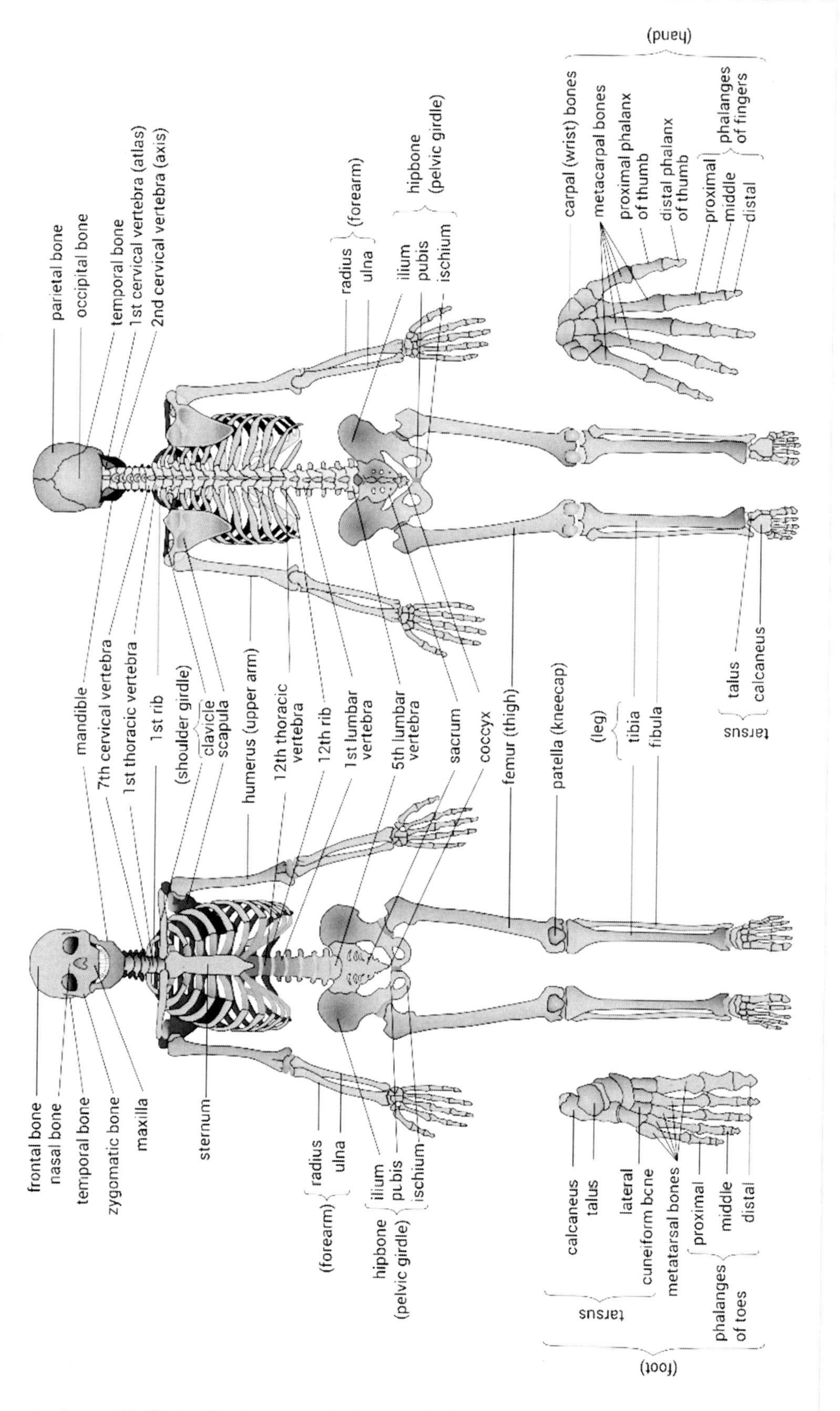
frontal bone
nasal bone
temporal bone
zygomatic bone
maxilla
sternum
radius
ulna
(forearm)
ilium
pubis
ischium
hipbone
(pelvic girdle)
calcaneus
talus
lateral
cuneiform bone
metatarsal bones
proximal
middle
distal
tarsus
phalanges
of toes
(foot)
mandible
7th cervical vertebra
1st thoracic vertebra
1st rib
(shoulder girdle)
clavicle
scapula
humerus (upper arm)
12th thoracic
vertebra
12th rib
1st lumbar
vertebra
5th lumbar
vertebra
sacrum
coccyx
femur (thigh)
patella (kneecap)
(leg)
tibia
fibula
talus
calcaneus
tarsus
parietal bone
occipital bone
temporal bone
1st cervical vertebra (atlas)
2nd cervical vertebra (axis)
radius
ulna
(forearm)
ilium
pubis
ischium
hipbone
(pelvic girdle)
carpal (wrist) bones
metacarpal bones
proximal phalanx
of thumb
distal phalanx
of thumb
proximal
middle
distal
phalanges
of fingers
(hand)

Bone is made of collagen fibers and calcium inorganic minerals, mostly in the form of hydroxyapatite, calcium carbonate, and phosphate salts. The inorganic minerals are strong but brittle, and the collagen fibers are weak but flexible, so the combination makes bone resistant to shattering. There are two types of bone: compact and spongy. **Compact bone**, also called **cortical bone**, has a basic functional unit, called the **Haversian system**. **Osteocytes**, or bone cells, are arranged in concentric circles around a central canal, called the Haversian canal, which contains blood vessels.

While Haversian canals run parallel to the surface of the bone, perforating canals, also known as the **canals of Volkmann**, run perpendicularly between the central canal and the surface of the bone. The concentric circles of bone tissue that surround the central canal within the Haversian system are called **lamellae**. The spaces that are found between the lamellae are called **lacunae**. The Haversian system is a reservoir for calcium and phosphorus for blood. **Spongy** bone or **cancellous** bone, in contrast to compact bone, is lightweight and porous. It has a branching network of parallel lamellae, called **trabeculae**. Although spongy bone forms an open framework inside the compact bone, it is still quite strong.

Different bones have different ratios of compact-to-spongy bone, depending on their functions. The outside of the bone is covered by the **periosteum**, which has four major functions. It isolates and protects bones from the surrounding tissue, provides a place for attachment of the circulatory and nervous system structures, participates in growth and repair of the bone, and attaches the bone to the deep fascia. The **endosteum** is found inside the bone; it covers the trabeculae of the spongy bone and lines the inner surfaces of the central canals.

One major function of the skeletal system is to provide structural support for the entire body. It provides a framework for the soft tissues and organs to attach to. The skeletal system also provides a reserve of important nutrients, such as calcium and lipids. Normal concentrations of calcium and phosphate in body fluids are partly maintained by the calcium salts stored in bone. Lipids that are stored in yellow bone marrow can be used as a source of energy. Yellow bone marrow also produces some white blood cells. Red bone marrow produces red blood cells, most white blood cells, and platelets that circulate in the blood. Certain groups of bones form protective barriers around delicate organs. The ribs, for example, protect the heart and lungs, the skull encloses the brain, and the vertebrae cover and protect the spinal cord.

Special Senses

The **special senses** include vision, hearing and balance, smell, and taste. They are distinguished from general senses in that special senses have **special somatic afferents** and **special visceral afferents**, both a type of nerve fiber relaying information to the CNS, as well as specialized organs devoted to their function. Touch is the other sense that is typically discussed, but unlike the special senses, it relays information to the CNS from all over the body and not just one particular organ; **skin**, the largest organ of the body, is the largest contributor to tactile information, but touch receptors also include **mechanoreceptors**, **nociceptors** for pain, and **thermoreceptors** for heat. Tactile messages are carried via **general somatic afferents** and **general visceral afferents**. Various touch receptors exist in the body such as the following:

- **Pacinian corpuscles:** detect rapid vibration in the skin and fascia
- **Meissner's corpuscles:** respond to light touch and slower vibrations
- **Merkel's discs:** respond to sustained pressure
- **Ruffini endings:** detect deep touch and tension in the skin and fascia

Urinary System

The **urinary system** includes the kidneys, ureters, urinary bladder, and the urethra. It is the main system responsible for getting rid of the organic waste products, excess water, and electrolytes that are generated by the body's other systems. The kidneys are responsible for producing **urine**, which is a fluid waste product containing water, ions, and small soluble compounds. The urinary system has many important functions related to waste excretion. It regulates the concentrations of sodium, potassium, chloride, calcium, and other ions in the plasma by controlling the amount of each that is excreted in urine. This also contributes to the maintenance of blood pH. It regulates blood volume and pressure by controlling the amount of water lost in the urine. It eliminates toxic substances, drugs, and organic waste products, such as urea and uric acid.

The Kidneys

Under normal circumstances, humans have two functioning **kidneys**. They are the main organs responsible for filtering waste products out of the blood and transferring them to urine. Kidneys are made of millions of tiny filtering units called **nephrons.** Nephrons have two parts: a **glomerulus**, which is the filter, and a **tubule.** As blood enters the kidneys, the glomerulus allows fluid and waste products to pass through it and enter the tubule. Blood cells and large molecules, such as proteins, do not pass through and remain in the blood. The filtered fluid and waste then pass through the tubule, where any final essential minerals are sent back to the bloodstream. The final product at the end of the tubule is **urine**.

Waste Excretion

Once urine accumulates, it leaves the kidneys. The urine travels through the ureters into the urinary **bladder**, a muscular organ that is hollow and elastic. As more urine enters the urinary bladder, its walls stretch and become thinner, so there is no significant difference in internal pressure. The urinary bladder stores the urine until the body is ready for urination, at which time the muscles contract and force the urine through the urethra and out of the body.

Chemical and Physical Foundations of Biological Systems

Foundational Concept 4: Complex living organisms transport materials, sense their environment, process signals, and respond to changes using processes understood in terms of physical principles.

Translational Motion, Forces, Work, Energy, and Equilibrium in Living Systems

Translational Motion

People have been studying the movement of objects since ancient times, sometimes prompted by curiosity, and sometimes by necessity. On Earth, items move according to specific guidelines and have motion that is fairly predictable. In order to understand why an object moves along its path, it is important to understand what role forces have on influencing an object's movements. The term **force** describes an outside influence on an object. Force does not have to refer to something imparted by another object. Forces can act upon objects by touching them with a push or a pull, by friction, or without touch like a magnetic force or even gravity. Forces can affect the motion of an object.

In order to study an object's motion, the object must be locatable and describable. When locating an object's position, it can help to locate it relative to another known object, or put it into a **frame of reference.** This phrase means that if the placement of one object is known, it is easier to locate another object with respect to the position of the original object.

The measurement of an object's movement or change in position (x), over a change in time (t) is an object's **speed.** The measurement of speed with direction is **velocity**. A "change in position" refers to the difference in location of an object's starting point and an object's ending point. In science, a change is represented by the Greek letter Delta, Δ.

Equation:

$$velocity\ (v) = \frac{\Delta x}{\Delta t}$$

Position is measured in meters, and time is measured in seconds. The standard measurement for velocity is meters per second (m/s).

$$\frac{meters}{second} = \frac{m}{s}$$

The measurement of an object's change in velocity over time is an object's **acceleration**. Gravity is considered to be a form of acceleration.

Equation:

$$acceleration\ (a) = \frac{\Delta v}{\Delta t}$$

Velocity is measured in meters per second and time is measured in seconds. The standard measurement for acceleration is meters per second per second (m/s^2).

$$\frac{\frac{meters}{second}}{second} = \frac{meters}{second^2} = \frac{m}{s^2}$$

For example, consider a car traveling down the road. The speed can be measured by calculating how far the car is traveling over a certain period of time. However, since the car is traveling in a direction (north, east, south, west), the distance over time is actually the car's velocity. It can be confusing, as many people will often interchange the words speed and velocity. But if something is traveling a certain distance, during a certain time period, in a direction, this is the object's velocity. Velocity is speed with direction.

The change in an object's velocity over a certain amount of time is the object's acceleration. If the driver of that car keeps pressing on the gas pedal and increasing the velocity, the car would have a change in velocity over the change in time and would be accelerating. The reverse could be said if the driver were depressing the brake and the car was slowing down; it would have a negative acceleration, or be decelerating. Since acceleration also has a direction component, it is possible for a car to accelerate without changing speed. If an object changes direction, it is accelerating.

Motion creates something called **momentum**. This is a calculation of an object's mass multiplied by its velocity. Momentum can be described as the amount an object wants to continue moving along its current course. Momentum in a straight line is called **linear momentum**. Just as energy can be transferred and conserved, so can momentum.

For example, a car and a truck moving at the same velocity down a highway will not have the same momentum, because they do not have the same mass. The mass of the truck is greater than that of the car, therefore the truck will have more momentum. In a head-on collision, the vehicles would be expected to slide in the same direction of the truck's original motion because the truck has a greater momentum.

The amount of force that acts on an object during a length of time is referred to as the **impulse**. If the length of time can be extended, the impulse will be less, due to the conservation of momentum.

Consider another example, when catching a fast baseball, it helps soften the blow of the ball to follow through, or cradle the catch. This technique is simply extending the time of the application of the force of the ball, so the impact of the ball does not hurt the hand. As a final example, if a martial arts expert wants to break a board by executing a hand chop, he or she needs to exert a force on a small point on the board extremely quickly. Lengthening the time of the impact (slowing down the movement) will likely not break the board and may also cause injury.

Types of Motion

Newton's Three Laws of Motion

Sir Isaac Newton spent a great deal of time studying objects, forces, and how an object's motion responds to forces. Newton made great advancements in the ability to describe and predict the motion of objects by applying his mathematical models to different situations. Through his extensive research, Newton is credited for summarizing the basic laws of motion for objects on Earth. These laws are as follows:

1. **The law of inertia:** An object in motion remains in motion, unless acted upon by an outside force. An object at rest remains at rest, unless acted upon by an outside force. Simply put, **inertia** is the natural tendency of an object to continue what it is already doing; an outside force would have to act upon the object to make it change its course. This includes an object that is sitting still. The inertia of an object is relative to its momentum. For example, if a car is driving at a constant speed in a constant direction (also called a constant velocity), it

would take a force in a different direction to change the path of the car. Conversely, if the car is sitting still, it would take a force greater than that of friction from any direction to make that stationary car move.

2. $\boldsymbol{F = ma}$: The **force** (F) on an object is equal to the mass (m) multiplied by the acceleration (a) on that object. **Mass** (m) refers to the amount of a substance and acceleration (a) refers to a rate of velocity over time. In the case of an object on Earth, the acceleration due to gravity (a constant) is used for acceleration (a), and the force calculated by F = ma is called **weight** *(W)*. It is important to discern that an object's mass (measured in kilograms, kg) is not the same as an object's weight (measured in Newtons, N). Weight is the mass times the gravity. The gravity on the Earth's moon is considerably less than the gravity on Earth. Therefore, the weight of an object on the Earth's moon would be considerably less than the weight of the object on Earth. In each case, a different value for acceleration/gravity would be used in the equation F = ma.

Example: If a raisin is dropped into a bowl of pudding, it would make a small indentation and stick in the pudding a bit, but if a grapefruit is dropped into the same bowl of pudding, it would splatter the pudding out of the bowl and most likely hit the bottom of the bowl. Even though both items are accelerating at the same rate (due to gravity), the mass of the grapefruit is larger than that of the raisin; therefore, the force with which the grapefruit hits the bowl of pudding is considerably larger than the force from the raisin hitting the bowl of pudding.

3. **For every action, there is an equal and opposite reaction:** If someone pounds a fist on a table, the reactionary force from the table causes the person to feel a sharp force on the fist. The magnitude of the force felt on the fist increases the harder that the person pounds on the table. It should be noted that action/reaction pairs occur simultaneously. As the fist applies a force on the table, the table instantaneously applies an equal and opposite force on the fist. If an ice skater attempts to push on a heavy sled sitting in front of them the skater will be pushed in the direction opposite of their push on the sled; the push the skater is experiencing is equal and opposite to the force he or she is exerting on the sled. This is a good example of how the icy surface helps to lessen the effects of friction and allows the reactionary force to be more easily observed.

Force

Forces are anything acting upon an object either in motion or at rest; this includes friction and gravity. These forces are often depicted by using a **force diagram** or **free body diagram**. A force diagram shows an object as the focal point, with arrows denoting all the forces acting upon the object. The direction of the head of the arrow indicates the direction of the force. The object at the center can also be exerting forces on things in its surroundings; these forces would be displayed in the diagram.

Equilibrium

If an object is in constant motion or at rest (its acceleration equals zero), the object is said to be in **equilibrium**. Equilibrium does not imply that there are no forces acting upon the object, but that all of the forces are balanced in order for the situation to continue in its current state.

Note that both an object that is resting on top of a mountain peak or one that is traveling at a constant velocity down the side of that mountain describe situations in which an object is in a state of equilibrium.

Falling Objects

Objects falling within the Earth's atmosphere are all affected by gravity. Their rate of acceleration will be that of gravity. If two objects are dropped from a great height at the exact same time, regardless of mass, theoretically, they should hit the ground at the same time because gravity acts upon them at the same rate. In actuality, if this were attempted, the shape of the objects and external factors such as air resistance would affect their rates of fall and cause a discrepancy in when each object lands.

Consider the traditional illustration of this principle: A feather and a rock are released at the same time in regular air versus in a vacuum. In the open atmosphere, the feather would slowly loft down to the ground, due to the effects of air resistance, while the rock would quickly drop to the ground. If the feather and the rock were both released at the same time in a vacuum, they would both hit the bottom at the same time. The rate of fall is not dependent upon the mass of the item or any external factors in a vacuum (there is no air resistance in a vacuum), therefore, only gravity would affect the rate of fall. Gravity affects every object on the Earth with the same rate of acceleration (approximately 9.8 m/s^2).

Circular Motion

An **axis** is an invisible line on which an object can rotate. This is most easily observed with a toy top. There is actually a point (or rod) through the center of the top on which the top can be observed to be spinning. This is called the axis.

When objects move in a circle by spinning on their own axis, or because they are tethered around a central point (also an axis), they exhibit circular motion. Circular motion is similar in many ways to linear (straight line) motion; however, there are a few additional points to note. A spinning object is always accelerating because it is always changing direction. The force causing this constant acceleration on or around an axis is called **centripetal force** and is often associated with centripetal acceleration. Centripetal force always pulls toward the axis of rotation. An imaginary reactionary force, called **centrifugal force**, is the outward force felt when an object is undergoing circular motion. This reactionary force is not the real force; it just feels like it is there. For this reason, it has also been referred to as a "fictional force." The true force is the one pulling inward, or the centripetal force.

The terms *centripetal* and *centrifugal* are often mistakenly interchanged. If the centripetal force acting on an object moving with circular motion is removed, the object will continue moving in a straight line tangent to the point on the circle where the object last experienced the centripetal force. For example, when a traditional style washing machine spins a load of clothes to expunge the water from the load, it rapidly spins the machine barrel. A force is pulling in toward the center of the circle (centripetal force). At the same time, the wet clothes, which are attempting to move in a straight line, are colliding with the outer wall of the barrel that is moving in a circle. The interaction between the wet clothes and barrel wall causes a reactionary force to the centripetal force and this expels the water out of the small holes that line the outer wall of the barrel.

Conservation of Angular Momentum

An object moving in a circular motion also has momentum; for circular motion, it is called **angular momentum**. This is determined by rotational inertia, rotational velocity, and the distance of the mass from the axis or center of rotation. When objects exhibit circular motion, they also demonstrate the **conservation of angular momentum**, meaning that the angular momentum of a system is always constant, regardless of the placement of the mass. Rotational inertia can be affected by how far the mass of the object is placed with respect to the axis of rotation. The greater the distance between the mass and the axis of rotation, the slower the rotational velocity. Conversely, if the mass is closer to the axis of rotation, the rotational velocity is faster. A change in one affects the other, thus conserving the angular momentum. This holds true as long as no external forces act upon the system.

For example, ice skaters spinning in on one ice skate extends their arms out for a slower rotational velocity. When skaters bring their arms in close to their bodies (which lessens the distance between the mass and the axis of rotation), their rotational velocity increases and they spin much faster. Some skaters extend their arms straight up above their head, which causes an extension of the axis of rotation, thus removing any distance between the mass and the center of rotation, which maximizes their rotational velocity.

Another example is when a person selects a horse on a merry-go-round: the placement of their horse can affect their ride experience. All of the horses are traveling with the same rotational speed, but in order to travel along the same plane as the merry-go-round turns, a horse on the outside will have a greater linear speed because it is further away from the axis of rotation. Essentially, an outer horse has to cover a lot more ground than a horse on the inside in order to keep up with the rotational speed of the merry-go-round platform. Thrill seekers should always select an outer horse.

Energy

The term **energy** typically refers to an object's ability to perform work. This can include a transfer of heat from one object to another, or from an object to its surroundings. Energy is usually measured in Joules.

Potential energy (Gravitational Potential Energy, or **PE):** This is stored energy, or energy due to an object's height above the ground.

Kinetic energy (KE): This is the energy of motion. If an object is moving, it has some amount of kinetic energy.

Consider a rollercoaster car sitting still on the tracks at the top of a hill. The rollercoaster has all potential energy and no kinetic energy. As it travels down the hill, the energy transfers from potential energy into kinetic energy. At the bottom of the hill, where the car is going the fastest, it has all kinetic energy, but no potential energy. If energy lost to the environment (friction, heat, sound) it ignored, the amount of potential energy at the top of the hill equals the amount of kinetic energy at the bottom of the hill.

Mechanical Energy

Mechanical energy is the sum of the potential and kinetic energy in a system, minus energy lost to non-conservative forces. Often, the effects of non-conservative forces are small enough that they can be ignored. The total mechanical energy of a system is always conserved. The amount of potential energy and the amount of kinetic energy can vary to add up to this total, but the total mechanical energy in the situation remains the same.

$$ME = PE + KE\ (Mechanical\ Energy = Potential\ Energy + Kinetic\ Energy)$$

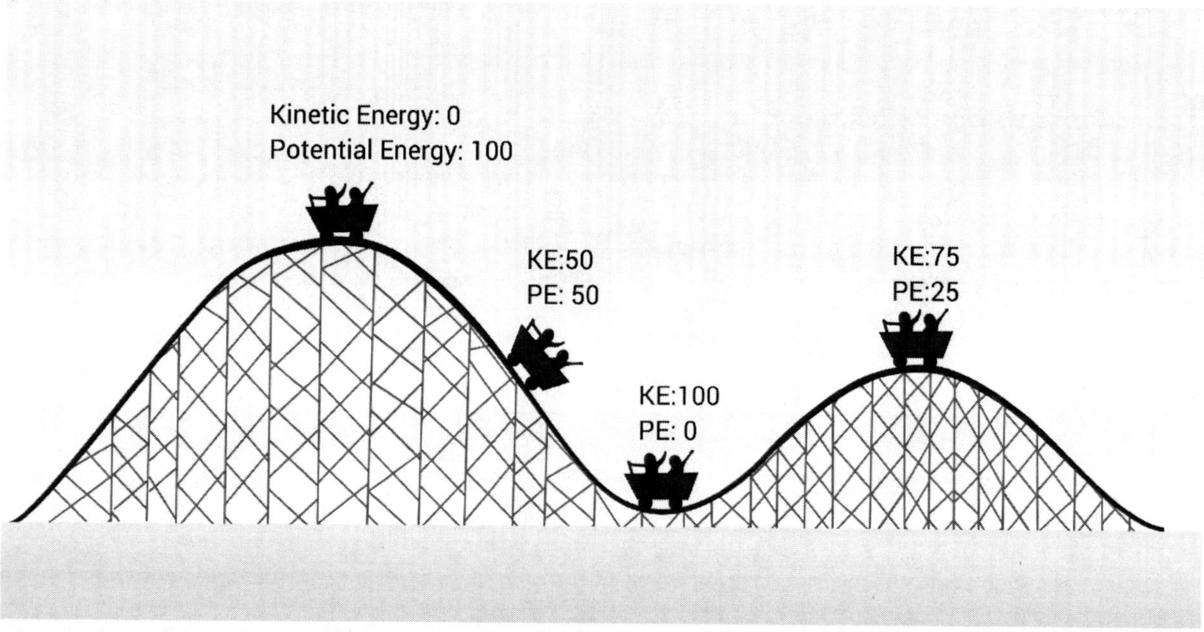

There is a fundamental law of thermodynamics (the study of heat and movement) called **Conservation of Energy.** This law states that energy cannot be created nor destroyed, but rather, energy is transferred to different forms. For instance, a car pushed beginning at one end of a street will not continue down that street forever; it will gradually come to a stop some distance away from where it was originally pushed. This does not mean the energy has disappeared or has been exhausted; it means the energy has been transferred to different mediums surrounding the car.

The frictional force from the road on the tires dissipates some of the energy, the air resistance from the movement of the car dissipates some of the energy, the sound from the tires on the road dissipates some of the energy, and the force of gravity pulling on the car dissipates some of the energy. Each value can be calculated such as measuring the sound waves from the tires, measuring the temperature change in the tires, measuring the distance moved by the car from start to finish, etc. It is important to understand that many processes factor into such a small situation, but all situations follow the conservation of energy.

As in the earlier example, the rollercoaster at the top of a hill has a measurable amount of potential energy, and when it rolls down the hill, it converts most of that energy into kinetic energy. There are still additional factors like friction and air resistance working on the rollercoaster that dissipate some of the energy, but energy transfers in every situation.

Importance of Fluids for the Circulation of Blood, Gas Movement, and Gas Exchange

Fluids

In addition to the behavior of solid particles acted on by forces, it is important to understand the behavior of fluids. **Fluids** include both liquids and gasses. The best way to understand fluid behavior is to contrast it with the behavior of solids.

First consider a block of ice, which is solid water. If it is set down inside a large box it will exert a force on the bottom of the box due to its weight as shown on the left, in Part A of the figure. The solid block exerts a pressure on the bottom of the box equal to its total weight divided by the area of its base:

$$Pressure = \frac{Weight\ of\ block}{Area\ of\ base}$$

That pressure acts only in the area directly under the block of ice.

If the same mass of ice is melted, it behaves much differently. It still has the same weight because its mass hasn't changed; however, the volume has increased.

The Behavior of Solids and Liquids Compared

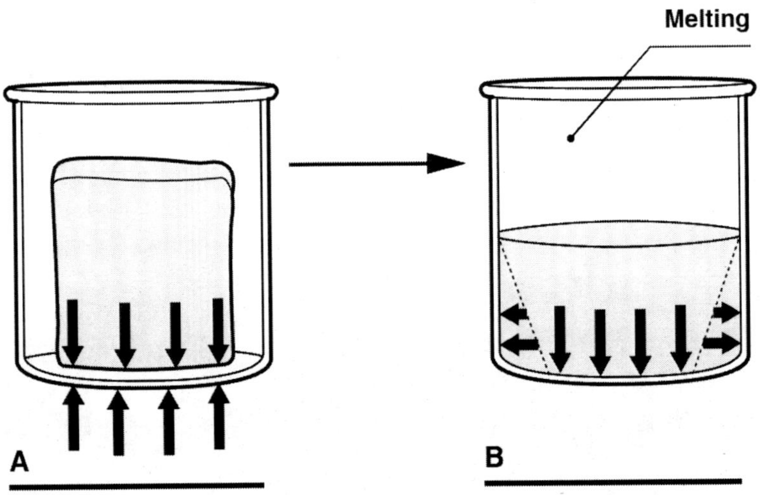

Forces exerted by a block of ice on its container

Forces exerted by a water on its container

The melted ice (now water) conforms to the shape of the container. This means that the fluid exerts pressure not only on the base, but on the sides of the box at the water line and below. Actually, pressure in a liquid is exerted in all directions, but all the forces in the interior of the fluid cancel each other out, so that a net force is only exerted on the walls. Note also that the pressure on the walls increases with the depth of the water.

The fact that the liquid exerts pressure in all directions is part of the reason some solids float in liquids. Consider the forces acting on a block of wood floating in water, as shown in the figure below.

The block of wood is submerged in the water and pressure acts on its bottom and sides. The weight of the block tends to force it down into the water. The force of the pressure on the left side of the block just cancels the force of the pressure on the right side.

There is a net upward force on the bottom of the block due to the pressure of the water acting on that surface. This force, which counteracts the weight of the block, is known as the **buoyant** force.

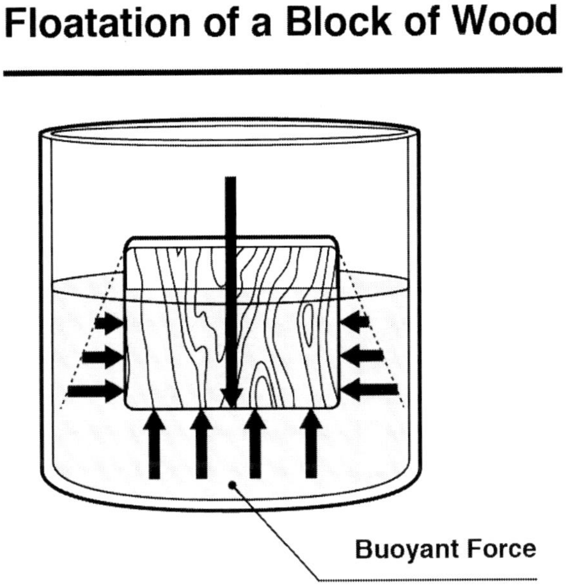

The block will sink to a depth such that the buoyant force of the water (equal to the weight of the volume of fluid displaced) just matches the total weight of the block. This will happen if two conditions are met:

1. The body of water is deep enough to float the block
2. The density of the block is less than the density of the water

If the body of water is not deep enough, the water pressure on the bottom side of the block won't be enough to develop a buoyant force equal to the block's weight. The block will be "beached," just like a boat caught at low tide.

If the density of the block is greater than the density of the fluid, the buoyant force acting on the bottom of the boat will not be sufficient to counteract the total weight of the block. That's why a solid steel block will sink in water.

If steel is denser than water, how can a steel ship float? The steel ship floats because it's hollow. The volume of water displaced by its steel shell (hull) is heavier than the entire weight of the ship and its contents (which includes a lot of empty space). In fact, there's so much empty space within a steel ship's hull that it can bob out of the water and be unstable at sea if some of the void spaces (called "ballast tanks") aren't filled with water. This provides more weight and balance (or "trim") to the vessel.

The discussion of buoyant forces on solids holds for liquids as well. A less dense liquid can float on a denser liquid if they're **immiscible** (do not mix). For instance, oil can float on water because oil isn't as dense as the water. Fresh water can float on salt water for the same reason.

Pascal's Law

Pascal's law states that a change in pressure, applied to an enclosed fluid, is transmitted undiminished to every portion of the fluid and to the walls of its containing vessel. This principle is used in the design of hydraulic jacks.

A force (F_1) is exerted on a small "driving" piston, which creates pressure on the hydraulic fluid. This pressure is transmitted through the fluid to a large cylinder. While the pressure is the same everywhere in the oil, the pressure action on the area of the larger cylinder creates a much higher upward force (F_2).

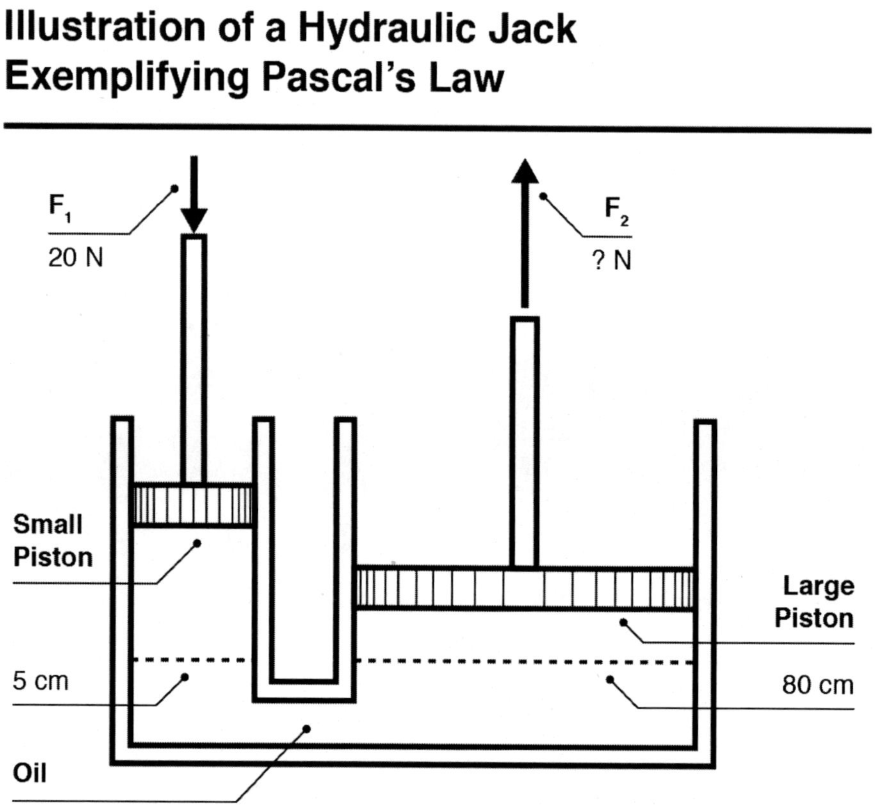

Looking again at the figure above, suppose the diameter of the small cylinder is 5 centimeters and the diameter of the large cylinder is 80 centimeters. If a force of 20 newtons (N) is exerted on the small driving piston, what's the value of the upward force F_2? In other words, what weight can the large piston support?

The pressure within the system is created from the force F_1 acting over the area of the piston:

$$P = \frac{F_1}{A} = \frac{20 \text{ N}}{\pi \, (0.05 \text{ m})^2/4} = 10{,}185 \text{ Pa}$$

The same pressure acts on the larger piston, creating the upward force F_2:

$$F_2 = P \times A = 10{,}185 \text{ Pa} \times \pi \times (0.8 \text{ m})^2/4 = 5{,}120 \text{ N}$$

Flow Rate

Because a liquid has no internal shear strength, it can be transported in a pipe or channel between two locations. A fluid's "rate of flow" is the volume of fluid that passes a given location in a given amount of time and is expressed in m^3/s. The **flow rate** (Q) is determined by measuring the **area of flow** (A) in m^2, and the **flow velocity** (v) in m/s:

$$Q = v \times A$$

This equation is called the **Continuity Equation**. It's one of the most important equations in engineering. For example, the figure below shows a pipe with an inside diameter of 1,200 millimeters running full with a velocity of 1.6 m/s (measured by a **sonic velocity meter**). What's the flow rate?

Using the Continuity Equation, the flow is obtained by keeping careful track of units:

$$Q = v \times A = 1.6\frac{m}{s} \times \frac{\pi}{4} \times \left(\frac{1{,}200 \text{ mm}}{1{,}000 \text{ mm/m}}\right)^2 = 1.81 \text{ m}^3/\text{s}$$

For more practice, imagine that a pipe is filling a storage tank with a diameter of 100 meters. How long does it take for the water level to rise by 2 meters?

Since the flow rate (Q) is expressed in m^3/s, and volume is measured in m^3, then the time in seconds to supply a volume (V) is $\frac{V}{Q}$. Here, the volume required is:

$$Volume\ Required = Base\ Area \times Depth = \frac{\pi}{4}100^2 \times 2 \text{ m} = 15{,}700 \text{ m}^3$$

Thus, the time to fill the tank another 2 meters is 15,700 m^3 divided by 1.81 m^3/s which equals 8,674 seconds or 2.4 hours.

It's important to understand that, for a given flow rate, a smaller pipe requires a higher velocity.

The energy of a flow system is evaluated in terms of potential and kinetic energy, the same way the energy of a falling weight is evaluated. The total energy of a fluid flow system is divided into potential energy of elevation, and pressure and the kinetic energy of velocity. **Bernoulli's Equation** states that, for a constant flow rate, the total energy of the system (divided into components of elevation, pressure, and velocity) remains constant. This is written as:

$$Z + \frac{P}{\rho g} + \frac{v^2}{2g} = \text{Constant}$$

Each of the terms in this equation has the dimensions of meters. The first term is the **elevation energy**, where Z is the elevation in meters. The second term is the **pressure energy**, where P is the pressure, ρ is the density, and g is the acceleration of gravity. The dimensions of the second term are also in meters. The third term is the **velocity energy**, also expressed in meters.

For a fixed elevation, the equation shows that, as the pressure increases, the velocity decreases. In the other case, as the velocity increases, the pressure decreases.

The use of the Bernoulli Equation is illustrated in the figure below. The total energy is the same at Sections 1 and 2. The area of flow at Section 1 is greater than the area at Section 2. Since the flow rate is the same at each section, the velocity at Point 2 is higher than at Point 1:

$$Q = V_1 \times A_1 = V_2 \times A_2$$

$$V_2 = V_1 \times \frac{A_1}{A_2}$$

Finally, since the total energy is the same at the two sections, the pressure at Point 2 is less than at Point 1. The tubes drawn at Points 1 and 2 would actually have the water levels shown in the figure: the pressure at each point would support a column of water of a height equal to the pressure divided by the unit weight of the water ($h = \frac{P}{\rho g}$).

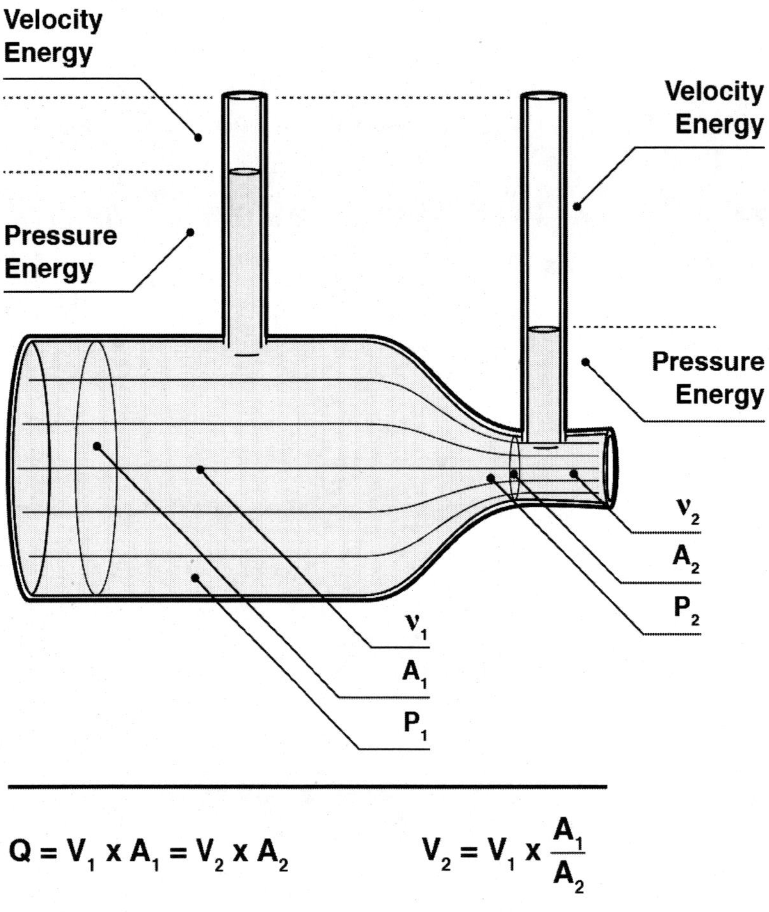

Ideal Gases

According to **kinetic molecular theory**:

- Gas particles have **Brownian**, or random, motion (consistent with the second law of thermodynamics)
- Particles travel in a straight line until they hit another object and change direction
- Volume of a gas particle is virtually zero

- There are no attractive or repulsive forces between gas particles, and there are no unaccounted chemical or physical interactions between particles
- There are elastic collisions of the gas with its container and other particles: particles don't slow down and are constantly moving
- Movement, or kinetic energy, is a function of temperature. As temperature increases, kinetic energy increases. Average kinetic energy is equal to temperature in **Kelvin**.

Collision theory is closely related to kinetic molecular theory. Based on the fact that as temperature increases, movement increases, its premise is that reactions happen faster as temperature increases due to increased reactant collisions with each other and with catalysts. Of note, from a biological perspective, there is a limit to this temperature increase because, if it is a reaction involving biological protein catalysts (enzymes), the enzyme will eventually denature, "cook," and lose functionality.

A whole field of study on particle movement in gas laws has evolved over time to create the **ideal gas law:**

$$PV = nRT$$

Scientists' contributions on advancements in ideal gas laws are referenced in this chart:

Charles' Law	Direct: As temperature increases, volume increases (Pressure and Number of moles held constant)	$\frac{V_1}{T_1} = \frac{V_2}{T_2}$
Gay Lussac's Law	Direct: As temperature increases, pressure increases (Volume and Number of moles held constant)	$\frac{P_1}{T_1} = \frac{P_2}{T_2}$
Boyle's Law	Inverse: As pressure increases, volume decreases (Temperature and Number of moles held constant)	$P_1V_1 = P_2V_2$
Avogadro's Law	Direct: As the Number of moles of gas increase, gas volume increases (Pressure and Temperature held constant)	$\frac{V_1}{n_1} = \frac{V_2}{n_2}$
Combined Law	Combination of Boyle's and Charles' Law	$\frac{P_1V_1}{T_1} = \frac{P_2V_2}{T_2}$
Joule's Law	The internal energy of a gas depends only on temperature. At a constant temperature, the internal energy is equal to zero.	$\frac{U}{T}$

Gas questions can also require stoichiometry, where Avogadro's constants will be useful:

$$1 \text{ mole of a gas at standard temperature and pressure (STP)} = 22.4 \text{ L (STP is 1 atm and } 0^\circ\text{C)}$$

$$1 \text{ mole of any substance} = 6.022 \times 10^{23} \text{ particles}$$

Example problem:

Given the combustion equation $C_3H_6 + 9O_2 \rightarrow 6CO_2 + 6H_2O$, how many liters of CO_2 are produced if 173 g of oxygen are involved and the reaction happens at STP? The molar mass of O_2 is 32 g/1 mole

173g O_2	1 mol O_2	6 mol CO_2	22.4 L CO_2	= 80.7 L
	32g O_2	9 mol O_2	1 mol CO_2	

Heat capacity, which is the ratio of heat change to temperature change, or $\frac{Q}{T}$, is another parameter involving gas behavior. Much like specific heat, substances that have large heat capacities don't change as much with temperature increases, but particles with small heat capacities will heat up much faster with the same temperature increase.

Heat capacity multiplied by temperature change (when volume is constant) is equal to a substance's **internal energy**. Heat capacity times a temperature change (when pressure is constant) is equal to **enthalpy**.

Real Gases

The ideal gas law makes two key assumptions:

- All gas particles have a volume of zero, even though protons, neutrons, and electrons actually do have mass, albeit very little
- All gas particles have no repulsive and attractive forces so collisions are elastic. As kinetic energy decreases, this becomes less and less true

At small volumes, gas particles are very close together. Therefore, the volume occupies a greater ratio of space, and renders incorrect the collision theory's assumption that gas particles have no mass. At high pressures, the volume that the particles occupy is so small and the particles are so close that there is an increase in intermolecular bonding, rendering the second postulate of collision theory incorrect.

Van der Waals derived the following formula to account for these effects:

$$\left[P + \frac{an^2}{V^2}\right](V - nb) = nRT$$

In this equation, *b* is a constant equal to the actual volume occupied by 1 mole of the particles. If the volume is very large in comparison to the volume taken up by the actual particles, the volume variable will be consistent with that proposed in the ideal gas law.

Van der Waals made another correction since a real gas' pressure is greater than the ideal equation proposes. Both constants, *a,* and *b*, are physical properties of the gas and *a* is a proportionality factor that corrects for intermolecular forces.

Fugacity is a measure of a real gas' behavior in proportion to what would be expected if the gas behaved like an ideal gas. It involves an assumption that the real and ideal gas have the same chemical potential.

$$\varphi = \frac{f}{P}$$

As pressure decreases, gas particles behave more like ideal gases; so, as pressure decreases, the fugacity coefficient, φ, increases. An ideal gas has a fugacity coefficient of one.

Electrochemistry and Electrical Circuits and Their Elements

Electrical Nature of Common Materials

Generally, an **atom** carries no net charge because the positive charges of the protons in the nucleus balance the negative charges of the electrons in the outer shells of the atom. This is considered to be electrically **neutral**. However, since electrons are the only portion of the atom known to have the freedom to "move," this can cause an object to become electrically charged. This happens either through a gain or a loss of electrons. **Electrons** have a negative charge, so a gain creates a net negative charge for the object. On the contrary, a loss of electrons creates a positive charge for the object.

This charge can also be focused on specific areas of an object, causing a notable interaction between charged objects. For example, if a person rubs a balloon on a carpet, the balloon transfers some of is electrons to the carpet. So, if that person were to hold a balloon near their hair, the electrons in the "neutral" hair would make the hair stand on end. This is due to the electrons wanting to fill the deficit of electrons on the balloon. Unless electrically forced into a charged state, most natural objects in nature tend toward reestablishing and maintaining a neutral charge.

When dealing with charges, it is easiest to remember that like charges repel each other and opposite charges attract each other. Therefore, negatives and positives attract, while two positives or two negatives will repel each other. Similarly, when two charges come near each other, they exert a force on one another. This is described through **Coulomb's Law:**

$$F = k\frac{q_1 q_2}{r^2}$$

In this equation, F is equal to the force exerted by the interaction, k is a constant ($k = 8.99\ x\ 109\ \mathrm{N\ m^2/C^2}$), q_1 and q_2 are the measure of the two charges, and r is the distance between the two charges.

When materials readily transfer electricity or electrons, or can easily accept or lose electrons, they are considered to be good conductors. The transferring of electricity is called **conductivity**. If a material does not readily accept the transfer of electrons or readily loses electrons, it is considered to be an **insulator.** For example, plastic is an insulator because it does not transfer electricity. Copper wire, on the other hand, easily transfers electricity; therefore, it is a good **conductor**.

Basic Electrical Concepts

In an electrical circuit, the flow from a power source, or the voltage, is "drawn" across the components in the circuit from the positive end to the negative end. This flow of charge creates an electric **current** (I), which is the time (t) rate of flow of net charge (q). It is measured with the formula:

$$I = \frac{q}{t}$$

Current is measured in amperes (amps). There are two main types of currents:

1. **Direct current (DC):** a unidirectional flow of charges through a circuit
2. **Alternating current (AC):** a circuit with a changing directional flow of charges or magnitude

Every circuit will show a loss in voltage across its conducting material. This loss of voltage is from resistance within the circuit and can be caused by multiple factors, including resistance from wiring and components such as light bulbs and switches. To measure the resistance in a given circuit, **Ohm's law** is used:

$$Resistance = \frac{Voltage}{current} = R = \frac{V}{I}$$

Resistance (R) is measured in Ohms (Ω).

Components in a circuit can be wired **in series** or **in parallel.** If the components are wired in series, a single wire connects each component to the next in line. If the components are wired in parallel, two wires connect each component to the next. The main difference is that the voltage across those in series is directly related from one component to the next. Therefore, if the first component in the series becomes inoperable, no voltage can get to the other components. Conversely, the components in parallel share the voltage across each other and are not dependent on the prior component wired to allow the voltage across the wire.

To calculate the resistance of circuit components wired in series or parallel, the following equations are used:

Resistance in series:

$$R_{total} = R_1 + R_2 + R_3 + \ldots$$

Resistance in parallel:

$$R_{total} = \frac{1}{R_1} + \frac{1}{R_2} + \frac{1}{R_3} + \ldots$$

To make electrons move so that they can carry their charge, a change in voltage must be present. On a small scale, this is demonstrated through the electrons traveling from the light switch to a person's finger. This might happen in a situation where a person runs their socks on a carpet, touches a light switch, and receives a small jolt from the electrons that run from the switch to the finger. This minor jolt is due to the deficit of electrons created by rubbing the socks on the carpet, and then the electrons going into the ground. The difference in charge between the switch and the finger caused the electrons to move.

If this situation were to be created on a larger and more sustained scale, the factors would need to be more systematic, predictable, and harnessed. This could be achieved through batteries/cells and generators. Batteries or cells have a chemical reaction that occurs inside, causing energy to be released and charges to be able to move freely. Batteries generally have nodes (one positive and one negative), where items can be hooked up to complete a circuit and allow the charge to travel freely through the item. Generators convert mechanical energy into electric energy using power and movement.

Basic Properties of Magnetic Fields and Forces

Consider two straight rods that are made from magnetic material. They will naturally have a negative end (**pole**) and a positive end (pole). These charged poles react just like any charged item: opposite charges attract and like charges repel. They will attract each other when arranged positive pole to negative pole. However, if one rod is turned around, the two rods will now repel each other due to the alignment of negative to negative and positive to positive. These types of forces can also be created and amplified by using an electric current. For example, sending an electric current through a stretch of wire creates an electromagnetic force around the wire from the charge of the current. This force exists as long as the flow of electricity is sustained. This magnetic force can also attract and repel other items with magnetic properties. Depending on the strength of the current in the wire, a greater or smaller magnetic force can be generated around the wire. As soon as the current is stopped, the magnetic force also stops.

How Light and Sound Interact with Matter

Optics and Waves

Electromagnetic Spectrum

The movement of light is described like the movement of waves. Light travels with a wave front, has an **amplitude** (height from the neutral), a cycle or **wavelength**, a **period**, and **energy**. Light travels at approximately 3.00×10^8 m/s and is faster than anything created by humans thus far.

Light is commonly referred to by its measured **wavelengths**, or the distance between two successive crests or troughs in a wave. Types of light with the longest wavelengths include radio, TV, and micro, and infrared waves. The next set of wavelengths are detectable by the human eye and create the **visible spectrum.** The visible spectrum has wavelengths of 10^{-7} m, and the colors seen are red, orange, yellow, green, blue, indigo, and violet. Beyond the visible spectrum are shorter wavelengths (also called the **electromagnetic spectrum**) containing ultraviolet light, X-rays, and gamma rays. The wavelengths outside of the visible light range can be harmful to humans if they are directly exposed or are exposed for long periods of time.

Basic Characteristics and Types of Waves

A **mechanical wave** is a type of wave that passes through a medium (solid, liquid, or gas). There are two basic types of mechanical waves: longitudinal and transverse.

A **longitudinal wave** has motion that is parallel to the direction the waves travel. This can best be visualized by compressing one side of a tethered spring and then releasing that end. The movement travels in a bunching/un-bunching motion across the length of the spring and back.

A **transverse wave** has motion that is perpendicular to the direction the waves travel. The particles on a transverse wave do not move across the length of the wave; instead, they oscillate up and down, creating peaks and troughs.

A wave with a combination of both longitudinal and transverse motion can be seen through the motion of a wave on the ocean—with peaks and troughs, and particles oscillating up and down.

Mechanical waves can carry energy, sound, and light, but they need a medium through which transport can occur. An electromagnetic wave can transmit energy without a medium, or in a vacuum.

A more recent addition in the study of waves is the **gravitational wave**. Its existence has been proven and verified, yet the details surrounding its capabilities are still somewhat under inquiry. Gravitational waves are purported to be ripples that propagate as waves outward from their source and travel in the curvature of space/time. They are thought to carry energy in a form of radiant energy called **gravitational radiation**.

Basic Wave Phenomena

When a wave crosses a boundary or travels from one medium to another, certain things occur. If the wave can travel through one medium into another medium, it experiences **refraction**. This is the bending of the wave from one medium to another due to a change in density of the mediums, and thus, the speed of the wave changes. For example, when a pencil is sitting in half of a glass of water, a side view of the glass makes the pencil appear to be bent at the water level. What the viewer is seeing is the refraction of light waves traveling from the air into the water. Since the wave speed is slowed in water, the change makes the pencil appear bent.

When a wave hits a medium that it cannot penetrate, it is bounced back in an action called **reflection**. For example, when light waves hit a mirror, they are reflected, or bounced, off the mirror. This can cause it to seem like there is more light in the room, since there is a "doubling back" of the initial wave. This same phenomenon also causes people to be able to see their reflection in a mirror.

When a wave travels through a slit or around an obstacle, it is known as **diffraction.** A light wave will bend around an obstacle or through a slit and cause what is called a **diffraction pattern**. When the waves bend around an obstacle, it causes the addition of waves and the spreading of light on the other side of the opening.

Dispersion is used to describe the splitting of a single wave by refracting its components into separate parts. For example, if a wave of white light is sent through a dispersion prism, the light appears as its separate rainbow-colored components, due to each colored wavelength being refracted in the prism.

When wavelengths hit boundaries, different things occur. Objects will absorb certain wavelengths of light and reflect others, depending on the boundaries. This becomes important when an object appears to be a certain color. The color of an object is not actually within that object, but rather, in the wavelengths being transmitted by that object. For example, if a table appears to be red, that means the table is absorbing all other wavelengths of visible light except those of the red wavelength. The table is reflecting, or transmitting, the wavelengths associated with red back to the human eye, and so it appears red.

Interference describes when an object affects the path of a wave, or another wave interacts with a wave. Waves interacting with each other can result in either constructive interference or destructive interference, based on their positions. With **constructive interference**, the waves are in sync with each other and combine to reinforce each other. In the case of **deconstructive interference**, the waves are out of sync and reduce the effect of each other to some degree. In **scattering**, the boundary can change the direction or energy of a wave, thus altering the entire wave. **Polarization** changes the oscillations of a wave and can alter its appearance in light waves. For example, polarized sunglasses remove the "glare" from sunlight by altering the oscillation pattern observed by the wearer.

When a wave hits a boundary and is completely reflected, or if it cannot escape from one medium to another, it is called **total internal reflection**. This effect can be seen in the diamonds with a brilliant cut. The angle cut on the sides of the diamond causes the light hitting the diamond to be completely reflected back inside the gem, making it appear brighter and more colorful than a diamond with different angles cut into its surface.

The **Doppler effect** applies to situations with both light and sound waves. The premise of the Doppler effect is that, based upon the relative position or movement of a source and an observer, waves can seem shorter or longer than they actually are. When the Doppler effect is noted with sound, it warps the noise being heard by the observer. This makes the pitch or frequency seem shorter or higher as the source is approaching, and then longer or lower as the source is getting farther away. The frequency/pitch of the source never actually changes, but the sound in respect to the observer makes it seem like the sound has changed. This can be observed when a siren passes by an observer on the road. The siren sounds much higher in pitch as it approaches the observer and then lower after it passes and is getting farther away.

The Doppler effect also applies to situations involving light waves. An observer in space would see light approaching as being shorter wavelengths than the light actually is, causing it to look blue. When the light wave gets farther away, the light would appear red because of the apparent elongation of the wavelength. This is called the **red-blue shift**.

Basic Optics

When reflecting light, a mirror can be used to observe a virtual (not real) image. A **plane mirror** is a piece of glass with a coating in the background to create a reflective surface. An image is what the human eye sees when light is reflected off the mirror in an unmagnified manner. If a **curved mirror** is used for reflection, the image seen will not be a true reflection. Instead, the image will either be enlarged or miniaturized compared to its actual size. Curved mirrors can also make the object appear closer or farther away than the actual distance the object is from the mirror.

Lenses can be used to refract or bend light to form images. Examples of lenses are the human eye, microscopes, and telescopes. The human eye interprets the refraction of light into images that humans understand to be actual size.

Microscopes allow objects that are too small for the unaided human eye to be enlarged enough to be seen. **Telescopes** allow objects to be viewed that are too far away to be seen with the unaided eye. **Prisms** are pieces of glass that can have a wavelength of light enter one side and appear to be divided into its component wavelengths on the other side. This is due to the ability of the prism to slow certain wavelengths more than others.

Sound

Sound travels in waves and is the movement of vibrations through a medium. It can travel through air (gas), land, water, etc. For example, the noise a human hears in the air is the vibration of the waves as they reach the ear. The human brain translates the different **frequencies** (pitches) and intensities of the vibrations to determine what created the noise.

A **tuning fork** has a predetermined frequency because of the length and thickness of its tines. When struck, it allows vibrations between the two tines to move the air at a specific rate. This creates a specific tone, or note, for that size of tuning fork. The number of vibrations over time is also steady for that tuning fork and can be matched with a frequency. All pitches heard by the human ear are categorized by using frequency and are measured in Hertz (cycles per second).

The level of sound in the air is measured with sound level meters on a **decibel (dB)** scale. These meters respond to changes in air pressure caused by sound waves and measure sound intensity. One decibel is $1/10^{th}$ of a *bel*, named after Alexander Graham Bell, the inventor of the telephone. The decibel scale is logarithmic, so it is measured in factors of 10. This means, for example, that a 10 dB increase on a sound meter equates to a 10-fold increase in sound intensity.

Atoms, Nuclear Decay, Electronic Structure, and Atomic Chemical Behavior

Atoms, Elements, and Compounds

Atoms are the building blocks of elements, and they are made up of protons, electrons, and neutrons. **Protons** are positively charged, and **electrons** are negatively charged. **Neutrons** have no charge. The protons and neutrons cluster together in the central part of the atom: the **nucleus**. The electrons circle the nucleus in an orbit within certain energy levels called **shells**. The outside shell of electrons is called the **valence shell**, and the number of electrons in the valence shell can be determined by which group the element belongs to on the periodic table. For example, an element in Group 6 or 16 will have six electrons in its valence shell.

Neutral atoms have an equal number of protons and electrons. Usually, atoms also have at least the same number of neutrons as protons. However, different **isotopes** of an element can exist that have the same number of protons but a different number of neutrons. For example, carbon (C) has three known naturally occurring isotopes: carbon-

12 (^{12}C) has six protons and six neutrons, carbon-13 (^{13}C) has six protons and seven neutrons, and carbon-14 (^{14}C) has six protons and eight neutrons.

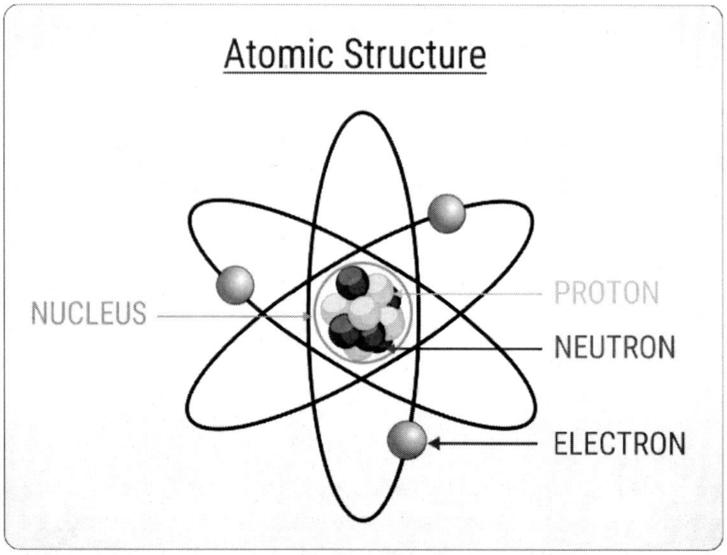

The **atomic number** of an element is based on the number of protons. The simplest element is hydrogen (H), which only has one proton and, therefore, one electron. At 75 percent, hydrogen is the most abundant element in the entire universe. Helium (He) is the second most abundant element in the universe at 23 percent, followed by oxygen (O) at 1 percent. The remaining 1 percent of the universe is made up of all the other elements combined.

Molecules and compounds are mixtures of elements. All compounds are classified as molecules, but not all molecules are classified as compounds. **Molecules** are mixtures that are made up of two or more atoms. **Compounds** are molecules that are made up of a combination of two or more elements. For example, water (H_2O) is a molecule and a compound because it is made up of two hydrogens atoms and one oxygen atom.

The **periodic table** is the most important reference for chemistry. Elements are arranged periodically from left to right and from top to bottom by their atomic numbers. Each row indicates a different **period**, and each column indicates a different **group**. Groups are named from 1–18, sometimes identified as Groups 1A–8A for the **main group** elements and Groups 1B–8B for the **transition** elements. The periodic table also demonstrates a variety of additional trends.

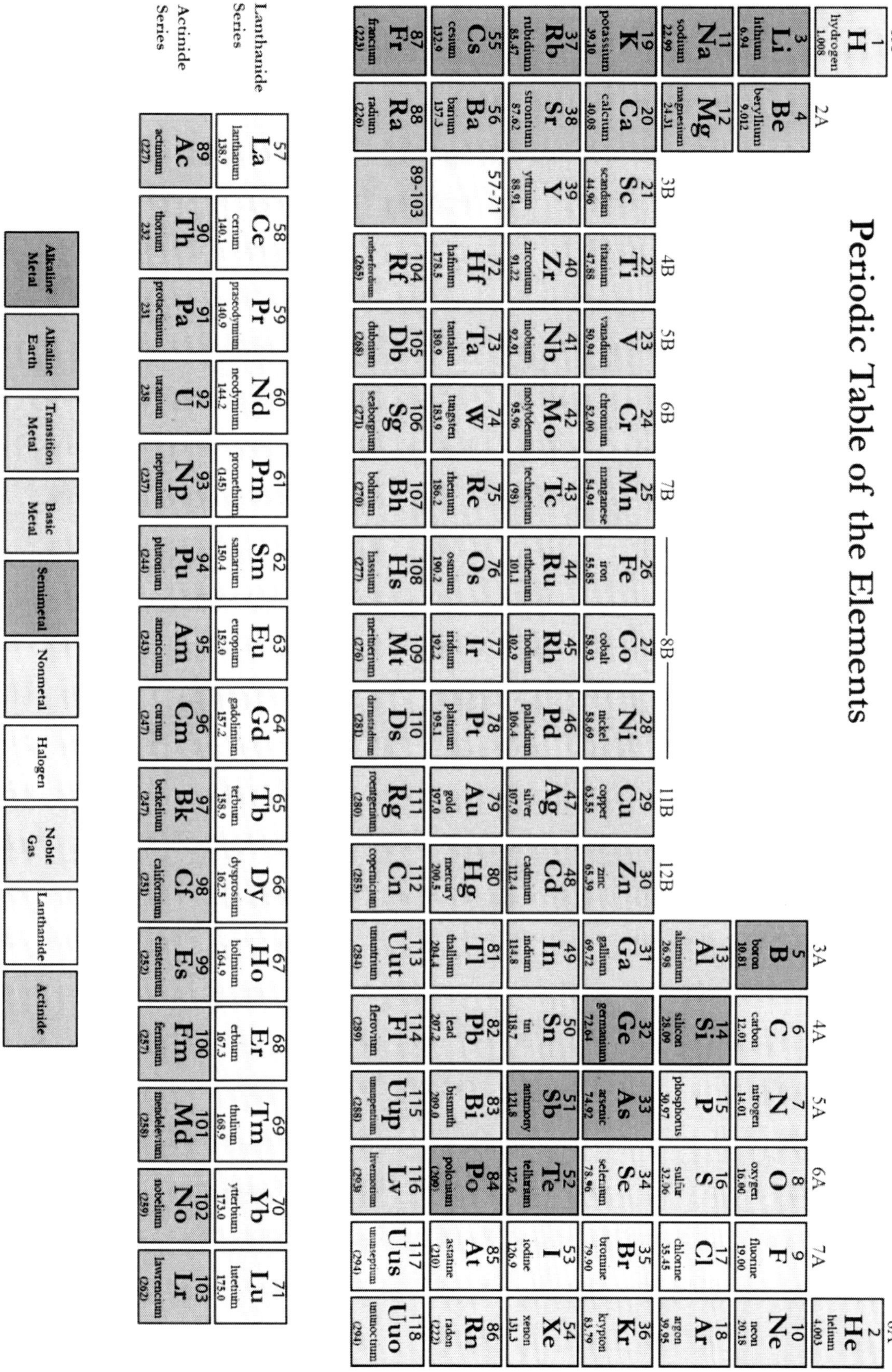
Periodic Table of the Elements
1A 2A 3B 4B 5B 6B 7B 8B 11B 12B 3A 4A 5A 6A 7A 8A
1 H hydrogen 1.008
2 He helium 4.003
3 Li lithium 6.94
4 Be beryllium 9.012
5 B boron 10.81
6 C carbon 12.01
7 N nitrogen 14.01
8 O oxygen 16.00
9 F fluorine 19.00
10 Ne neon 20.18
11 Na sodium 22.99
12 Mg magnesium 24.31
13 Al aluminum 26.98
14 Si silicon 28.09
15 P phosphorus 30.97
16 S sulfur 32.06
17 Cl chlorine 35.45
18 Ar argon 39.95
19 K porassium 39.10
20 Ca calcium 40.08
21 Sc scandium 44.96
22 Ti titanium 47.88
23 V vanadium 50.94
24 Cr chromium 52.00
25 Mn manganese 54.94
26 Fe iron 55.85
27 Co cobalt 58.93
28 Ni nickel 58.69
29 Cu copper 63.55
30 Zn zinc 65.39
31 Ga gallium 69.72
32 Ge germanium 72.64
33 As arsenic 74.92
34 Se selenium 78.96
35 Br bromine 79.90
36 Kr krypton 83.80
37 Rb rubidium 85.47
38 Sr strontium 87.62
39 Y yttrium 88.91
40 Zr zirconium 91.22
41 Nb niobium 92.91
42 Mo molybdenum 95.96
43 Tc technetium (98)
44 Ru ruthenium 101.1
45 Rh rhodium 102.9
46 Pd palladium 106.4
47 Ag silver 107.9
48 Cd cadmium 112.4
49 In indium 114.8
50 Sn tin 118.7
51 Sb antimony 121.8
52 Te tellurium 127.6
53 I iodine 126.9
54 Xe xenon 131.3
55 Cs cesium 132.9
56 Ba barium 137.3
57-71
72 Hf hafnium 178.5
73 Ta tantalum 180.9
74 W tungsten 183.9
75 Re rhenium 186.2
76 Os osmium 190.2
77 Ir iridium 192.2
78 Pt platinum 195.1
79 Au gold 197.0
80 Hg mercury 200.5
81 Tl thallium 204.4
82 Pb lead 207.2
83 Bi bismuth 209.0
84 Po polonium (209)
85 At astatine (210)
86 Rn radon (222)
87 Fr francium (223)
88 Ra radium (226)
89-103
104 Rf rutherfordium (265)
105 Db dubnium (268)
106 Sg seaborgium (271)
107 Bh bohrium (270)
108 Hs hassium (277)
109 Mt meitnerium (276)
110 Ds darmstadtium (281)
111 Rg roentgenium (280)
112 Cn copernicium (285)
113 Uut ununtrium (284)
114 Fl flerovium (289)
115 Uup ununpentium (288)
116 Lv livermorium (293)
117 Uus ununseptium (294)
118 Uuo ununoctium (294)
Lanthanide Series
57 La lanthanum 138.9
58 Ce cerium 140.1
59 Pr praseodymium 140.9
60 Nd neodymium 144.2
61 Pm promethium (145)
62 Sm samarium 150.4
63 Eu europium 152.0
64 Gd gadolinium 157.2
65 Tb terbium 158.9
66 Dy dysprosium 162.5
67 Ho holmium 164.9
68 Er erbium 167.3
69 Tm thulium 168.9
70 Yb ytterbium 173.0
71 Lu lutetium 175.0
Actinide Series
89 Ac actinium (227)
90 Th thorium 232
91 Pa protactinium 231
92 U uranium 238
93 Np neptunium (237)
94 Pu plutonium (244)
95 Am americium (243)
96 Cm curium (247)
97 Bk berkelium (247)
98 Cf californium (251)
99 Es einsteinium (252)
100 Fm fermium (257)
101 Md mendelevium (258)
102 No nobelium (259)
103 Lr lawrencium (262)
Alkaline Metal
Alkaline Earth
Transition Metal
Basic Metal
Semimetal
Nonmetal
Halogen
Noble Gas
Lanthanide
Actinide

Chemistry of the Main Group Elements

The main group elements of the periodic table comprise Groups 1 and 2 (also known as Groups 1A and 2A) and Groups 13 to 18 (also known as Groups 3A to 8A). These groups contain the most abundant elements, and various trends in physical and chemical properties exist within the main group elements.

Electronic Structures of the Main Group Elements

The main group elements are those in Groups 1 and 2 (*s* block) and 13–18 (*p* block). They are grouped in columns according to how many electrons they have in their valence shell. The main group element's chemistry revolves around interactions with the *s* and *p* orbitals.

Elements in Group 1 have one *s* electron in their valence shell. Group 2 elements have two *s* electrons. Remembering that *s* shells only hold two electrons, Group 13 elements must therefore have two valence electrons in an *s* orbital and one electron in a *p* orbital, and so on, until reaching Group 18 elements, which have two valence electrons in an *s* orbital and six valence electrons in a *p* orbital.

The following diagram can be used along with the diagonal rule to work out the electronic structures of elements:

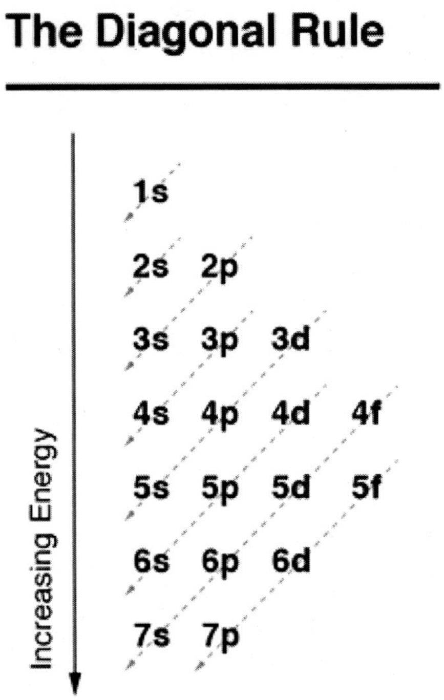

Example: Beryllium (Be) is in Group 2, with an atomic number of $Z = 4$. This means that it has four protons and, if neutral, four electrons.

- To write the electron configuration for an atom with four electrons, the first arrow would need to be followed to find that the non-valence electrons are 1s2—two non-valence electrons in an *s* orbital.
- Then, the second arrow would need to be followed to find that the valence shell is 2s2—two electrons in an *s* orbital—for a total of four electrons.
- The valence shell is always represented by the highest principal quantum number that is seen in the electron configuration. In this case, it's 2.

Occurrences and Recovery of the Main Group Elements

Group 1 elements—hydrogen and the **alkali metals**—are powerful reductants, with lithium being the strongest reductant. They are not found in their pure form in nature and must be stored in oil due to their high reactivity with air and water. Most of the Group 1 elements can be isolated through electrolysis of their molten salts. Rubidium and cesium can be isolated via reacting their hydroxide salts with a reductant. Group 1 elements can also be recovered using a multistep process from their silicate ores.

Group 2 elements—the **alkaline earth metals**—are only found in compounds in nature. They are soft, silver metals that are less reactive than Group 1 elements. Beryllium (Be) is rare on Earth and in the universe. It was first discovered in 1798 from a chemical reaction involving aluminum silicates. Magnesium (Mg) is the 8th most abundant element in the Earth's crust and was first discovered via the electrolysis of magnesia and mercury oxide. Calcium (Ca) is the 5th most abundant element in the Earth's crust and was first isolated from the electrolysis of lime and mercuric acid. Radium (Ra), after oxidizing, is a white or black highly-radioactive solid and was discovered in a pitchblende uranium ore. It is a breakdown product of uranium.

Group 13 is the **boron family**. Some of these elements can be found in their pure form naturally. Boron (B) forms compounds, such as borax, in the Earth's crust. Aluminum (Al) is the most abundant element in the Earth's crust. It was historically difficult to isolate due to its high melting point.

Group 14 comprises the **carbon family**. Carbon (C) is one of the most common elements on Earth and is the distinguishing feature of an organic compound. Silicon (Si), which is classified as a metalloid, is the second most common element in the Earth's crust and is the backbone of the mineral and computing world. It can be found in sand. Germanium (Ge) is similar to silicon, and it is found in coal, ore, and germanite. It forms grey-white crystals. Tin (Sn) is a soft metal that is either gray or white in color, depending on temperature. Lead (Pb) is a soft, malleable metal similar to tin.

Group 15 is the **nitrogen family**. Nitrogen (N) only makes up 0.002% of the Earth's crust, but it makes up around 78% of the Earth's atmosphere. It has no color or taste. Phosphorus (P) is found in compounds, especially from apatite ores. It is nonmetallic and is the 11th most abundant element on Earth. It exists in allotropic forms—white phosphorus or red phosphorus are the most common. Arsenic (As) is a very poisonous metalloid, formed mostly through heating sulfides that contain arsenic. Antimony (Sb) is another metalloid mostly obtained from sulfide ores. Bismuth (Bi) is metallic and is mostly obtained as a by-product of refining other metals.

Group 16 is the **oxygen family** and these elements are essential for life. The elements in this group can be found in nature in both combined and free forms. Oxygen (O) exists as a colorless, odorless gas in nature and is the most abundant element on Earth. It is usually obtained via fractional distillation. Sulfur (S) is a yellow, odorless solid at room temperature, and it is the 16th most abundant element in the Earth's crust. It exists in various forms, including sulfide and sulfates. It is mined using the Frasch process from quicksand or under water. Selenium (Se), classified as a nonmetal, is either a red or black solid or a red or grey crystal. Selenium is rarely found in nature, except when it bio-accumulates in some plants, and is usually obtained through a refining process involving copper. Tellurium (Te) is usually found as a telluride of gold. Polonium (Po) is a rare radioactive metal that does not exist in nature.

Group 17 is the **halogen family**, and all of these non-metallic elements are toxic. Fluorine (F), a yellow gas at room temperature, was first isolated from hydrofluoric acid. It exists as F_2 naturally and is the most abundant halogen in the Earth's crust. Chlorine (Cl) was first isolated from hydrochloric acid. It is a light green gas at room temperature. Bromine (Br) is a red-brown liquid at room temperature. Iodine, a violet solid at room temperature, was first discovered in seaweed treated with sulfuric acid. Astatine (At), which is radioactive, is a black-metallic solid at room temperature and is the only member of the halogen group that is not diatomic.

Group 18 is the **noble gases**. They are on the far right of the periodic table and used to be known as the inert gases. They were first discovered after removing all oxygen and nitrogen from a container of air.

Physical and Chemical Properties of Main Group Elements and Their Compounds

Group 1, the alkali metals—apart from hydrogen (H)—are very reactive due to their single valence electron. They can react vigorously with water to form alkaline solutions and their reactivity increases from top to bottom in the group. Group 1 elements are soft and are shiny, but dull quickly after reacting with oxygen or water. They can react with halogens (Group 17), forming **ionic halides**, and with heavy chalcogens (Group 16), forming **metal chalcogenides**. They can also react with oxygen to form various compounds, such as peroxides and superoxides. All alkali metals also react with hydrogen.

Group 2, the alkaline earth metals, are similar in some ways to Group 1 metals, but they are less reactive, are harder, and have a higher melting point.

Group 13, the boron family, are metals with three electrons in their outermost shell. Boron (B) prefers an oxidation state of $+3$, and aluminum is the most important member of the boron family in terms of its uses. Aluminum also usually adopts a $+3$-oxidation state and is a soft, malleable metal that is silver in color. Aluminum does not react with water due to an **anodizing effect**—a protective layer of $\mathrm{Al_2 0_3}$, which protects against oxidization. Gallium (Ga) and indium (In) also prefer an oxidation state of $3+$, whereas thallium (Tl) most commonly has an oxidation state of $+1$.

Group 14 is the carbon family. Each element in this group contains only two electrons in its outer *p* orbital. The Group 14 elements tend to adopt oxidation states of $+4$, or, for the heavier compounds, $+2$. Carbon can, and often does, form double and triple bonds with itself or other elements, but the heavier elements in this group can only form single bonds. Metallic properties increase down the group. Carbon (C) is not a metal. Silicon (Si) and germanium (Ge) are metalloids. Tin (Sn) and lead (Pb) are metals. Carbon exists in three allotropes—graphite, diamond, and fullerenes—each of which has different physical properties. Graphite has lubricating properties. Diamond is hard and can dissipate heat well, and **fullerenes**—carbon rings joined together into more complex structures like buckeyballs—can be used to create carbon nanotubes.

Group 15 is the nitrogen family. All Group 15 elements have the outer electron shell configuration of ns^2np^3. Group 15 elements generally follow the periodic trends: decreasing electronegativity going down the group, decreasing ionization energy, increasing atomic radii, decreasing electron affinity, increasing melting and boiling points, and increasing metallic character. Nitrogen (N) and phosphorus (P) are nonmetals. Arsenic (As) is a highly poisonous metalloid, and antimony (Sb) is a metalloid. Bismuth (Bi) is metallic. Group 15 elements exist in various different oxidation states.

Group 16 is the oxygen family—also called the **chalcogen family**. These elements have two electrons in the outermost *s* orbital and four in the outermost *p* orbital. Periodic table trends are generally followed in this group, and the most common oxidation state is -2, although $+2$, $+4$, and $+6$ states are also possible for some members. At room temperature, oxygen (O) is a gas, sulfur (S) is a yellow solid, selenium (Se) is a red/black amorphous solid or red/grey crystal, tellurium (Te) is a silver / white metalloid, and polonium (Po) is a rare, highly toxic, radioactive compound.

Group 17 is the halogens. They are the most reactive nonmetals due to their electron configuration p^5—almost full, which is very reactive. They react with most metals to produce **salts** (ionic compounds), such as copper chloride and sodium chloride. Halogens exist in all states of matter. At room temperature, iodine (I) and asinine (At) are solids, bromine (Br) is a liquid, and fluorine (F) and chlorine (Cl) are gases.

Group 18 is the noble gases. They have a full octet in their outer energy level, making them very stable. For example, neon (Ne) has an electron configuration of $2s^2 2p^6$. All end in p^6, which is a very stable electron configuration. Helium and neon, in particular, have very low reactivity.

Chemistry of the Transition Elements

Electronic Structures of the Transition Elements

The **transition elements** are those located in the d-block of the periodic table. Their electronic structure relies on the behavior of the *d* orbitals; they are characterized by partially-filled *d* subshells. Therefore, transition metals can be found in various oxidation states, since it is easier for transition metals compared to alkali metals, for example, to lose electrons. This is because they have five *d* orbitals. However, they usually adopt a single oxidation state based on stability.

The d-block elements are described as having a *d* orbital energy level (n) of $n - 1$. For example, although the first row of the transition metals is on row four of the periodic table, the energy of the *d* orbital is:

$$n - 1 = 4 - 1 = 3$$

However, the energy of the *s* orbitals is still $n = 4$. Therefore, the electron configuration for iron (Fe) in its ground state is $[\mathrm{Ar}]4s^2 3d^6$.

The **ground state** electron configuration for transition elements follows $ns^2 nd^x$ for all elements except two important exceptions: chromium (Cr) and copper (Cu). These have a $4s^1$ instead of a $4s^2$ because they are both 1 *d*-electron short of being either full or half-full, so the *d* orbital takes one from the *s* orbital. Therefore, chromium has a ground state electron configuration of $[\mathrm{Ar}]4s\hat{}3d^5$ because it takes less energy to maintain an electron in the half-filled *d* subshell than the full *s* subshell.

For transition metals that are charged, the electrons from the *s* orbital move to the *d* orbital to form either $ns^0 nd^x$ or $ns^1 nd^x$. The *s* orbital electrons lose their charge first because they have higher energy.

Occurrences and Recovery of Transition Elements

Some transition elements occur naturally in their metallic state. For example, gold, silver, and copper have been used historically for coins since the Bronze Age. Iron was used heavily in the Iron Age to make tools; it occurs almost exclusively in oxidized forms like $\mathrm{Fe_2O_3}$ (rust). Usually, transition elements are extracted from minerals found in ores. Most elements can be isolated by electrolysis or by reduction with an active metal—for example, calcium. Carbon may also be used as a reducing agent to obtain transition elements from their ions. Generally, **isolation** involves three processes:

1. Preliminary treatment, such as crushing or grinding
2. Smelting, which is extraction of the metal in the molten state
3. Refining, by distillation for low boiling metals, or by electrolysis

Physical and Chemical Properties of the Transition Elements and Their Compounds

Common characteristics of transition elements and their compounds include the following:

- Most transition elements are solids at room temperature.
- Most have high density, high melting and boiling points.
- They conduct electricity well.

- They form monatomic ions with a 2+ charge. However, they can form other ions with different charges. In compounds, they often have higher oxidation states.
- Most transition metals can react with hydrogen, nitrogen, carbon, and boron to form hydrides (e.g., TiH_2), nitrides (e.g., TiN), carbides (e.g., TiC), and borides (e.g., TiB_2).
- They can often be used as catalysts.
- They are paramagnetic when they have unpaired *d* electrons.
- They form coordination compounds, often brightly colored.
- They have some periodic trends in common.
- The two heaviest elements of each group of the transition elements generally have similarities in chemical behaviors.
- They become increasingly polarized across the *d*-block.

Coordination Chemistry

Coordination chemistry involves the formation of complex or coordination compounds. The molecules have a metal as a central ion, which is bound to other neutral or negatively-charged ligands—such as atoms, ions, or molecules—that donate electrons to the metal. An example of a metal complex is $[Co(NH_2CH_2CH_2NH_2)_2ClNH_3]^{2+}Cl_2{}^{2-}$. Many transition metal-containing compounds are coordination complexes.

A feature of many transition metal complexes is their interesting bright colors, which is caused by the absorption of light causing electronic transitions.

The **inner coordination sphere**—or **first sphere**—contains the central metal that is directly bound to the ligands. The **outer coordination sphere**—or **second sphere**—contains other ions that are attached to the complex ion. The properties of complex compounds are different from the properties of individual atoms or individual ligands.

Coordination refers to the coordinate covalent bonds—known as **dipolar bonds**—between a central metal and ligands. The coordination number can be described as the number of donor atoms attached to the central metal. The most common coordination numbers are 2, 4 and 6. If the ligands are Lewis bases that donate a single pair of electrons—described as **monodentate**—then the number of donor atoms is the same as the number of ligands. But if the ligands are **bidentate**—Lewis bases that donate two pairs of electrons—then the number of donor atoms is not equal to the number of ligands. For example, the complex $Pt(en)_2{}^{2+}$ has a coordination number of 4, rather than 2, because it contains two bidentate ligands, for a total of four donor atoms.

Different coordination numbers result in different structural arrangements called **geometries.** The most common are as follows:

- For two-coordinated structures: linear
- For three-coordinated structures: trigonal planar
- For four-coordinated structures: tetrahedral or square planar
- For five-coordinated structures: trigonal bipyramidal or square pyramidal
- For six-coordinated structures: octahedral (orthogonal)
- For seven-coordinated structures: pentagonal bipyramidal, capped octahedral, or capped trigonal prismatic
- For eight-coordinated structures: square antiprismatic or dodecahedral
- For nine-coordinated structures: tri-capped trigonal prismatic (triaugmented triangular prism) or capped square antiprismatic

Half-life

Half-life ($t_{1/2}$) describes the time taken for half of the radioactive material to decay. Half-life is linked to the isotope undergoing radioactive decay. For example, the isotope of carbon—carbon-14 (^{14}C)—can undergo beta decay to nitrogen-14 (^{14}N). Carbon-14 has a half-life of 5,730 years. This means that if one started with 100g of carbon-14, then after 5,730 years, 50g of carbon-14 would be left over, and 50g of nitrogen-14 would be produced. After an additional 5,730 years—11,460 years in total—there would be 25 g of carbon-14 and 75 g of nitrogen-14. Because half-life is constant, it can be used in carbon dating to work out the age of certain organic objects.

The following equation can be used to work out the fraction of parent material that remains after radioactive decay (where *n* equals the number of half-lives elapsed):

$$\text{Fraction remaining} = \frac{1}{2^n}$$

Nuclear Chemistry

Traditional chemical reactions involve the electrons in the valence shell surrounding an atom's nucleus. **Nuclear chemistry**, however, deals with changes in the atom's nucleus itself. Several types of changes in an atom's nucleus can produce different types of radiation. The three major types of radiation are alpha, beta, and gamma decay.

- **Alpha (α) radiation** involves the emission from an atom's nucleus of an alpha particle. Because alpha particles are made up of two protons and two neutrons—very similar to a helium nucleus—when an atom emits an alpha particle, its atomic mass will decrease by four, and its atomic number will decrease by two. This means that the element will turn into a different element, otherwise known as a transmutation.
- **Beta (β) radiation** is when a neutron transmutes into a proton and an electron. The electron is then emitted from the nucleus. When a beta particle is emitted, the atom's mass won't change, but the atomic number increases by one.
- **Gamma (γ) radiation** involves electromagnetic energy emission from the nucleus. Electromagnetic energy is very similar to light; no particles are lost during this type of radiation, and no transmutation occurs. Gamma radiation typically happens at the same time as alpha or beta decay. X-rays are a common type of gamma radiation.

Foundational Concept 5: The principles that govern chemical interactions and reactions form the basis for a broader understanding of the molecular dynamics of living systems.

The Unique Nature of Water and its Solutions

Water

Most cells are primarily composed of water and live in water-rich environments. Since water is such a familiar substance, it is easy to overlook its unique properties. Chemically, water is made up of two hydrogen atoms bonded to one oxygen atom by covalent bonds. The three atoms join to make a V-shaped molecule. Water is a polar molecule, meaning it has an unevenly distributed overall charge due to an unequal sharing of electrons. Due to oxygen's electronegativity and its more substantial positively-charged nucleus, hydrogen's electrons are pulled closer to the oxygen. This causes the hydrogen atoms to have a slight positive charge and the oxygen atom to have a slight negative charge. In a glass of water, the molecules constantly interact and link for a fraction of a second due to intermolecular bonding between the slightly positive hydrogen atoms of one molecule and the slightly negative oxygen of a different molecule. These weak intermolecular bonds are called **hydrogen bonds**.

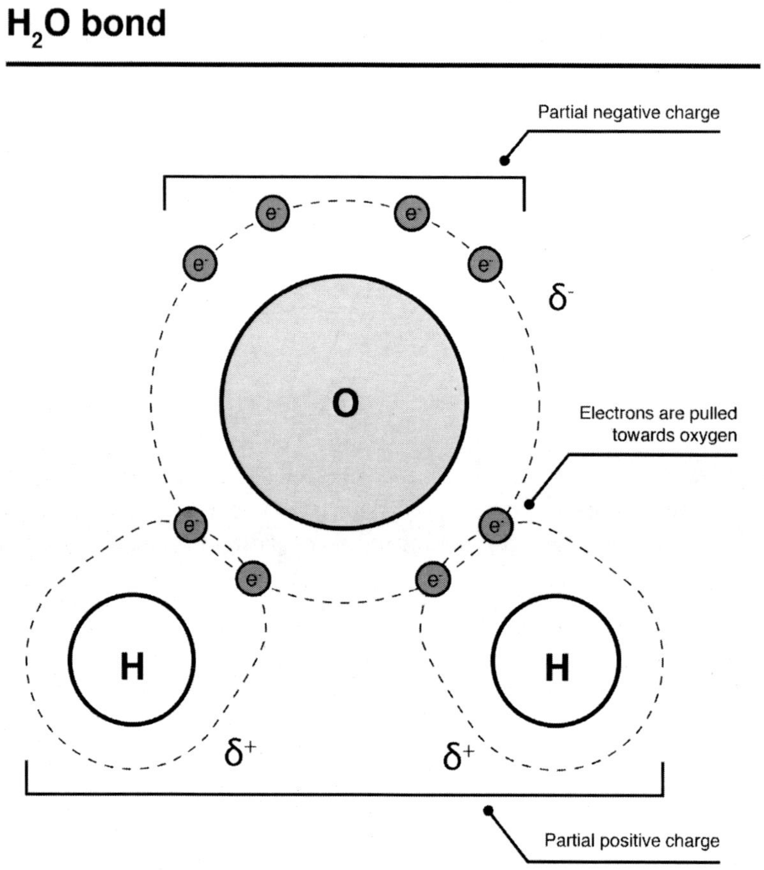

Water has several important qualities, including: cohesive and adhesive behaviors, temperature moderation ability, expansion upon freezing, and diverse use as a solvent.

Cohesion is the interaction of many of the same molecules. In water, cohesion occurs when there is hydrogen bonding between water molecules. Water molecules use this bonding ability to attach to each other and can work against gravity to transport dissolved nutrients to the top of a plant. A network of water-conducting cells can push water from the roots of a plant up to the leaves. The cohesive behavior of water also causes surface tension. If a glass of water is slightly overfull, water can still stand above the rim. This is because of the unique bonding of water molecules at the surface—they bond to each other and to the molecules below them, making it seem like it is covered with an impenetrable film. A raft spider can actually walk across a small body of water due to this surface tension. In contrast to cohesion in which water molecules are attracted to other water molecules, **adhesion** is the attraction of two different substances, in this case, water with something else. For example, water molecules can form a weak hydrogen bond with, or adhere to, plant cell walls to help fight gravity.

Another important property of water is its ability to moderate temperature. Water can moderate the temperature of air by absorbing or releasing stored heat into the air. Water has the distinctive capability of being able to absorb or release large quantities of stored heat while undergoing only a small change in temperature. This is because of the relatively high **specific heat** of water, where specific heat is the amount of heat it takes for one gram of a material to change its temperature by 1 degree Celsius. The specific heat of water is one calorie per gram per degree Celsius, meaning that for each gram of water, it takes one calorie of heat to raise the temperature of water by 1 degree Celsius.

When the temperature of water is reduced to freezing levels, water displays another interesting property: It expands instead of contracts. Most liquids become denser as they freeze because the molecules move more slower and stay closer together. Water molecules, however, form hydrogen bonds with each other as they move together. As the temperature lowers and they begin to move slower, these bonds become harder to break apart. When water freezes into ice, molecules are frozen with hydrogen bonds between them and they take up about 10 percent more volume than in their liquid state. The fact that ice is less dense than water is what makes ice float to the top of a glass of water.

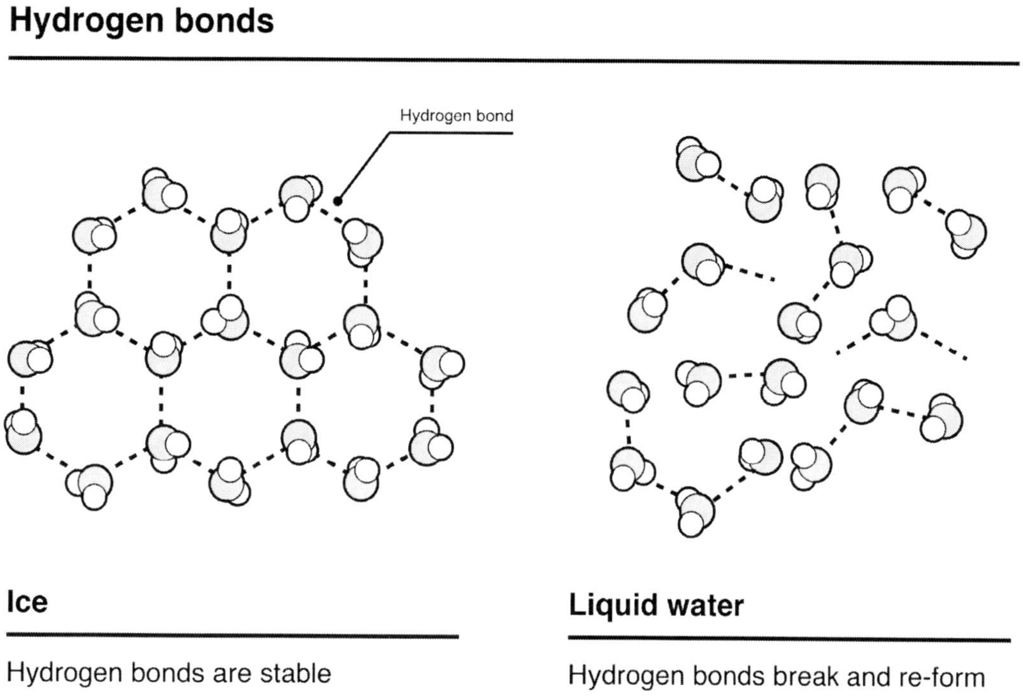

Lastly, the **polarity** of water molecules makes water a versatile solvent. Ionic compounds, such as salt, are made up of positively and negatively charged atoms, called **cations** and **anions**, respectively. Cations and anions are easily dissolved in water because of their individual attractions to the slight positive charge of the hydrogen atoms or the slight negative charge of the oxygen atoms in water molecules. Water molecules separate the individually charged atoms and shield them from each other so they don't bond to each other again and create a homogenous solution of the cations and anions. Non-ionic compounds, such as sugar, have polar regions, so they are easily dissolved in water. For these compounds, the water molecules form hydrogen bonds with the polar regions (hydroxyl groups) to create a homogenous solution. Any substance that is attracted to water is termed **hydrophilic.** Substances that repel water are termed **hydrophobic**.

Concepts of Acids and Bases

All liquids have either acidic or basic traits. When hydrogen ions (H^+) are released in a liquid, it becomes acidic. Conversely, when hydroxide ions are released in a liquid (OH^-), it becomes basic. These are the two ions that determine whether a solution is an acid or a base.

Brønsted-Lowry Approaches

In the **Brønsted-Lowry Theory** of acids and bases (alkalines), the **acid** is a proton donor (a hydrogen ion), and the **base** is a proton acceptor. Acids and bases can be described using what is known as the pH scale. The pH scale ranges from 0-14. A pH of 7 is **neutral**, while values less than seven are acidic and those greater than seven are alkaline (basic).

Acids and basis can be divided into strong and weak categories. The strength of an acid can be measured using the following equation:

$$K_a = \frac{[H^+][A^-_{weak}]}{[HA_{weak}]}$$

When K_a is large, it is a strong acid (e.g., HCL Ka = 1×103). An acid with a small K_a is a weak acid (e.g., H_2O $K_a = 1.8 \times 10^{-16}$). The strength of a base can be measured using the following formula:

$$K_b = \frac{[HB^+][OH^-]}{[B]}$$

In Brønsted theory, every acid has a conjugate base, and every base has a conjugate acid.

Lewis Theory

In the **Lewis Theory** of acids and bases, bases can donate pairs of electrons, and acids accept pairs of electrons. This means that in Lewis theory, a **Lewis acid** is any substance that can accept a pair of non-bonding electrons. A good example of a Lewis acid is the hydrogen ion H^+ because it can accept a lone pair of electrons.

In contrast, a **Lewis base** is any substance that can donate a pair of electrons to a Lewis acid. A good example of a Lewis base is hydroxide (OH^-) because it can donate a lone pair of electrons. When Lewis acids and bases combine, they form a **Lewis adduct**.

Solution and Solubility

Different Types of Solutions

A **solution** is a homogenous mixture of more than one substance. A **solute** is another substance that can be dissolved into a substance called a **solvent.** If only a small amount of solute is dissolved in a solvent, the solution formed is said to be **diluted**. A solution is considered **concentrated** if a large amount of solute is dissolved into the solvent. For example, water from a typical, unfiltered household tap is diluted because it contains other minerals in very small amounts.

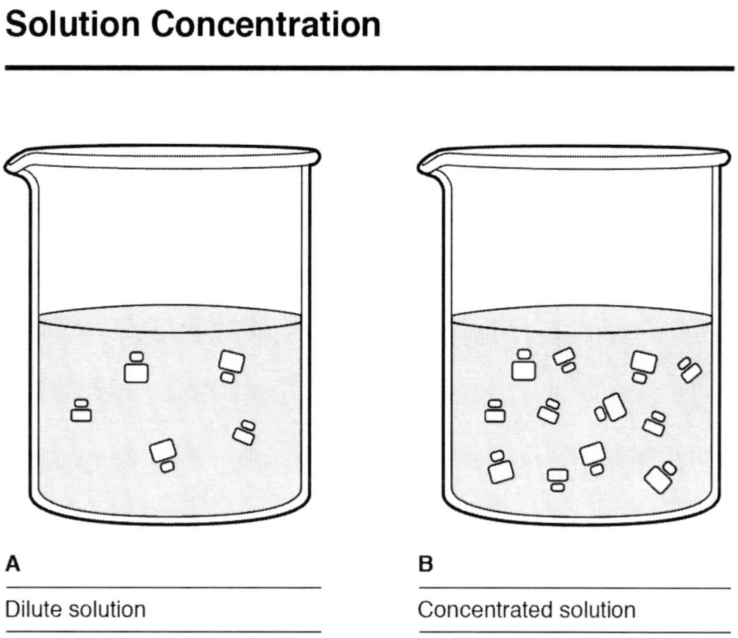

If more solute is being added to a solvent, but not dissolving, the solution is called **saturated.** For example, when hummingbirds eat sugar-water from feeders, they prefer it as sweet as possible. When trying to dissolve enough sugar (solute) into the water (solvent), there will be a point where the sugar crystals will no longer dissolve into the solution and will remain as whole pieces floating in the water. At this point, the solution is considered saturated and cannot accept more sugar. This level, at which a solvent cannot accept and dissolve any more solute, is called its **saturation point**. In some cases, it is possible to force more solute to be dissolved into a solvent, but this will result in crystallization. The state of a solution on the verge of crystallization, or in the process of crystallization, is called a **supersaturated** solution. This can also occur in a solution that seems stable, but if it is disturbed, the change can begin the crystallization process.

Although the terms *dilute*, *concentrated*, *saturated*, and *supersaturated* give qualitative descriptions of solutions, a more precise quantitative description needs to be established for the use of chemicals. This holds true especially for mixing strong acids or bases. The method for calculating the concentration of a solution is done through finding its **molarity**. In some instances, such as environmental reporting, molarity is measured in **parts per million** (ppm). Parts per million, is the number of milligrams of a substance dissolved in one liter of water. To find the molarity, or the amount of solute per unit volume of solution, for a solution, the following formula is used:

$$c = \frac{n}{V}$$

In this formula, c is the molarity (or unit moles of solute per volume of solution), n is the amount of solute measured in moles, and V is the volume of the solution, measured in liters.

Example:

What is the molarity of a solution made by dissolving 2.0 grams of NaCl into enough water to make 100 mL of solution?

To solve this, the number of moles of NaCl needs to be calculated:

First, to find the mass of NaCl, the mass of each of the molecule's atoms is added together as follows:

$$23.0 \text{ g (Na)} + 35.5 \text{ g (Cl)} = 58.8 \text{ g NaCl}$$

Next, the given mass of the substance is multiplied by one mole per total mass of the substance:

$$2.0 \text{ g NaCl} \times \frac{1 \text{ mol NaCl}}{58.5 \text{ g NaCl}} = 0.034 \text{ mol NaCl}$$

Finally, the moles are divided by the number of liters of the solution to find the molarity:

$$\frac{0.034 \text{ mol NaCl}}{0.100 \text{ L}} = 0.34 \text{ M NaCl}$$

To prepare a solution of a different concentration, the *mass solute* must be calculated from the molarity of the solution. This is done via the following process:

Example:

How would you prepare 600.0 mL of 1.20 M solution of sodium chloride?

To solve this, the given information needs to be set up:

$$1.20 \text{ M NaCl} = \frac{1.20 \text{ mol NaCl}}{1.00 \text{ L of solution}}$$

$$0.600 \text{ L solution} \times \frac{1.20 \text{ mol NaCl}}{1.00 \text{ L of solution}} = 0.72 \text{ moles NaCl}$$

$$0.72 \text{ moles NaCl} \times \frac{58.5 \text{ g NaCl}}{1 \text{ mol NaCl}} = 42.12 \text{ g NaCl}$$

This means that one must dissolve 42.12 g NaCl in enough water to make 600.0 L of solution.

Factors Affecting the Solubility of Substances and the Dissolving Process

Certain factors can affect the rate in dissolving processes. These include temperature, pressure, particle size, and **agitation** (stirring). As mentioned, the **ideal gas law** states that $PV = nRT$, where P equals pressure, V equals volume, and T equals temperature. If the pressure, volume, or temperature are affected in a system, it will affect the entire system. Specifically, if there is an increase in temperature, there will be an increase in the dissolving rate. An increase in the pressure can also increase the dissolving rate. Particle size and agitation can also influence the dissolving rate, since all of these factors contribute to the breaking of intermolecular forces that hold solute particles together. Once these forces are broken, the solute particles can link to particles in the solvent, thus dissolving the solute.

A **solubility curve** shows the relationship between the mass of solute that a solvent holds at a given temperature. If a reading is on the solubility curve, the solvent is **full (saturated)** and cannot hold anymore solute. If a reading is above the curve, the solvent is **unstable (supersaturated)** from holding more solute than it should. If a reading is below the curve, the solvent is **unsaturated** and could hold more solute.

If a solvent has different electronegativities, or partial charges, it is considered to be **polar**. Water is an example of a polar solvent. If a solvent has similar electronegativities, or lacking partial charges, it is considered to be **non-polar**. Benzene is an example of a non-polar solvent. Polarity status is important when attempting to dissolve solutes. The phrase "like dissolves like" is the key to remembering what will happen when attempting to dissolve a solute in a solvent. A polar solute will dissolve in a like, or polar solvent. Similarly, a non-polar solute will dissolve in a non-polar solvent. When a reaction produces a solid, the solid is called a **precipitate**. A **precipitation reaction** can be used for removing a **salt** (an ionic compound that results from a neutralization reaction) from a solvent, such as water. For water, this process is called **ionization**. Therefore, the products of a **neutralization reaction** (when an acid and base react) are a salt and water.

When a solute is added to a solvent to lower the freezing point of the solvent, it is called **freezing point depression.** This is a useful process, especially when applied in colder temperatures. For example, the addition of salt to ice in winter allows the ice to melt at a much lower temperature, thus creating safer road conditions for driving. Unfortunately, the freezing point depression from salt can only lower the melting point of ice so far and is ineffectual when temperatures are too low. This same process, with a mix of ethylene glycol and water, is also used to keep the radiator fluid (antifreeze) in an automobile from freezing during the winter.

Titration

Solution Stoichiometry

Solution stoichiometry deals with quantities of solutes in chemical reactions that occur in solutions. The quantity of a solute in a solution can be calculated by multiplying the molarity of the solution by the volume. Similar to chemical equations involving simple elements, the number of moles of the elements that make up the solute should be equivalent on both sides of the equation.

When the concentration of a particular solute in a solution is unknown, a **titration** is used to determine that concentration. In a titration, the solution with the unknown solute is combined with a standard solution, which is a solution with a known solute concentration. The point at which the unknown solute has completely reacted with the known solute is called the **equivalence point**. Using the known information about the standard solution, including the concentration and volume, and the volume of the unknown solution, the concentration of the unknown solute is determined in a balanced equation. For example, in the case of combining acids and bases, the equivalence point is reached when the resulting solution is neutral. HCl, an acid, combines with NaOH, a base, to form water, which is neutral, and a solution of Cl^- ions and Na^+ ions. Before the equivalence point, there are an unequal number of cations and anions and the solution is not neutral.

Precipitation Titrations

A titration in which the end point is determined by formation of a precipitate is called a **precipitation titration**. The most common precipitation titrations are **argentometric** (*Argentum* means silver in Latin). These reactions involve a silver ion with a titrant of silver nitrate ($\mathrm{AgNO_3}$). Silver nitrate is a useful titrant because it reacts very quickly. All products in these titrimetric precipitations are silver salts. A very simple argentometric precipitation titration is often performed to determine the amount of chlorine in seawater, as the chlorine anion is present most abundantly. The reaction is as follows

$$\mathrm{AgNO_3\ (aq) + NaCl\ (aq) \rightarrow AgCl\ (s) + NaNO_3\ (aq)}$$

Silver chloride is almost completely insoluble in water, so it precipitates out of solution. A selective indicator, potassium chromate ($\mathrm{K_2CrO_4}$), is added to determine when the reaction is complete. When all of the chloride ions from the sample have precipitated, silver ions then react with chromate ions to form $\mathrm{Ag_2CrO_4}$, which is orange in color. The volume of the sample, amount of titrant required to complete the precipitation, molar mass of the reacting species, and the density of the sample provide sufficient information to calculate the concentration of chloride ions.

Titration curves are useful in providing a graphical account of what occurs before, during, and after the equivalence point. Argentometric titration curves are sigmoidal when the concentration function is plotted on the y-axis and the reagent volume is plotted on the x-axis. An example is shown below:

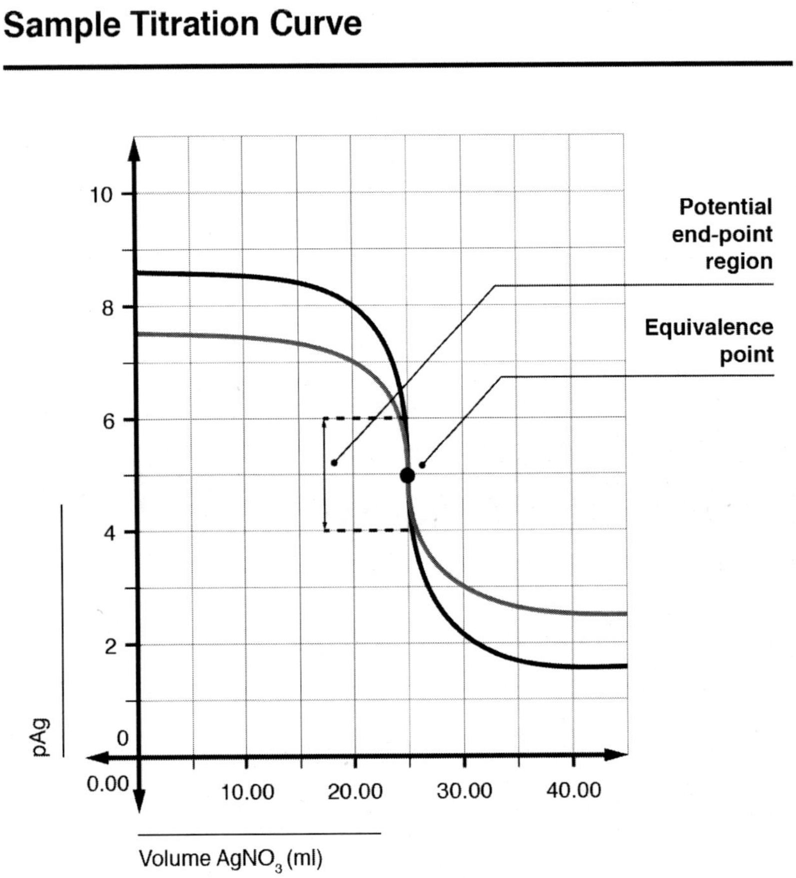

Note that at the equivalence point, there is a sharp drop in reagent concentration, and then beyond the equivalence point, the concentration decreases gradually. Around the equivalence point, small volumes of titrant added cause dramatic changes in the concentration of the analyte and reagent. At equivalence, the molar concentrations of sample cation/titrant anion and sample anion/titrant cation are equal.

Nature of Molecules and Intermolecular Interaction

Ionic Substances

Ionic compounds are those that are held together by **ionic bonds**—also known as **electrostatic forces**—through the transfer of electrons. Ionic substances are neutral overall, but they are balanced out by their **cations**—positively-charged ions and **anions**—negatively-charged ions. Ionic bonds usually form between metals and nonmetals. Most rocks and minerals are ionic compounds, including pyrite (FeS_2).

An example of an ionic compound is sodium chloride, which is held together by ionic bonds, due to sodium (Na^+) having a positive charge and chloride having a negative charge (Cl^-). The sodium ion is positively charged because sodium (Na) only has one electron in its valence shell. Therefore, sodium donates this electron easily to become a positively-charged ion (Na^+). Similarly, chloride (Cl) has seven electrons in its valence shell and accepts an electron easily to become a negatively-charged ion (Cl^-).

Lattice Geometries

Ionic compounds are held together in a specific, endlessly-repeating pattern, known as a **lattice**. The structure of the lattice depends on the ions present in the compound. The size of the lattice depends on how many single molecules are present. A single crystal of table salt, for example, is formed by a lattice of trillions of sodium chloride (NaCl) molecules.

Sodium and chloride ions alternate with each other in each of the x, y, and z dimensions to form a cube-like structure:

Sodium Chloride Lattice

6:6 Coordinated

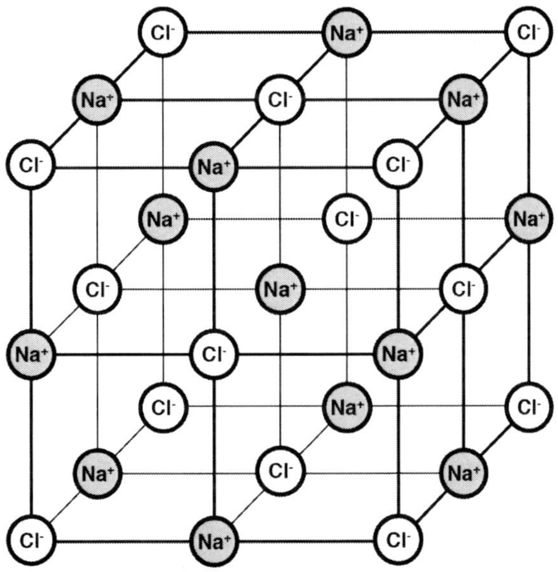

The sodium ion in the middle is joined to six chloride ions. If the chloride ion was centered, it would also be joined to six sodium ions. Therefore, sodium chloride is described as **6:6 coordinated**.

The type of lattice depends on how many attractions are possible between the ions. One sodium ion can only accept six chloride ions before the chloride ions start to repel each other from being too close to one another. If the chloride ions were to repel each other, the entire crystal structure would become unstable.

Different types of lattices are possible depending on the ions present. The compound zincblende (ZnS), for example, has a coordination of four for each ion, so it is said to be **4:4 coordinated.**

Lattice Energies

When two ions with opposite charges are attracted to each other and bond together, energy is released. This is called the **lattice energy**. Single ions need less energy to stay together in a crystal lattice.

The two main factors affecting lattice energy are the charges on the ions and the ionic radii. As the charges on ions increase in magnitude, the bonds become stronger. For example, a bond between a -2 anion and a $+3$ cation would be much stronger than a bond between a -1 anion and a $+1$ cation.

Lattice energy (U) is always a positive number and can be calculated as follows:

$$U = k' \frac{(q_1)(q_2)}{r_o}$$

The constant k' depends on the type of lattice and valence electron configurations; (q_1) and (q_2) are the charges on the ions, and r_o is the internuclear distance.

Two ionic compounds may have the exact same lattice arrangement but have different lattice energies. For example, sodium chloride (NaCl) and magnesium oxide (MgO) have the same crystal structure but different lattice energies. In magnesium oxide, $+2$ ions are bonded to -2 ions, but in sodium chloride, $+1$ ions are being attracted to -1 ions. A salt with a metal cation with a $+2$ charge and a nonmetal anion with a -2 charge will have a lattice energy four times greater than a salt with single charges, if the ions are of similar sizes.

Ionic Radii

Ionic radii can be defined as the radius of an atom's ion. When ions are small, the valence shell is closer to the nucleus, and the nucleus has a stronger pull. The nucleus can also affect nearby atoms, having a similar pull. This results in smaller ions having stronger bonds.

Radius/Ratio Effects

The **radius ratio** of any given pair of ions is defined as the ionic radius of the smaller ion divided by the ionic radius of the larger ion. Often, the smaller ion is the cation, and the larger ion is the anion. The lattice structure for crystals of simple 1:1 compounds (NaCl) depends on the radius ratio of the ions that are present. If the radius of the positive ion is greater than 73% of the negative ion, an 8:8 coordination is possible. If the radius of the positive ion is between 41 – 73% of the negative ion, a 6:6 coordination is possible.

Covalent Molecular Substances

Covalent bonds occur between two or more nonmetal atoms and are very strong bonds. They are formed by the sharing of electrons in the valence shells and often follow the octet rule. The **octet rule** is a common observation that many main group elements tend to bond in such a way that they have a total of eight electrons in their valence shells. This electron configuration is the same as a noble gas.

Lewis Diagrams

Lewis diagrams—also called **electron dot diagrams**—are used to represent covalent bonds. The diagram was named after Gilbert Lewis, an American physical chemist who discovered the structure of covalent bonds.

Lewis diagrams show the electrons in the valence shell of an atom. In other words, they show the electrons that are available for covalent bonding. The procedure for drawing Lewis diagrams is as follows:

- Work out the number of available electrons.
- If the compound has more than two atoms, the least electronegative atom goes in the center—remembering that hydrogen (H) must go on the outside.
- Place two electrons between atoms to form a chemical bond—usually represented with a dash.
- Complete the octets of electrons on the outside of the atom. Valence shells need eight electrons, except for hydrogen (H), which only needs two. There are some exceptions to this rule; for example, beryllium (Be) is happy with just four electrons in its valence shell and boron (B) with just six electrons in its valence shell.
- If all of the electrons are used up but the octets still haven't been filled, electrons can be moved from outer atoms, forming double or triple bonds.

An example to consider is carbon dioxide, CO_2. Carbon (C) is in Group 14 of the periodic table, so it has four valence electrons. Oxygen (O) is in Group 16, so it has six valence electrons. The total is ten electrons. The least electronegative atom is carbon, so it should be put in the center of the Lewis diagram, with the two oxygens on either side. Then, two of the ten electrons should be put between the carbon and oxygens to form covalent bonds, and then, the valence shells should be filled up. It is important to note that there aren't enough electrons to fill the octets. However, using two pairs of electrons to form double bonds fills the valence shell and yields the Lewis Dot structure below:

Lewis Diagram

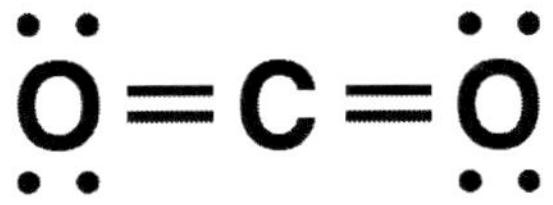

Valence Bond Theory

In **valence bond theory**, electrons are treated in a quantum mechanics fashion. Valence bond theory is good for describing the shapes of covalent compounds. Instead of electrons being pinpointed to an exact location, it's possible to map out a region of space—known as **atomic orbitals**—that the electron may inhabit. In valence bond theory, electrons are treated as excitations of the **electron field**, which exists everywhere. When energy is given to an electron field, electrons are said to exist inside a **wave function**—a mathematical function describing the probability an electron is in a certain place at any given time. Standing waves are created when energy is given to a wave function. Electrons function as standing waves around a nucleus.

There are two things to consider in valence bond theory: the overlapping of the orbitals and the potential energy changes in a molecule as the atoms get closer or further apart. For example, the Lewis structure of H_2 would be H – H, but this doesn't describe the strength of the bond. The electron cloud in the nucleus of one atom is interacting with the cloud of electrons in the nucleus of another atom. If the potential energy was mapped out as a function of distance between the two atoms, something like this would be obtained:

Potential Energy versus Internuclear Distance Between Two Atoms

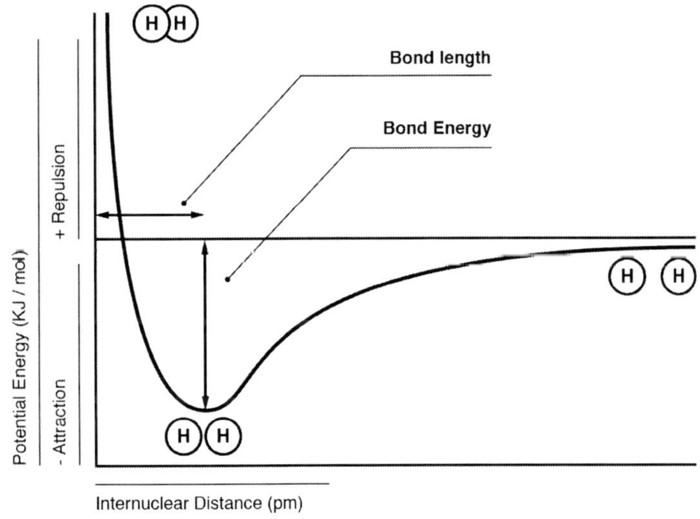

The two atoms approach this minimum value at a distance known as the **bond energy**. The link that corresponds to this is the equilibrium bond length—a happy medium corresponding to a minimum in potential energy. This minimum of energy is achieved when the atomic orbitals are overlapping and so contain two **spin-paired electrons**—when the two atoms' orbitals are overlapping each other. A greater amount of energy is needed to separate those two atoms when they are overlapped.

Molecular Orbitals

Atomic orbitals explain the behavior of a single electron or pairs of electrons in an atom. They are regions of space in which the electrons are more likely to spend their time. Every orbital can contain two electrons, and the orbital is at its lowest energy when it has two electrons. One electron spins up, and one spins down. The standard atomic orbitals are known as *s*, *p*, *d*, and *f* orbitals.

- The simplest of the orbitals is the ***s* orbital**: the inner orbital of any atom or the outer orbital for light molecules, such as hydrogen and helium. The *s* orbital is spherical in shape and can contain two electrons.
- After the *s* orbital is filled, the ***p* orbitals** are filled. There are three *p* orbitals, one on each of the x-, y-, and z-axes. Each *p* orbital can contain two electrons for a total of six electrons.
- After the *p* orbitals are filled, the ***d* orbitals** are filled next. There are five *d* orbitals, for a total of ten electrons.
- The ***f* orbitals** are next; there are seven *f* orbitals, which can contain a total of fourteen electrons.

Each shell/energy level has an increasing number of subshells available to it:

- The first shell only has the *1s* subshell, so it has two electrons.
- The second shell has the *2s* and *2p* subshells, so it has $(2 + 6)$ eight electrons.
- The third shell has the *3s, 3p* and *3d* subshells, so it has $(2 + 6 + 10)$ 18 electrons.
- The fourth shell has the *4s, 4p, 4d* and *4f* subshells, so it has $(2 + 6 + 10 + 14)$ 32 electrons.

To find the maximum number of electrons per shell, the formula $2n^2$ is used, where n is the shell number. For example, elements in the third period have three subshells—space for up to 18 electrons—but will only have up to eight valence electrons. This is because the *3d* orbitals aren't filled (i.e., the elements from the third period don't completely fill their third shell).

Any element in the periodic table can be written in terms of its electron configuration. For instance, Calcium (Ca), which is in the 4th period on the periodic table and has an atomic number of 20, would be written as $1s^2 2s^2 2p^6 3s^2 3p^6 4s^2$. However, it's important to remember that the transition metals do not follow this rule because quantum energy level rules allow for some of their shells to remain unfilled. For example, the transition metal scandium (Sc), which has an atomic number of 21, has the electron configuration $1s^2 2s^2 2p^6 3s^2 3p^6 3d^1 4s^2$, and the *d* subshell is not filled.

In **molecular orbital theory**, the assumption is that bonding, non-bonding, and anti-bonding orbitals—which have different energies—are formed when atoms are brought together. For N atomic orbitals in a molecule, the assumed result would be N molecular orbitals, which can be described by wave functions.

For example, for a molecule that has two atomic orbitals, two molecular orbitals must be formed: one bonding and one anti-bonding. The molecular orbitals would be separated by a certain energy. A molecule that has three atomic orbitals would form one bonding, one non-bonding, and one anti-bonding molecular orbital. A molecule that has ten atoms would form five anti-bonding and five bonding molecular orbitals.

Sigma bonds (σ bonds) are formed by direct overlapping of atomic orbitals, and they are the strongest type of covalent bond. Sigma bonds are symmetrical around the bond axis. Common sigma bonds—where z is the axis of the bond—are $s + s$, $p_z + p_z$, $s + p_z$, and ${d_z}^2 + {d_z}^2$.

In contrast, **pi bonds (π bonds)** are usually weaker than sigma bonds and are a type of covalent bond where two ends of one *p* orbital overlap the two ends of another *p* orbital. *d* orbitals can also form pi bonds.

Generally, single bonds are sigma bonds, and multiple bonds consist of one sigma bond plus one pi bond. A **double bond** is one sigma bond plus one pi bond. A *triple bond* consists of one sigma bond and two pi bonds. For example, ethylene has **delta bonds (δ bonds)** that are formed from four ends of one atomic orbital overlapping with four ends of another atomic orbital.

Hybridization

Sometimes, the *s*, *p*, *d*, and *f* orbitals do not fully explain where an electron will be at any given time. This is where hybrid orbitals come in. **Hybrid orbitals** are combinations of the standard atomic orbitals. For instance, if the *s* and *p* orbitals hybridize, instead of being two different kinds of orbitals, they become four identical orbitals. When the *s* orbital hybridizes with all three *p* orbitals, it's called sp^3 hybridization, and it forms a tetrahedral shape. This is the type of hybridization that occurs in H_2O. The description used depends on the properties of the compound, including its numbers of lone pairs of electrons.

Bond Energies

The **bond energy** can be described as the amount of energy required to break apart one mole of covalently-bonded gases. Bond energies are measured in kilojoules per mole of bonds (kJ/mol). Again, one mole of something is equal to Avogadro's number: $6.02214078 \times 10^{23}$. To calculate the number of moles of something, some simple formulas can be used:

$$\text{Moles} = \text{mass (g)} \,/\, \text{Relative mass (grams per mole)}$$

Example: How many moles are there in 30 grams of helium?

On the periodic table, Helium's relative mass is approximately two. Using this information and the formula yields this result:

$$\text{Moles} = \frac{30}{2} = 15 \text{ moles}$$

During a chemical reaction, some bonds are broken, and some are formed. Bonds do not break or form spontaneously—they require energy to be added or released. The energy needed to break a bond is the **bond energy**. Generally, the shorter the bond length, the greater the bond energy.

When atoms combine to make bonds and form a compound, energy is always released, normally as heat. Certain types of bonds have similar bond energies, despite each molecule being different. For example, all C-H bonds will have a value of roughly 413 kJ/mol. There are published lists of average bond energies for reference.

Using bond energies, it is possible to calculate the **enthalpy change** within a system. When a chemical reaction occurs, there will always be an accompanying change in energy. Energy is released to make bonds, so the enthalpy when breaking bonds is positive. Conversely, energy is also required to break bonds. Thus, the enthalpy change within a system is negative because energy is released when forming bonds.

- Some reactions are **exothermic**—where energy is released during the reaction, usually in the form of heat—because the energy of the products is lower than the energy of the reactants. In exothermic reactions, energy can be thought of as a **product.**
- Some reactions are **endothermic**—where energy is absorbed from the surroundings because the energy of the reactants is lower than the energy of the products. In endothermic reactions, energy can be thought of as a **reactant**.

It's possible to look at two sides of a chemical reaction and work out whether energy is gained or lost during the formation of the products, thus determining whether the reaction is exothermic or endothermic. Here is an example:

Two moles of water forming two moles of hydrogen and one mole of oxygen:

$$2H_2O(g) \rightarrow 2H_2 \ + \ O_2(g)$$

The sum on the reactant's side (2 moles of water) is equal to four lots of H-O bonds, which is:

$$4 \times 460 \text{ kJ/mol} = 1840 \text{ kJ/mol}$$

This is the input.

The sum on the product's side is equal to 2 moles of $\mathrm{H-H}$ bonds and 1 mole of $\mathrm{O=O}$ bonds, which is $2 \times 436.4 \text{ kJ/mol}$ and,

$$1 \times 498.7 \text{ kJ/mol} = 1371.5 \text{ kJ/mol}$$

This is the output.

The total energy difference is:

$$1840 - 1371.5 = +468.5 \text{ kJ/mol}$$

Because the energy difference is positive, it means that the reaction is endothermic and that the reaction will need energy to be carried out.

Covalent and van der Waals Radii

The **covalent radius (rcov)** is the length of one half of the bond length when two atoms of the same kind are bonded through a single bond in a neutral molecule. The sum of two covalent radii from atoms that are covalently bonded should, theoretically, be equal to the covalent bond length:

$$rcov(AB) = r(A) + r(B)$$

The van der Waals radius, rv, can be defined as half the distance between the nuclei of two non-bonded atoms of the same element when they are as close as possible to each other without being in the same molecule or being covalently bonded. The covalent radii changes depending on the environment that an atom is in and whether it is single, double, or triple bonded, but average values exist for use in calculations. The van der Waals radii also changes based on the intermolecular forces present, but average values also exist. This information is useful for determining how closely molecules can pack into a solid.

Intermolecular Forces

Intermolecular forces are the forces of attraction or repulsion between molecules. They are responsible for various properties that are exhibited by some materials, including surface tension, friction, and viscosity. They can be split into two groups:

- **Short-range forces:** when the centers of molecules are separated by three angstroms or less and tend to be repulsive
- **Long-range forces:** when the centers of molecules are separated by more than three angstroms and tend to be attractive, also known as van der Waals forces

Separation and Purification Methods

Chemical Separations

Frequently, a more rigorous physical separation or extraction technique is necessary to isolate the compound of interest, such as electrophoresis, solvent extraction, chelation, distillation, filtration, or chromatography, among many others. Separation methods take advantage of the differences in chemical or physical properties of matter, including size, mass, electron affinity, density, and polarity.

Electrophoresis

Electrophoresis is a technique that separates large molecules, based on relative size, using an electric current. When an electric current is applied to a gel matrix, the migration rate of nucleic acid molecules indicates their size, with shorter nucleic acids migrating more quickly and further through the minute openings in the gel matrix than larger ones.

Solvent Extraction

Solvent extraction is the process of selectively removing a solute from a liquid mixture, with the use of another immiscible solvent. It is a unique method in that it is an extraction between two liquid phases. The mixture containing the solute of interest is often aqueous and the extracting solvent is typically a non-polar organic solvent. After solvent extraction is complete, isolation of the solute or analyte is sometimes achieved through distillation or evaporation of the solvent. A commonly used recovery method is **back extraction**, where an aqueous solution containing a species known to react with the compound of interest, is mixed with the organic solvent.

Chelation

Chelation is the bonding between polydentate ligands and metal compounds and is associated with the heme complex. Chelation is performed as part of a procedure to separate trace amounts of metals from ore samples through a process called **leaching**. Ores are treated in solutions with varying pH, temperature, and chelating agents, to extract metals. Chelation is also used in the removal of toxic heavy metals, such as lead, from the human body. The patient suffering from metal poisoning is infused with a chelating agent that will bind to the metal in their system, and then those complexes are excreted by the body.

Distillation

Distillation separates liquid mixtures by taking advantage of the differences in the components' heat of vaporization. A simple distillation apparatus is equipped with a thermometer and consists of a distillation flask, a heat source, a condensing tube, and a receiving flask. The flask containing the mixture to be distilled is heated and the most volatile component evaporates first. The condensing tube contains water that circulates in a column to liquefy the vapor. Then, extracted condensate is collected in a suitable vessel.

Filtration

Solids and liquids are sometimes separated through **filtration**. Filtration equipment allows liquid to pass through a porous filter while capturing the solid material. Filters are often made of cellulose, carbon, glass, or polypropylene. Membrane filters with pores ranging in size from 0.001 to 10µm have been developed for the separation of microorganisms, viruses, and bacterium from a liquid medium.

Chromatography

Chromatography is a separation technique that isolates mixed compounds by taking advantage of the difference in their rate of movement through an appropriate medium. The basis for all chromatographic science is a mobile phase transporting the species of interest through a stationary phase. The stationary phase is where the separation of compounds takes place. There are two universally recognized categories of chromatography, planar chromatography and column chromatography.

Planar Chromatography

The stationary phase in **planar chromatography** is either paper, for **paper chromatography**, or a sheet of textile material treated with an adsorbent compound such as silica or cellulose, called **thin layer chromatography**. Planar chromatography takes advantage of capillary action to move the mobile phase-sample mixture through the stationary phase. The sample analytes move up the plate or paper at different rates based on polarity. Analytes that have a higher affinity for the mobile phase than the stationary phase will move more quickly up the paper or plate. The retention of the analytes is compared to the migration of the mobile phase.

Column Chromatography

The stationary phase in column chromatography is housed in a tube and the mobile phase is moved either by natural forces or by applied pressure. In **column chromatography**, the mobile phase may be liquid or gas. There are several different types of column chromatography.

Size exclusion chromatography (SEC) separates compounds by molecular weight and size. The column is uniformly porous and the column packing pore size is chosen based on the molecular size of the compounds to be separated. Some compounds may be too large to enter the pores inside the column and therefore, will not be retained on the column for any significant period of time. These will be the first to elute. The smallest of the compounds will elute last.

Normal and **reverse phase chromatography** separate analytes based on their polarities. Normal phase columns are typically packed with hydrophilic polar materials such as silica or alumina, while the mobile phase is a non-polar organic compound such as hexane. The least polar solutes will elute first in normal phase chromatography. In reverse phase chromatography, the opposite is true. The column is packed with non-polar materials, such as C_{18}, and the mobile phase is a polar solvent, such as water or acetonitrile. The least polar compounds will elute last in reverse phase chromatography.

Ion exchange chromatography (IEC) separates species based on the degree of their ionic charge and affinity for the charged column packing. IEC is effective in separating almost any charged molecule, regardless of molecular size. The mobile phase is typically a buffer consisting of an inorganic salt and other needed stabilizers. Anion exchange column packing is positively charged, whereas cation exchange column packing is negatively charged.

Chiral chromatography is a separation technique that resolves **optical isomers**, or **enantiomers**, from one another. Frequently, the stationary phase is treated with an appropriate chiral molecule to increase the affinity of one of the isomers to the stationary phase. The isomer that is preferentially attracted to the column packing will elute first.

Gas chromatography is used to separate and quantify materials that vaporize without changing physically. The mobile phase, in this case, is usually a neutral carrier gas such as helium. The stationary phase, as in liquid chromatography, is a column that is typically coated internally with an inert material such as fused silica or glass.

Structure, Function, and Reactivity of Biologically-Relevant Molecules

Biomolecules

Humans, animals, and plants are built with and require different biomolecules to function. **Biomolecules** are organic polymers that perform various functions in the human body. Among their many functions, biomolecules may do the following:

- Constitute the structure of human body
- Provide nutrition and energy to cells
- Perform various enzymatic reactions in the body
- Regulate the body defense mechanism
- Control genetic functions through heredity

Classes of important biomolecules include:

- Carbohydrates, such as starch (in animals) and cellulose (in plants)
- Proteins, such as nucleoprotein, plasma protein, hormones, enzymes, and antibodies
- Nucleic acids, such as ribonucleic acid (RNA) and deoxyribonucleic acid (DNA)

All biomolecules are **polymers**, which are repetitions of basic units called **monomers**. These polymers can be hydrolyzed into their respective monomers.

Carbohydrates are represented by a general formula, $(C_6H_{10}O_5)_n$, where $40 \leq n \leq 3000$. When hydrolyzed, starch produces the monosaccharide glucose $(C_6H_{12}O_6)$.

However, glucose remains stored as glycogen in the liver and muscle. Glycogen stores energy in the body.

$$n\, C_6H_{12}O_6 \xrightarrow{\text{Glycogen Synthase}} (C_6H_{10}O_5)_n$$

Where n = approx. 6000 - 30000

Proteins can be hydrolyzed under acidic condition to form amino acids.

$$\text{Protein} + nH_2O \xrightarrow{H^+} \text{Amino acids}$$

Nucleic acids are structurally associated with some proteins to form nucleoproteins. The hydrolysis of nucleic acids and nucleoproteins is illustrated below.

$$\text{Nucleoprotein} + nH_2O \xrightarrow{H^+} \text{Nucleic acid} + \text{Protein}$$

$$\text{Nucleic acid} + nH_2O \xrightarrow{H^+} \underset{\substack{purine \\ pyrimidine}}{\text{Base}} + \text{Pentose sugar} + H_3PO_4$$

Classification of Carbohydrates

Carbohydrates are classified into three categories:

1. **Monosaccharides:** Monosaccharides are the monomer unit for carbohydrates. They are the smallest unit. They are represented by a general formula $(CH_2O)_n$, where n = 3 – 6. Examples of monosaccharides are glucose (dextrose), fructose, and galactose.

2. **Disaccharides:** Disaccharides are two monosaccharides joined together. When hydrolyzed, disaccharides produce two molecules of monosaccharides. For example, hydrolyzing sucrose yields one molecule of glucose and one molecule of fructose. Hydrolyzing lactose yields a molecule of glucose and a molecule of galactose. Lastly, hydrolyzing maltose yields two molecules of glucose.

3. **Polysaccharides:** Polysaccharides are high molecular weight carbohydrates. When hydrolyzed, they produce many molecules of monosaccharides. Examples of polysaccharides are starch, glycogen, and cellulose.

Monosaccharides

Monosaccharides are named based on the number of carbon atoms in the molecule, such as triose (C3), tetrose (C4), pentose (C5), and hexose (C6). A monosaccharide with an aldehyde group is called an "aldose" and one with a ketone group is called a "ketose" (e.g., fructose).

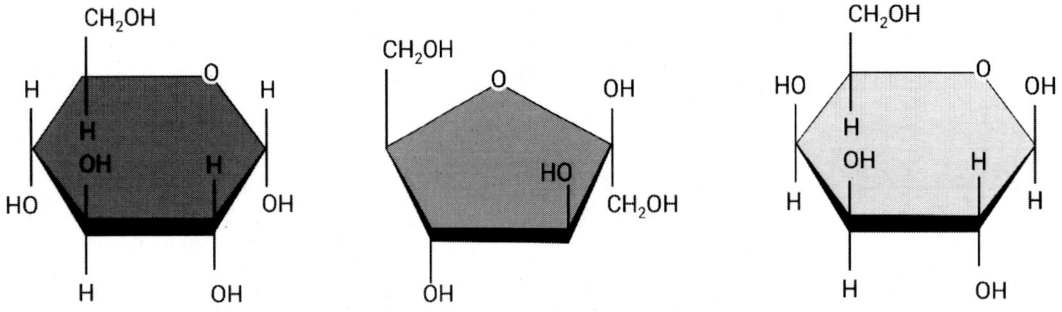

Glucose Fructose Galactose

Carbonyl compounds, aldehydes and ketones, can react with –OH group of an alcohol to form hemiacetal and acetal.

Glucose and fructose contain both carbonyl and hydroxyl groups, and therefore, they can form intramolecular hemiacetal to produce a cyclic structure. This hemiacetal formation takes place between the C1 and C5 carbons to form a stable heterocyclic structure. The cyclic structure forms a pyranose ring, which is a six-membered ring consisting of five C atoms and one O atom. In a cyclic structure, C1 might have $-\mathrm{OH}$ group at the right or left side, and therefore may be termed α-D-glucose and β-D-glucose, respectively.

Reducing sugars are ones with a free aldehyde or ketone groups, and they can act as reducing agents. All monosaccharides, including glucose, fructose, and galactose, are reducing sugars. Many disaccharides, including lactose and maltose (except sucrose), are also reducing sugars. The reducing sugars are able to reduce Fehling's solution and Tollens' reagent.

Fehling's solution is prepared by mixing a copper sulphate solution with potassium sodium tartrate in NaOH. When Fehling's solution is treated with a reducing sugar, the deep blue color of Fehling's solution fades and then forms a reddish precipitate.

When a solution of reducing sugar is heated with **Tollens' reagent**, silver is precipitated and forms silver mirror on the inner surface of the reaction vessel.

Lipids

Lipids are a class of biological molecules that are **hydrophobic**, meaning they don't mix well with water. They are mostly made up of large chains of carbon and hydrogen atoms, termed **hydrocarbon chains**. When lipids mix with water, the water molecules bond to each other and exclude the lipids because they are unable to form bonds with the long hydrocarbon chains. The three most important types of lipids are fats, phospholipids, and steroids.

Fats are made up of two types of smaller molecules: three fatty acids and one glycerol molecule. **Saturated fats** do not have double bonds between the carbons in the fatty acid chain, such as glycerol, pictured below. They are fairly straight molecules and can pack together closely, so they form solids at room temperature. **Unsaturated fats** have one or more double bonds between carbons in the fatty acid chain. Since they cannot pack together as tightly as saturated fats, they take up more space and are called oils. They remain liquid at room temperature.

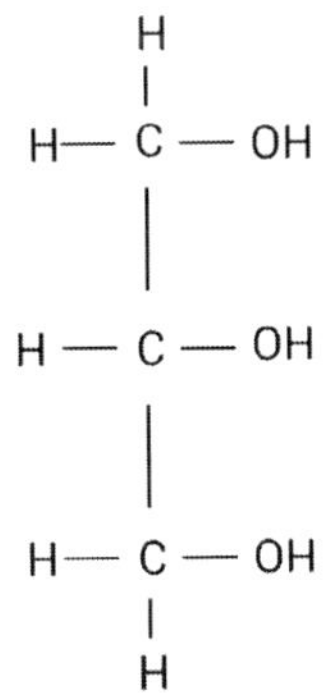

Glycerol

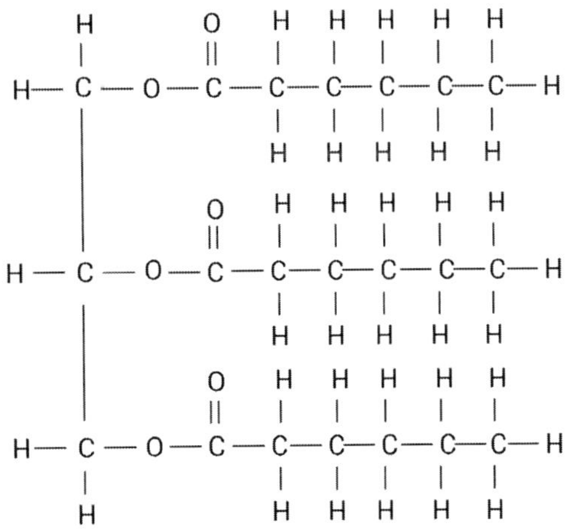

Triglyceride-Saturated

Phospholipids are made up of two fatty acid molecules linked to one glycerol molecule. When phospholipids are mixed with water, they inherently create double-layered structures, called bilayers, which shield their hydrophobic regions from the water molecules.

Steroids are lipids that consist of four fused carbon rings. They can mix in between the phospholipid bilayer cell membrane and help maintain its structure, as well as aid in cell signaling.

Proteins

Proteins are essential for almost all functions in living beings. The name *protein* is derived from the Greek word *proteios*, meaning **first** or **primary.** All proteins are made from a set of twenty amino acids that are linked in unbranched polymers. The combinations are numerous, which accounts for the diversity of proteins. Amino acids are linked by peptide bonds, while polymers of amino acids are called polypeptides. These polypeptides, either individually or in linked combination with each other, fold up to form coils of biologically-functional molecules, called proteins.

As mentioned previously, there are four levels of protein structure: primary, secondary, tertiary, and quaternary. The **primary structure** is the sequence of amino acids, similar to the letters in a long word. The **secondary structure** is beta sheets, or alpha helices, formed by hydrogen bonding between the polar regions of the polypeptide backbone. **Tertiary structure** is the overall shape of the molecule that results from the interactions between the side chains linked to the polypeptide backbone. **Quaternary structure** is the overall protein structure that occurs when a protein is made up of two or more polypeptide chains.

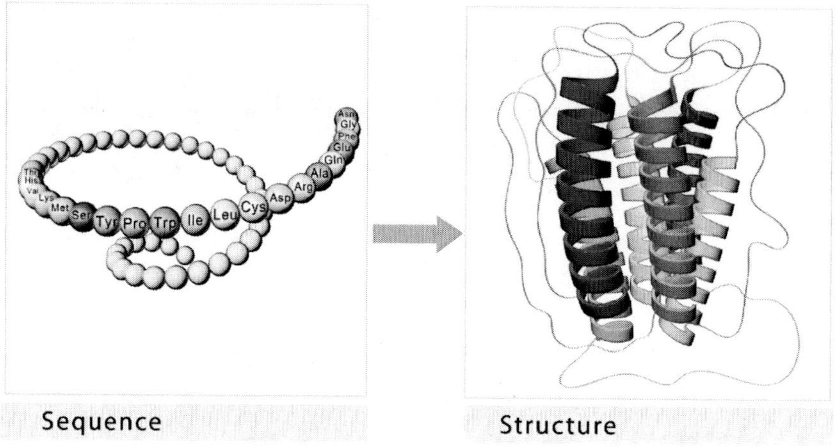

Nucleic Acids

Nucleic acids can also be called **polynucleotides** because they are made up of chains of monomers called **nucleotides.** Nucleotides consist of a five-carbon sugar, a nitrogen-containing base, and a phosphate group. There are two types of nucleic acids: deoxyribonucleic acid (DNA) and ribonucleic acid (RNA). Both DNA and RNA enable living organisms to pass on their genetic information and complex components to subsequent generations. While

DNA is made up of two strands of nucleotides coiled together in a double-helix structure, RNA is made up of a single strand of nucleotides that folds onto itself.

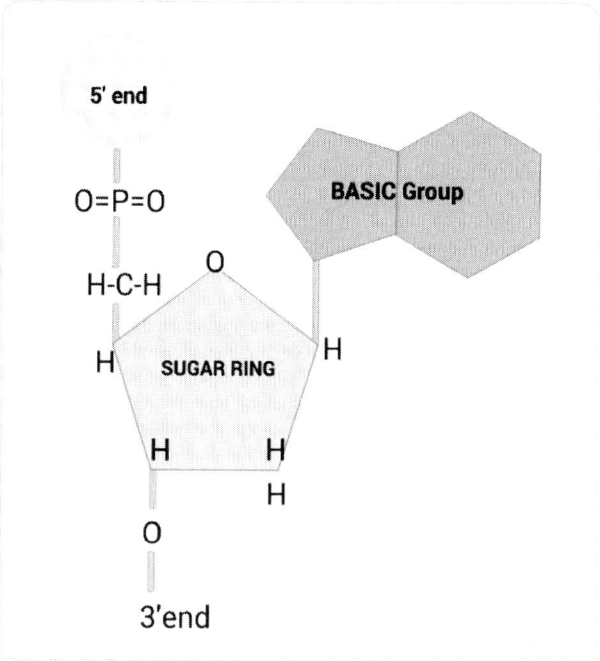

Principles of Chemical Thermodynamics and Kinetics

Gibbs Free Energy

Reactions must use energy to do work, and that available energy is called **Gibbs free energy** (G). Gibbs free energy, or G, represents the thermodynamic work potential for a system that is at a constant temperature and pressure (it may help to know that Gibbs free energy used to be called "available energy"). Free energy can be found by identifying the changes in enthalpy and entropy of a system.

$$\Delta H_{reaction} = \Delta H_{products} - \Delta H_{reactants}$$

$$\Delta S_{reaction} = \Delta S_{products} - \Delta S_{reactants}$$

A reaction can only be **spontaneous**, or occur without any influence of an outside force, if G is negative, and G depends on both entropy and enthalpy.

$$G = \Delta H - T\Delta S$$

T is in Kelvin and can never be negative

Gibbs Free Energy (G)

$G = \Delta H - T \Delta S$

Summary Spontaneous and Non-Spontaneous Reactions

	$\Delta H > 0$	$\Delta H < 0$
$\Delta S > 0$	**Spontaneity depends on T** spontaneous at higher temperatures	**Spontaneous at all temperatures**
$\Delta S < 0$	**Nonspontaneous** proceeds only with a continous input of energy	**Spontaneity depends on T** spontaneous at lower temperatures

Process	Products	Reactants	Sign	Meaning
Enthalpy	Lower #	Higher #	-	Exothermic (energy released)
Enthalpy	Higher #	Lower #	+	Endothermic (energy absorbed)
Entropy	Lower #	Higher #	+	More disorder
Entropy	Higher #	Lower #	-	Less disorder
BOLDED reactions are favorable				

In terms of **collision theory**:

- $H > 0$ and $S > 0$: If an endothermic reaction has high entropy and temperatures are low with slow particle movement, free energy (energy not invested into other chemical reactions) will be used up. However, if T is high enough, the extreme kinetic energy will make G negative and the reaction will be spontaneous.
- $H > 0$ and $S < 0$: If an endothermic reaction has low entropy, the reaction will require additional energy to proceed. This reaction has two unfavorable properties and will never be spontaneous.

- $H < 0$ and $S > 0$: If an exothermic reaction has high entropy, the reaction will always be spontaneous. It will never require additional energy since it has two favorable properties.
- $H < 0$ and $S < 0$: If an exothermic reaction has little random particle movement due to low temperatures, the reaction may not be spontaneous. Movement might be too low and slow for the reaction to proceed (collision theory).

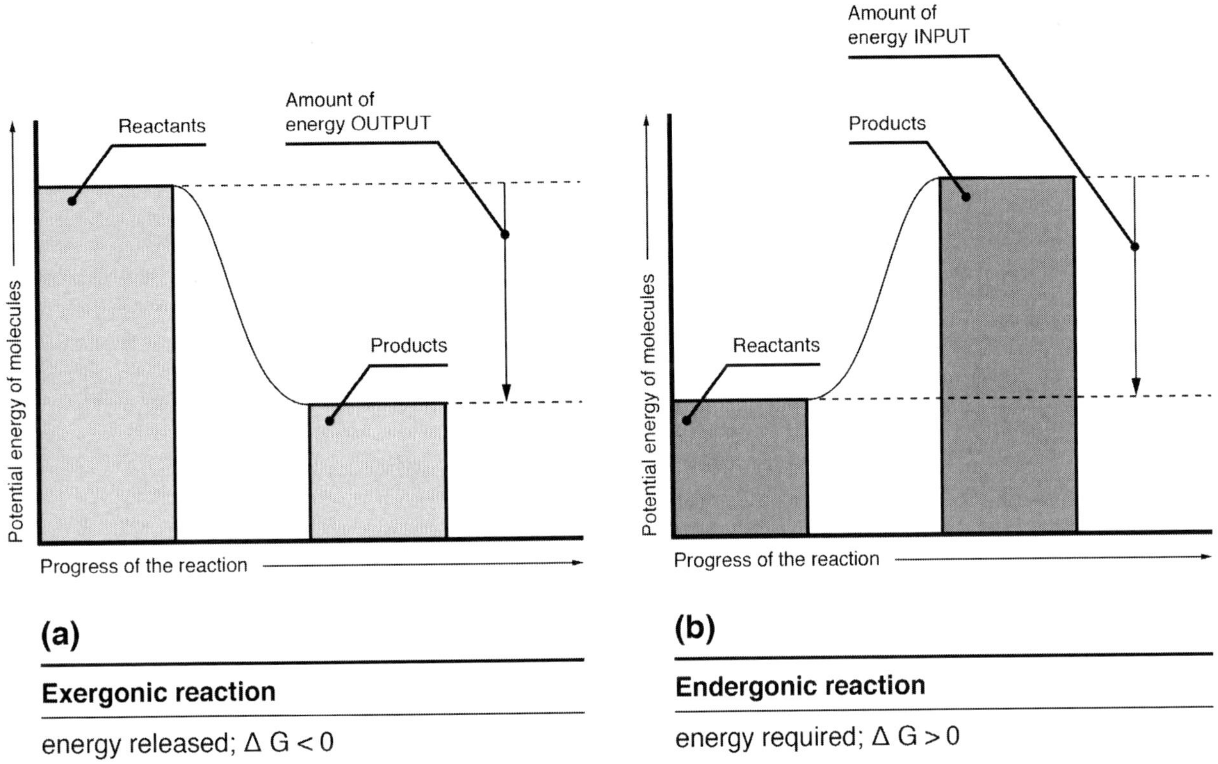

Helmholtz Free Energy

Helmholtz free energy measures available work from a closed thermodynamic system with a constant temperature. Although rarely used in thermodynamic chemistry, it is used under certain conditions, like in explosives research.

A is analogous to G and is equal to Helmholtz energy, which can be determined using the equation below.

$$A = U - TS$$

Like Gibbs, the reaction is spontaneous only when *A* is negative.

Chemical Potential

Chemical potential is free energy per system per number of moles (G per number of moles) and is referred to as molar free energy. In terms of kinetic theory, substances have higher chemical potential in areas where they are more concentrated because they have more potential to move in order to achieve equilibrium. The higher the concentration gradient, the larger the chemical potential. Also, the colder the temperature, the higher the chemical potential because the low temperatures keep molar concentration high due to movement limitations.

μ denotes chemical potential, which can be summarized in the equation:

$$\mu \equiv \left(\frac{\delta G}{\delta n}\right)_{T,p}$$

This simply restates what we already know: that chemical potential is equal to the change in free energy over the change in the number of moles.

Across the board, independent of which is held constant, gases have low chemical potential and solids have high chemical potential. Solids are the most compact and have the smallest molar volume. This also means that they are far more "concentrated" than liquids or gases, resulting in a very large concentration gradient. This large concentration gradient results in a large chemical potential. Gases, on the other hand, are already moving so quickly that their concentration gradient is very low. They will always have low chemical potential.

Also, across the board, the slope is greatest in the gas phase and smallest in the solid phase. This also makes sense because heating up solids has little effect on their movement due to intermolecular bonding, resulting in a low heat to movement ratio (slope). Liquids are easier to heat up because they have fewer intermolecular bonds due to their fluidity and mild kinetic energy, resulting in a medium heat to movement ratio (slope).

Gases, on the other hand, have negligible intermolecular bonding, and any heat input results in a quick increase in kinetic energy, resulting in a high heat to movement ratio (slope).

As pressure increases, gases will phase to liquid, then liquid to solid. Temperature increases are the opposite; as temperature increases, solid will phase to liquid then liquid to gas.

Chemical Equilibrium

$$\mathrm{N_2 + 3H_2 \leftrightarrow 2NH_3}$$

The driving force of reactions is G, and if it is a very large negative number, the reaction may go almost to completion. Equilibrium, as indicated by the double arrows in equations, does not mean that the reaction has stopped, as particles are moving and dynamic. It also does not mean that there are equal amounts of products and reactants. For example, spontaneous reactions will have more products since they are so favorable. Many reactions are reversible, so learning the conditions and factors that will cause a system to reach equilibrium can be useful.

Altered conditions affect equilibrium. For example, adding more reactants yields more products. Increasing the external pressure will affect the reaction depending on where the most gas particles are (as determined by coefficients). Greater pressures will cause the side with the greatest gas particles to react faster since they will be moving faster, pushing the direction of the reaction to the other side. Increasing temperature will always change the equilibrium constant (K) because K is dependent on temperature as shown in this equation (valid with reversible reactions that are at equilibrium):

$$\Delta G = -RTlnK$$

The **equilibrium constant** (K) is a value that expresses the ratio of the products over the reactants. If K is greater than one, there are more products at equilibrium (forward reaction is favored), while a value less than one indicates that the reverse reaction is favored. The equilibrium constant can be calculated using the molarity of each product (to the power of its coefficient) divided by the molarity of each reactant (to the power of its coefficient) as shown in the equation below:

$$aA + bB \leftrightarrow cC + dD$$

$$Kc = \frac{[C]^c[D]^d}{[A]^a[B]^b}$$

While K shows the equilibrium values, the reaction quotient Q shows how far away the reaction is from equilibrium. It is the same equation but shows the ratio of products over reactants at any given time. Eventually, once a reversible reaction reaches equilibrium, Q will be equal to K.

Gas equilibrium constants are measured in terms of **partial pressure**, rather than concentration, and the equation is:

$$Kp = \frac{[PC]^c[PD]^d}{[PA]^a[PB]^b}$$

The equilibrium constant for heterogeneous solutions is the same except no substances other than gases are included.

Catalysis describes the increase in the rate of a reaction caused by the addition of a catalyst. The addition of a catalyst causes reactions to speed up and require less activation energy. Only small amounts of catalysts are required, and they are not consumed by the reaction. Catalytic activity is indicated using the symbol z, and it is measured in mol/s. Catalysts usually react with one—or sometimes more than one—reactant, forming intermediates. Catalysts provide alternative mechanisms for chemical reactions that involve different transition states and lower activation energy.

Psychological, Social, and Biological Foundations of Behavior

Foundational Concept 6: Biological, psychological, and sociocultural factors influence the ways that individuals perceive, think about, and react to the world.

Sensing the Environment

Sensory Processing

Sensation

Humans understand the world around them through sensory processing. The human body has receptors that sense or detect different types of energy or stimuli and then process that information through the nervous system. This is the simplified process of sensation, such as that involved in touch and smell. The energy is converted to electrical signals and then transmitted to the brain through a series of action potentials travelling along the axons of millions of neural cells.

Thresholds

The **sensory threshold** is the amount or level of stimulus that is required for an individual to register a sensation. The absolute threshold refers to the smallest detectable level of any kind of sensory stimulus that an individual can detect 50% of the time during a given test. The **difference threshold**, or **Just Noticeable Difference (JND)** is the smallest difference between two stimuli that an individual can actually detect as being different 50% of the time during a given test.

Weber's Law

Ernst Weber was a German physician who observed that in order for the difference between two stimuli to be detected, the stimuli must differ by a constant proportion. This idea was then formulated into **Weber's Law**, which is written as $k = \Delta R/R$, where k is a different constant for each sensation, R is the amount of existing stimulation, and ΔR is the amount of stimulation that needs to be added for a JND.

Signal Detection Theory

The process of **signal detection** occurs when someone detects a stimulus and must distinguish it from background noise. Signal detection theory states that how an individual perceives a stimulus depends on the individual's physical and psychological state, as well as the intensity of the stimulus. For example, in a crowded parking lot, an individual may not notice the rustling of leaves on the ground, but on a quiet day, the sound of the rustling leaves would be more apparent and the individual may pay more attention to it, since there are fewer background noises.

Sensory Adaptation

Sensory adaptation occurs when there is constant exposure to a stimulus. Over time, an individual becomes less sensitive and more adaptable to that stimulus.

Psychophysics

Psychophysics is a field that studies an individual's relationship between physical stimuli and their psychological experience. Experiments are done that can be objectively measured and have quantitative outcomes, such as with threshold measurements.

Sensory Receptors

Different types of sensory receptors recognize different types of energy. For example, light receptors, which are located in the eyes, and sound receptors, which are located in the ears, convert their respective energy stimuli to neural activity through different specialized pathways.

Sensory Pathways

Each type of stimuli, such as touch, hearing, and vision, follows a different sensory pathway from the receptor to the brain. However, generally, all pathways have three long neurons called the primary, secondary, and tertiary neurons. The **primary neuron** has its cell body in the dorsal root ganglion of the spinal nerve. The **secondary neuron** has its cell body either in the spinal cord or in the brain stem. The **tertiary neuron** has its cell body in the thalamus. The pathway includes many breakpoints, or stations, each of which plays a different role in information processing. For example, if a painful sensation is felt on the finger, one station may cause the hand to withdraw from the stimuli and another station may cause the head to turn towards the source of the pain.

Types of Sensory Receptors

Different types of sensations are processed by different sensory receptors. Below is a list of the main sensory receptors found in the human body.

- **Mechanoreceptors:** Detect touch through contact with the body surface and detect sound through vibrations in the air or water. They are located in the skin, hair follicles, and ligaments.
- **Photoreceptors:** Detect vision through visible radiant energy
- **Thermoreceptors:** Detect warmth and cold through changes in skin temperature
- **Chemoreceptors:** Detect smell through substances dissolved in the air or water through the nasal cavity, and taste through substances that come in contact with the tongue

Vision

Structure and Function of the Eye

The **eye** is an elaborate organ that allows individuals to transduce light into neural signals and process their surrounding environment. Depending on their level of focus and concentration on an image, humans can see more or less detail on that object. The eye has many features that are similar to those of a camera. The **lens** allows the eye to focus light. The **ciliary muscles** bend the lens to change its shape and adjust the focus. The **cornea** is curved and bends the light rays so that they can form an image on the **retina** in the back of the eye. The amount of light that enters the eye is controlled by the **pupil**. The **optic nerve**, which is made up of the axons from the ganglion cells in the eye, then conveys the visual information to the brain.

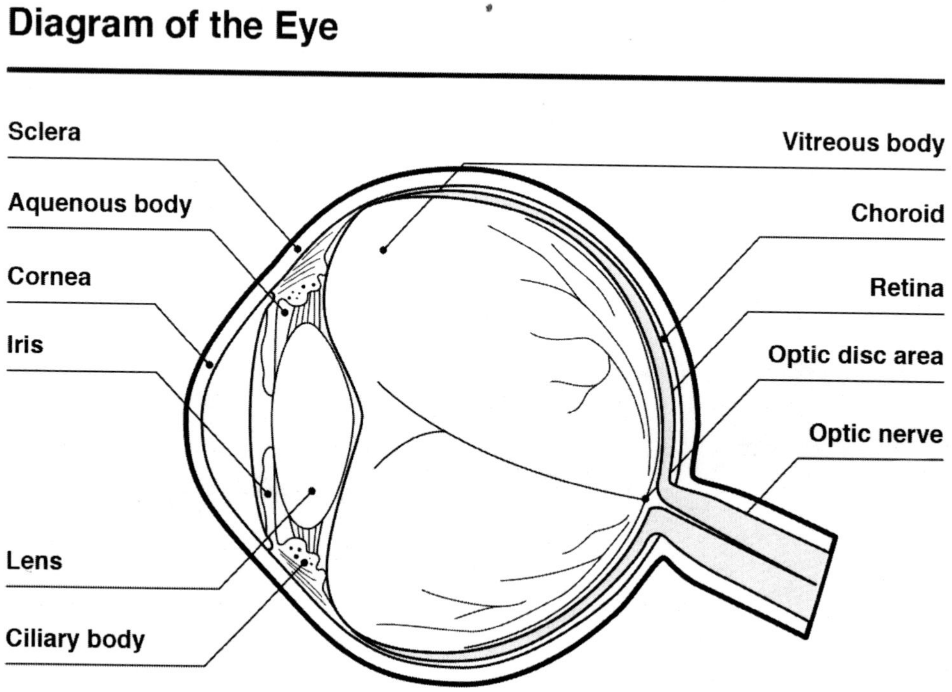

Visual Processing

Visual processing begins in the retina. Images that are taken in through the cornea and lens are transmitted upside down onto the retina. The two types of photoreceptors in the retina are called rods and cones. **Rods** are part of the scotopic system and can be stimulated with low light intensity. **Cones** are part of the photopic system and need strong light intensity to be stimulated. The **photopic system** is responsible for color vision. The signals that are produced from the processing that occurs in the retina are then transferred to ganglion cells, whose axons make up the optic nerve. Signals travel along these axons to the brain, where the visual information is processed, and the images are returned to their proper orientation.

Visual Pathways in the Brain

An individual's visual field is the entire area that they can see without moving their head. The visual cortex in the right hemisphere of the brain receives its input from the left half of the visual field and the visual cortex in the left hemisphere of the brain receives its input from the right half of the visual field. Some retinal ganglion cells have axons that lead to the superior colliculus in the brain, which helps coordinate the rapid movements of the eye towards a target. Others have axons that lead to the nuclei of the hypothalamus that control **circadian rhythms**, or the daily cycles of human behavior, or to the midbrain nuclei to control the size of the pupil and coordinate movement of the eyes or to map the visual space.

Parallel Processing

Parallel processing is the method by which the brain distinguishes incoming stimuli of differing quality. When processing visual stimuli, the brain divides what it sees into the categories of color, motion, shape, and depth. Each quality is analyzed individually but simultaneously and then combined for comprehension of the object.

Feature Detection

Feature detection is a process that starts gradually when an individual begins looking at an object. At first, the individual may look at the overall object, but as the neurons in the brain become more focused on the object, smaller details become more apparent. Feature detection allows the brain to become more selective in what it focuses on. For example, from a picture of a woman's face, the brain begins to see the curves, angles, and small lines of the face as the individual looks at the picture for a longer time.

Hearing

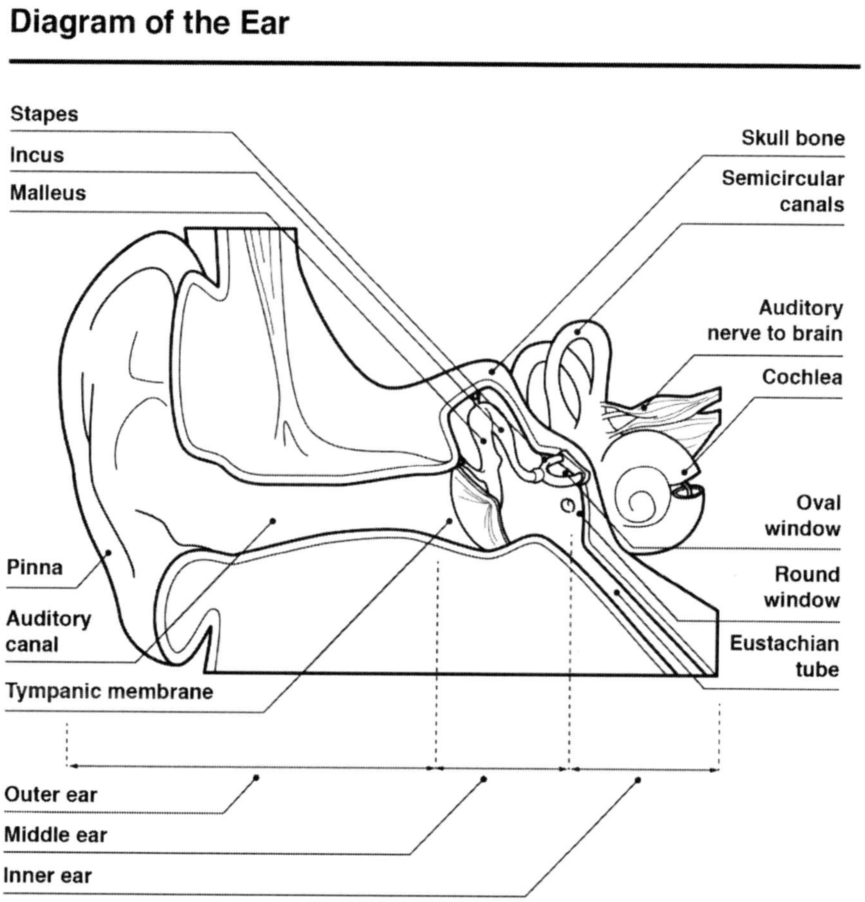

Structure and Function of the Ear

Each part of the ear plays a specific role in hearing. The **external ear** captures sound waves and sends them down the ear canal to the **eardrum**, or **tympanic membrane**. The shape of the external ear is important because it increases the efficiency of sounds within a certain frequency, especially those within the range important for speech perception, and helps with sound localization, so that individuals can identify where a sound is coming from. The **middle ear** consists of a chain of three small bones called **ossicles** that connect the tympanic membrane to the **oval window**, which is the opening of the inner ear. The ossicles are responsible for transferring and concentrating the mechanical stimuli of the tympanic membrane through the fluid of the middle ear to the auditory portion of the inner ear, which is called the **cochlea.** The inner ear has a structure called the **organ of Corti** that then converts the sound energy into neural activity. The organ of Corti has hairs on it that either convey messages to the brain or receive messages back from the brain.

Auditory Processing

Once a sound reaches the organ of Corti, it then travels as an electrical signal through the auditory ganglion cells and afferent nerves to the cochlear nuclei in the brainstem. There is a cochlear nucleus on each side of the brainstem, one for each ear. The signal then reaches ***the superior olivary nuclei***, which is the first location to receive signals from both ears. This helps greatly with auditory localization. Signals then travel to the inferior colliculus, the medial geniculate nucleus, and then to the auditory cortex. The neurons on this pathway are arranged in a very organized manner, dependent on the stimuli that they process. For example, cells that respond to high frequency sounds are at a distance from those that respond to low frequency sounds.

Sensory Reception by Hair Cells

Each ear contains about 3500 inner hair cells (IHCs) and 12,000 outer hair cells (OHCs). IHCs cannot regenerate, so damage to them causes a permanent decrease in hearing sensitivity. The IHC and OHC each have about 50 to 200 **stereocilia**, which are even smaller, stiff hairs protruding from them. Approximately 16 to 20 auditory nerve fibers come in contact with each IHC. The organ of Corti has two **afferent** nerve fibers, whose job is to convey messages from the hair cells to the brain, and two **efferent** nerve fibers, whose job is to convey messages from the brain to the hair cells. When fluid moves in the cochlea, the hair cells inside the organ of Corti start to bend in response to the vibrations that the fluid influx produces. The small movements then cause excitation of the hair cells and of the afferent axons. The sound stimulus is translated into electrical signals that are sent to the auditory brainstem and auditory cortex of the brain.

Other Senses

Somatosensation

Somatosensation is the reception and interpretation of sensory information that comes from specialized organs in the joints, ligaments, muscles, and skin. The somatosensory system consists of nerve cells, or sensory receptors, that respond to changes in these organs, including pressure, texture, temperature, and pain. Signals are sent along a chain of nerve cells to the spinal cord and then to the brain for information processing. Nociceptors are sensory receptors that detect pain in a range from acute and tolerable to chronic and intolerable. The skin is the largest organ in the somatosensory system. It contains three types of touch receptors: mechanoreceptors, thermoreceptors, and nociceptors. Muscles and joints contain mostly **proprioceptors**, which detect joint position and movement, as well as the direction and velocity of the movement.

Taste

Humans can detect five basic tastes with gustatory (taste nerve) cells: sweet, salty, sour, bitter, and umami. The human tongue has small projections, called **papillae**, that contain most of the taste receptor cells, or taste buds. Each papilla has one or more cluster of 50 to 150 taste buds. In addition to the taste buds, the papillae also contain pain receptors, which can sense spice for example, and touch receptors.

Taste buds are specific for one of the five taste sensations and are activated through different mechanisms. Below are descriptions of how each taste is sensed by the brain.

Salty

Salt-sensing taste buds are activated when sodium ions are transported across the membrane of the taste bud through sodium ion channels. The taste buds get partially depolarized, causing a release of neurotransmitters. This stimulates afferent neurons, which relay the stimulation information to the brain.

Sour

Sour tastes are sensed when sour foods or drinks release a hydrogen ion, which blocks the potassium channels of the taste bud membranes. The build-up of potassium in the cell leads to depolarization, neurotransmitter release, and stimulation information gets sent to the brain.

Sweet

The taste buds that sense sweetness have a more complicated stimulation pathway than those of the salty and sour taste buds. When sweet molecules bind to the receptors on their taste buds, a conformational change occurs in the molecule, which then activates a G-protein called **gustducin.** Several other proteins are activated along the pathway, which eventually leads to a blockage of potassium ion channels and an opening of a calcium ion channel. The influx of calcium to the cell causes a greater depolarization of the cell, release of neurotransmitters, and afferent neurons transmit the stimulation information to the brain.

Bitter

The bitter taste sensation has an even more complex pathway than that of sweetness. Bitterness is thought to the be the most sensitive of the tastes and is often perceived as sharp and unpleasant. In a similar pathway to the sweet taste, taste receptors are coupled to the G-protein gustducin. When a bitter substance is sensed, the gustducin breaks apart. Potassium ion channels are closed, calcium ion channels are opened, and the taste cell is depolarized. Neurotransmitters are released, and afferent neurons transmit stimulation information to the brain.

Umami

The taste of umami, which may be described as a meaty or savory flavor, was only relatively recently recognized as a separate taste. The receptors for umami react to glutamates and nucleotides, which are both found abundantly in meats and fermented foods. The fermenting process for many foods frees glutamic acid from proteins which creates ionic bonds with various cations to form different glutamates. Like with sweet and bitter flavors, when umami receptors bind to umami molecules, the receptors activate G proteins which are part of the pathway to sense umami via gustatory nerves.

Smell

Olfactory cells/chemoreceptors that detect specific chemicals

The dorsal portion of the nasal cavities is lined with an **olfactory epithelium**. This epithelium contains the receptor neurons that sense smell. If the olfactory epithelium is ever damaged, it has the capability to regenerate itself, including replacement of the receptor neurons. The chemical nature of odors is important for distinguishing between them because odors bind to olfactory receptors that are specific for a certain functional group of the odorant.

Pheromones

In addition to the main olfactory epithelium, the olfactory system has a **vomeronasal organ (VNO)**. Both organs are responsible for detecting pheromones, which are secreted chemicals that trigger a social reaction from members of the same species.

Olfactory Pathways in the Brain

The axons of the olfactory nerves terminate at the anterior end of the brain in a structure called the **olfactory bulb**. The olfactory bulb is organized into **glomeruli**, which are spherically-shaped neural circuits. The output from the bulb goes to the prepyriform area, the amygdala, and the hypothalamus within the brain for information processing.

Kinesthetic Sense

Kinesthetic sense is the sensation of movement and orientation. This sense is composed of information that comes from the sensory receptors in the inner ear regarding motion and orientation as well as in the stretch receptors that are in the muscles and ligaments, which provide information about stance. When the brain receives information regarding these movements, it can help to control and coordinate the body's actions, such as simultaneous walking and talking.

Vestibular Sense

Vestibular sense includes the sense of balance and spatial orientation. Combining these two things allows for the coordination of movement and balance. The receptors for the vestibular system are also found within the inner ear. This system allows the brain to understand how the body is moving and accelerating at each moment.

Perception

Perception is the interpretation of sensory information in order to understand the environment. It begins with an object stimulating one or more of the sensory organs in the body. For example, light stimulates the retina in the eye and odor molecules stimulate the receptors in the nasal cavity. In a process called transduction, this stimulation information is transformed into neural activity. These neural signals are then transmitted to the brain and processed there. The brain then creates a memory of this stimulus. When an unfamiliar object is encountered, the brain tries to collect as much information about the object as possible. When a familiar object is encountered again, the brain uses the senses to confirm that the object is indeed the familiar one.

Bottom-up and Top-down Processing

Bottom-up and **top-down** processing are two different methods of information processing. Sensory input is considered bottom-up processing while top-down processing involves the organization of information from many different sources and is considered a more complex process. Bottom-up processing can be described as a progression from individual elements to a complete picture. A stimulus is seen clearly, and the brain can make sense of the object using only the senses. Top-down processing involves the receipt of vague sensory information followed by the resolution of it using internal hypotheses and expectation interactions. The brain uses more than just the sensory areas to figure out what the stimulus is.

Perceptual Organization

Sensory organs help resolve different facets about an object. Depth perception is how a person judges their distance from an object. Each eye has a slightly different view on the same object, which can help distinguish where an object is located and what it fully looks like. The relative size of two objects can be distinguished by the differently sized images that are projected onto the retina. **Relative motion** can be determined by detecting that objects closer than the visual point of focus are moving in the opposite direction of the viewer's moving head and vice versa. **Perceptual constancy** is the idea that objects are stable and unchanging despite changes in sensory stimulation. The brain can identify familiar objects at any distance, from any angle, and with any illumination. Shape, color, and brightness are all perceived the same as they were originally. For example, a woman standing one hundred feet away appears small, but the brain knows what her actual height is and processes it as such.

Gestalt's Principles

Gestalt's principles are a set of principles that help explain perceptual organization. They are based on the idea that a whole is different than the sum of its parts. There are five parts to this set of principles:

1. **Law of Similarity:** Similar things tend to appear grouped together in both visual and auditory settings.

2. **Law of Pragnanz:** Objects in the environment are seen in a way that makes them appear as simple as possible. For example, the Olympics ring symbol is seen as five intertwined circles as opposed to a collection of curved and connected lines.

3. **Law of Proximity:** Objects that are near to each other tend to appear grouped together.

4. **Law of Continuity:** Points that are connected by a straight or curved line are seen in a way that follows the smoothest path.

5. **Law of Closure:** The brain often fills in the gap between separate objects to make a complete whole.

Making Sense of the Environment

Attention

Attention is the process of selectively focusing on particular information while ignoring other information that is present.

Selective Attention

Selective attention is the process by which the brain filters out large amounts of sensory information in order to focus on one single message. For example, someone who is filtering out a person talking to them while paying attention to the television would be using selective attention. When the brain becomes overloaded with sensory information, it begins to filter out the information that is unimportant and concentrate on what is needed and wanted.

There are several models that have been used to understand selective attention. One of the oldest models is the **spotlight model**. The idea behind this theory is that the visual field has an area of focus in the middle, an area of fringe around that, and a margin around the outer edge. Objects in the focus area are seen in high resolution while the objects located in the fringe area are a much lower resolution and are seen much more crudely. The cut off of the fringe area is referred to as the margin. Another model that builds on the spotlight model is called the **zoom-lens model**. This enhanced model incorporates the idea that if attention is being directed to a smaller focus area, the information being processed becomes sharper, or clearer, and can be processed faster.

Another theory of selective attention is the **bottleneck model**. This model explains how when the brain is overloaded with information, it has to find a way to choose what information to process first. This information is allowed through the bottleneck while the other information must wait to be processed. While some psychologists have hypothesized that the information that is waiting to get processed is completely ignored, others have proposed that it is actually just attenuated and if something important, like the person's name, were part of the message, the brain would begin to process that information.

Divided Attention

Divided attention is when a person is processing more than one piece of information at a time. This process occurs frequently, such as when driving and paying attention to speed, traffic, and traffic signals or when listening to music while doing homework. It is an important part of everyday life. Attention resources are limited, so the more resources that are devoted to one task, the less that are available for another simultaneous task.

Cognition

Cognition is the process of acquiring knowledge and then using thought, experience, and the senses to further understand it. Cognition is both conscious and unconscious and involves reasoning, problem solving, and decision-making skills.

Information-Processing Model

The **information-processing model** is a theory about the development of cognition in humans. Instead of having automatic responses to sensory information, humans process the information they receive and then make an informed decision about how to respond. The human mind has attention mechanisms for bringing in the information, working memory for processing and manipulating the information to better understand it, and long-term memory for storing the information for future use. As children grow and their brains continue to develop, the mind can process and respond to information more efficiently and maturely. While most of a person's cognitive abilities are based on their genetics, there are some influences from the environment, such as with behavior and learning.

Cognitive Changes in Late Adulthood

After the brain has fully developed, cognitive changes are seen again in late adulthood. As the brain ages, certain processes do not occur as fast or efficiently as during their peak performance time. The central nervous system begins to slow down, which affects the speed of information processing. The capacity of a person's working memory and their ability to recall specific events from the past or recently acquired information begins to decline.

Role of Culture in Cognitive Development

The environment and culture that surrounds a person can influence how they learn and process sensory information around them. It also affects their view on the world around them.

Influence of Heredity and Environment on Cognitive Development

Jean Piaget was a psychologist who believed that a child's cognitive development occurred from the genes they inherited. He theorized that children approached the world independently, without influence from their environment, so all children would develop universally.

In contrast, Lev Vygotsky was a psychologist who hypothesized that social interactions were a key influence in the continuous development and change seen in children's thoughts and behaviors. In different cultures, the same situation could elicit a different response from a child based on their previous interactions with a more knowledgeable person within that culture. This theory provides a basis for much more variable cognitive development.

Biological Factors that Affect Cognition

There are several biological factors that can affect cognitive development, including the sense organs, intelligence, heredity, and maturation. Proper development of the sense organs is important for proper cognitive development because the sense organs are responsible for detecting sensory information in the environment. Intelligence affects all aspects of mental capacity. Children with low intelligence are unable to take in sensory information properly, which causes their cognitive development to lag behind. Heredity includes the genes that are passed down from one generation to the next. A child's cognitive development will be similar to that of their parents. Lastly, as children mature, their interactions with the environment increase. These interactions are important influences in proper cognitive development.

Problem Solving and Decision-Making

Types of Problem Solving

Problem solving is the mental process of reaching a goal using complex logic to fill in the missing information that stands between a person's present condition and the goal. There are several different ways of attempting to solve a problem. Using the **problem-solving cycle**, a person would define the problem, develop a strategy to fix the problem, find the resources available for implementing the strategy, monitor progress, and then evaluate the solution for accuracy. Another method is the **GROW method**, in which *G* stands for goal, *R* stands for reality or the current situation, *O* stands for obstacles and options, and *W* stands for way forward or the path that the person would take to reach their goal. **PDCA** is another four-step approach that stands for planning, doing, checking, and acting.

Barriers to Effective Problem-Solving

There are five main barriers to effective problem solving: confirmation bias, mental set, functional fixedness, unnecessary constraints, and irrelevant information. **Confirmation bias** includes preconceived notions that make a person more willing to favor studies that align with their beliefs. **Mental set** describes a person's bias towards attempting to solve a problem in a way that has worked previously, even though a different method may be more efficient. **Functional fixedness** is a type of mental set in which a person will not use an object for any other purpose than its original function. **Unnecessary constraints** are when a person subconsciously places boundaries on a task at hand. **Irrelevant information** is information that is present along with a problem that is unrelated to the problem and will not help in solving the task.

Approaches to Problem Solving

There are many different strategies that can be used to solve a problem once it has been identified. The table below describes some of these options.

Technique	Description
Abstraction	Solving the problem in a model of the system before applying it to the real system
Analogy	Using a solution that solves an analogous problem
Brainstorming	Suggesting many solutions or ideas and combining and developing them until an optimum solution is found
Divide and Conquer	Breaking down a large, complex problem into smaller, solvable problems
Hypothesis Testing	Assuming a possible explanation to the problem and trying to prove (or, in some contexts, disprove) the assumption
Means-ends Analysis	Choosing an action at each step to move closer to the goal
Reduction	Transforming the problem into another problem for which solutions exist
Research	Employing existing ideas or adapting existing solutions to similar problems
Root Cause Analysis	Identifying the cause of a problem
Trial-and-Error	Testing possible solutions until the right one is found

Heuristics and Biases

Heuristics are approaches to problem solving that are practical but not necessarily optimal or perfect. They help people to form judgments about a situation and then make a decision. Biases occur when the heuristics deviate from logic and probability. Two examples of common biases are overconfidence and belief perseverance. **Overconfidence** occurs when a person has greater confidence in a piece of information than the actual objective accuracy of that information. **Belief perseverance** occurs when a person continues to maintain their belief despite the appearance of contradictory new information.

Intellectual Functioning

Intelligence is a person's innate ability to learn, recognize problems, and solve problems.

Theories of Intelligence

Different researchers have formed different theories of intelligence over time. Four main theories of intelligence are described below:

1. **General Intelligence:** Intelligence is a single, general cognitive ability that can be measured and expressed numerically. If a person does well on one cognitive test, he or she will likely do well on other tests as well.

2. **Primary Mental Abilities:** Intelligence is composed of seven different primary mental abilities including verbal comprehension, reasoning, perceptual speed, numerical ability, word fluency, associative memory, and spatial visualization.

3. **Multiple Intelligences:** There are eight different intelligences based on different skills and abilities including visual-spatial, verbal-linguistic, bodily-kinesthetic, logical-mathematical, interpersonal, musical, intrapersonal, and naturalistic.

4. **Triarchic Intelligence:** The three main parts of intelligence are analytical, creative, and practical.

Influence of Heredity and Environment on Intelligence

Both heredity and environment can influence intelligence. Speed of information processing depends on neurologic efficiency and is genetically controlled and will be similar between parents and biological children. Environmental factors such as nutrition, exposure to toxic substances, and access to enriching learning environments can also influence the development of intelligence. Malnutrition and exposure to toxic substances can affect brain development. Home and school environments that are not mentally enriching and do not support learning can cause cognitive abilities to diminish over time.

Variations in Intellectual Ability

The extreme variations of intellectual ability can be characterized as *mentally retarded* for lower ability and **intellectually gifted** for higher ability. A person with low intellectual ability has below average intellectual function and is limited in two or more adaptive skill areas. An intellectually gifted person has either a general or a specific high intellectual ability.

Consciousness

States of Consciousness

The mind has three main states of consciousness: conscious, subliminal, and unconscious. Each state is produced by a different wavelength in the brain and responsible for a different level of understanding and information processing. **Beta waves** operate at around 13-30 Hz and are associated with learning, worry, and activities that involve mental focus. For this reason, these wavelengths are involved in the conscious mind. **Alpha waves** are 8-13 Hz and are the wavelengths that predominate during relaxing or daydreaming; part of the subliminal mind. **Theta waves** are 4-8 Hz and involved in deeper relaxation, dreams and the REM phase of sleep, and also part of the subliminal, and somewhat unconscious, mind. Lastly, **delta waves** are up to 4 Hz. They are involved in deep sleep and the unconscious mind.

Alertness

Alertness is a heightened sense of awareness. It is an active state of attention in which a person is quick to react to stimuli.

Sleep

Sleep is an unconscious state of the mind. It is a time for the brain to process information and experiences that were learned during the day. It also helps transfer information to the long-term memory.

Stages of Sleep: There are four stages of non-**rapid eye movement** (REM) sleep that occur before REM sleep. Stage 1 includes the transition from being awake to being asleep. Stage 2 includes a slowing of the heart rate and breathing. Stage 3 is a deep sleep. Stage 4 is a very deep sleep with a transition to mostly delta brain waves. REM sleep is where dreams occur and the heart rate and breathing actually quicken.

Sleep Cycles and Changes to Cycles: Sleep cycles last from 90 to 110 minutes on average in adults. They begin with Stage 1 and then progress to REM sleep after about ninety minutes. The first REM sleep lasts about ten minutes and increases in length with each subsequent sleep cycle, with the final one lasting up to one hour.

Sleep and Circadian Rhythms: Although the pattern of sleep cycles is consistent from childhood through adulthood, the timing of sleep changes. A **circadian rhythm** is a biological process that follows a twenty-four-hour cycle.

Humans have an internal circadian pacemaker that makes them aware of the time of the day and when they should go to sleep and wake up. As a person develops and ages, the preferred time to go to sleep and wake up changes. Children tend to go to sleep early in the evening, adolescents tend to stay up late into the night, and adults tend to go to sleep at the end of the evening or early in the night.

Dreaming: **Dreams** are a series of thoughts and images that occur in a person's mind while they are asleep. They mostly occur during the REM stage of sleep. There are several theories as to why people dream including memory consolidation, emotional regulation, and threat simulation.

Sleep–Wake Disorders: Sleep is essential for restoration and repair of the body as well as for processing of the information received during the waking hours. There are many different types of sleep-wake disorders that are disruptive to getting a proper night of sleep, such as insomnia, restless leg syndrome, narcolepsy, and breathing-related sleep disorders.

Hypnosis and Meditation

Hypnosis is a state of consciousness that involves reducing awareness of a person's surroundings and focusing attention on one specific piece of information. **Hypnotherapy** is the use of hypnosis to help solve a psychological problem, such as sleep disorders.

Meditation is the act of focusing on quiet thoughts and disregarding the surrounding environment. It can help to calm the mind before bedtime and help eliminate sleep disorders.

Consciousness-Altering Drugs

Consciousness-altering drugs, or **psychoactive drugs**, are pharmaceutical substances that produce changes in mood, perception, and consciousness.

Types of Consciousness-Altering Drugs and Their Effects on the Nervous System and Behavior

1. **Anxiolytics:** Decrease anxiety; used to sedate the central nervous system

2. **Euphoriants:** Induce a state of intense elation and alter perception; increase the activity of certain neurotransmitters

3. **Stimulants:** Stimulate the mind and cause a person to wake up; enhance the activity of certain neurotransmitters in the brain

4. **Depressants:** Induce a calm state of mind, reduce anxiety, and can alter perception; can induce sleep

5. **Hallucinogens:** Produce distinct alterations in perception, time, and emotional states; disrupt the interaction of nerve cells and serotonin, which helps regulate behavior and perception

Drug Addiction and the Reward Pathway in the Brain

The reward pathway in the brain is responsible for the feeling of pleasure in response to an enjoyable experience. It engages all five senses and then motivates a person to repeat the enjoyable activity to feel pleasure again. Drugs, such as psychoactive substances, bypass the senses and start the pathway directly in the brain, causing a large release of dopamine and an abnormally intense feeling of pleasure. The brain then adjusts for this overabundance of dopamine by reducing the number of dopamine receptors, causing a low feeling to follow the immense high. Addiction causes the person to crave the feeling of intense pleasure again and the cycle of drug use to continue.

Memory

Memory is the process by which information is encoded, stored, and retrieved by the brain.

Encoding

Process of Encoding Information

Encoding begins with perception of stimuli through the senses. From these sensations, a short-term memory is created. The information is sent to the sensory area of the cortex and then to the hippocampus in the brain. The hippocampus analyzes the information and decides whether to store it in the long-term memory.

Processes that Aid in Encoding Memories

New memories can be encoded easier if they can be associated with memories that are already stored in the brain. Elaboration is a strategy of organization that allows new information to associate with long-term memories. The use of **mnemonics** is a type of elaboration. Rhymes, acronyms, and acrostics are all examples of mnemonics that make remembering information easier. The association of images with words also aids in memory encoding.

Storage

Types of Memory Storage

The **sensory memory** is responsible for holding sensory information about objects that a person encounters. It can recall that information very quickly, even after observing the object for a very short length of time. The sensory memory is an automatic response and is out of conscious control. The **working**, or **short-term, memory** has a limited amount of storage. It is responsible for holding, processing, and manipulating information when it first reaches the brain for just a few minutes at longest. This memory aids in reasoning and decision-making. The **long-term memory** holds information indefinitely and has a very large capacity. It is generally outside of a person's awareness, but the memories stored here can be recalled to the working memory when needed.

Semantic Networks and Spreading Activation

Semantic networks are formed when a piece of knowledge is better understood by linking together several different concepts. Spreading activation is a method for searching a semantic network to retrieve a specific piece of information.

Retrieval

Recall, Recognition, and Relearning

There are two main methods of accessing memories: recall and recognition. **Recall** is the retrieval of information that had been previously encoded and stored in the brain. **Recognition** is mostly an unconscious process in which an event or object is associated with a previously stored memory. Relearning involves learning information again that has been previously learned. This process can make retrieving information in the future easier and can improve the strength of memories.

Retrieval Cues

Retrieval cues are stimuli that aid in memory retrieval from the long-term memory. They can be external, like the smell of a candle that reminds you of a childhood memory, or internal, like a feeling of sadness that reminds you of a death in the family.

The Role of Emotion in Retrieving Memories

Memories that are emotionally charged are usually easier to recall. Memories associated with strong emotions, pleasant or unpleasant, are remembered better than less emotional events that occurred at the same time. Positive memories often contain more details, which aids in retrieval.

Processes that Aid Retrieval

Exercising can help increase a person's heart rate and get the blood flowing to the brain, which in turn enlarges the hippocampus, a vital part of the brain for memory.

Forgetting

Aging and Memory

Normal aging causes a decline in memory abilities and cognitive tasks. The brain is slower to encode new memories as well as to recall previously-stored memories.

Memory Dysfunctions

Memory dysfunction occurs when there is damage to the neurological structures of the brain that work towards the storage, retention, and recollection of memories. They can be progressive like Alzheimer's disease and Korsakoff's syndrome or immediate, such as in the case of a head injury. Alzheimer's disease is a neurodegenerative disease that starts with short-term memory loss and advances to disorientation and behavioral issues. Korsakoff's syndrome is a result of a deficiency of thiamine in the brain, most often caused by alcoholism, that results in severe memory loss as well an inability to create new memories.

Decay

The **theory of decay** proposes that memories fade from the brain over time. It becomes harder to retrieve them as the strength of the memory wears away.

Interference

Retroactive interference theory proposes that when a person learns something new and there is an overlap or interaction with a past learned behavior, it becomes harder to retrieve the old knowledge. **Proactive interference theory** proposes that past memories inhibit a person's full ability to retain new memories.

Memory Construction and Source Monitoring

Since the brain has a limited capacity for storage of memories, there is a theory that proposes memories are not stored as whole entities, but rather, as pieces of data that can be pieced together to create the whole memory. Every time a memory is recalled, it is newly reconstructed. Unfortunately, this allows room for error with each memory. **Source-monitoring errors** occur when a memory is attributed to the wrong source, such as learning new information from a friend but later stating that a person read about it in the newspaper. It can be due to limited encoding of source information or by a disruption in the judgment process when deciding on the source.

Changes in Synaptic Connections Underlie Memory and Learning

Neural Plasticity

Neural plasticity is the ability of the brain to change throughout a person's lifetime. The neural synapses in the brain that are important for learning and memories are constantly changing size and shape and making new connections to accommodate the new information.

Memory and Learning

When new memories are made or new behavior is learned, the brain stores the information by changing the strength of some of its synapses. The memories are encoded within these synapses. Different types of memories are stored in different types of neurons.

Long-Term Potentiation

Long-term potentiation is an enhancement in the signal transmission between two neurons that results from the repeated pairing and stimulation of the neurons. The strength of the action potential is boosted, there is an increase in the number of receptors on the dendrite, and sometimes the amount of available neurotransmitters is increased as well.

Language

Language is a set of sounds and symbols that have distinct meaning and that are used for communication. There are approximately 5000 to 7000 different languages used by humans across the world. Infants are born with the ability to distinguish between sounds found in all languages. However, by about seven months of age, they begin to concentrate on the language or languages that are spoken to them the most. New languages are easiest to learn before the age of seven and become harder to learn through adolescence and then adulthood.

Theories of Language Development

There are several theories that exist about language development. The **learning theory** proposes that both adults and children learn best through repetition and external reinforcement in the form of encouragement or critique. In the case of language, infants and adults have conversations even before the infant has the ability to speak; the interactions between them build structure of language in infants that prepares them for the time when they are ready to speak.

The **nativist theory** states that children are born with a genetic ability to learn the laws of language, such as sentence structure and grammar principles. Being around people who are speaking and using these laws allows children to utilize their innate ability as they begin to speak themselves. This theory also supports the idea of *universal grammar*, which is the idea that all languages have the same basic underlying structure and that specific languages just utilize this structure with different patterns.

The **interactionist theory of language** relies on the idea that social interaction is important for language development. A child first observes language interaction between other people and then develops the same behavior within themselves. When a child is first learning to speak, the adult leads the conversation but as the interactions continue and the child's skills grow, the child can speak more independently.

Influence of Language on Cognition

Language affects the cognitive process in a person. Linguistic relativity is a theory that the language that a person speaks shapes how they view and think about the world around them. Thoughts are often unable to be directly translated between different languages, so the meaning of those thoughts becomes different in the different cultures. Linguistic determinism is the idea that the structure of a language is limited, and therefore limits the knowledge and thought processes that shape that language and the people who speak it.

Brain Areas that Control Language and Speech

Different areas of the brain are responsible for different parts of language processing. Four levels of language comprehension and their associated brain activation are described below.

1. Passive exposure to written words activates the posterior area of the left hemisphere of the brain.

2. Passive exposure to spoken words activates the temporal lobes.

3. Oral repetition of words activates the motor cortex on both sides of the brain, the supplementary motor cortex, and a portion of the cerebellum and insular cortex.

4. Generation of a verb that is associated with a presented noun activates language-related regions in the left hemisphere, including Broca's area.

Responding to the World

Emotion

Emotion is a state of mind or instinctive feeling that is derived from the situation or mood that a person is in.

Three Components of Emotion

There are three components of emotion. The **cognitive** part of emotion is how a person experiences the emotion and verbally describes how they are feeling. The **physiological** part is the part of emotion that is expressed through bodily responses, such as tears that come when a person feels sad. The **behavioral** component is how a person's actions change in response to an emotion. For example, a person may become defensive in response to a threat.

Universal Emotions

There are six emotions that are universally recognized in all cultures: fear, anger, happiness or joy, surprise, disgust, and sadness. Each has a distinct facial expression and physiological response associated with it as well.

- **Fear:** A feeling induced by perceived danger or threat
- **Anger:** A strong emotional response to a perception of threat, hurt, or provocation
- **Happiness** or **Joy:** A feeling of great pleasure and positive emotions
- **Surprise:** A feeling of astonishment from something unexpected
- **Disgust:** A feeling of repulsion in response to something unpleasant or offensive
- **Sadness:** An emotional pain associated with a feeling of loss, helplessness, or disappointment

Adaptive Role of Emotion

Emotions cause humans to be adaptive and respond to how they are feeling. They provide motivation for action and change. For example, if a person does not study and ends up doing poorly on a test, he or she feels sad. This sadness motivates the person to study more for the next test in order to avoid feeling sad again. The same motivation exists for feelings of happiness—activities that elicit feelings of pleasure are likely to be pursued and repeated. Charles Darwin believed that the adaptive nature of emotions allowed humans to survive and reproduce in line with his theory of natural selection.

Theories of Emotion

James–Lange Theory

The **James-Lange theory of emotion** proposes that emotions are felt in response to bodily changes that are already occurring. It is the body's response to a stimulus that triggers the emotional response. For example, the hair on the back of a person's neck stands up before the feeling of fear is processed in the brain and then physically experienced with awareness.

Cannon–Bard Theory

The **Cannon-Bard theory** proposes that the role of emotion is to help a person deal with changes in the environment. It focuses on the connection between emotion and the autonomic nervous system, which comprises the sympathetic nervous system and the parasympathetic nervous system. The sympathetic nervous system makes changes such as increasing heart rate, increasing breathing rate, and causing reflex actions, and the parasympathetic nervous system works at a slower rate to dampen or inhibit physiological responses. The Cannon-Bard theory proposes that the brain is oversees which emotion is an appropriate response to the stimulus that is being processed. The cerebral cortex simultaneously decides on the emotion and activates the sympathetic nervous system so that the body is ready for an immediate response once the decision is made.

Schachter–Singer Theory

There are two parts to the **Schachter-Singer theory of emotion**: the physiological arousal and the cognitive label. The theory proposes that when an emotion is felt, a physiological change is felt first. Then, the person searches the environment for clues to help identify the cause of the physiological change and label the emotion. Identification of emotion in this manner can lead to misinterpretation of the feelings a person is experiencing, which is a realistic scenario.

The Role of Biological Processes in Perceiving Emotion

Brain Regions Involved in the Generation and Experience of Emotions

Different regions of the brain are activated by the generation and experience of different emotions. The **amygdala** is responsible for intense affective emotions, such as love and fear. They **hypothalamus** is involved with the feelings of both pleasure and rage. The **cingulate gyrus** is a part of the brain that coordinates present sights and smells with previous emotions. It also regulates feelings of aggression.

The Role of the Limbic System in Emotion

The **limbic system** is a complex set of structures in the brain, including the hypothalamus, hippocampus, and amygdala, among others. It is involved in the recognition of emotion and the formation of emotional memories. Although each structure of the complex system is responsible for a different part of the emotion-eliciting process, the whole system works together as one to connect the cognitive, physiological, and behavioral components of emotions.

Emotion and the Autonomic Nervous System

The generation, recognition, expression, and experience of emotion are largely mediated by the autonomic nervous system. There are two types of patterned activity that are exhibited by the autonomic nervous system in response to emotions: coherence and specificity. **Coherence** is the organization and coordination of activity within the autonomic nervous system as well as between the autonomic nervous system and other response systems, such as facial expressions and cognitive emotional experience. **Specificity** is the idea that each emotion activates a different response and activity from the autonomic nervous system.

Physiological Markers of Emotion

Changes in the autonomic nervous system are the most obvious physiological signs of emotion. This system controls the smooth muscle, cardiac muscle, and glands in the body and mediates increases and decreases in heart rate, increased and decreased blood flow to the face, which results in blushing or turning pale, and sweating, among many other things.

Stress

Stress is the emotional strain that a person feels from circumstances that are demanding or that do not provide assurance of a positive outcome.

The Nature of Stress

Appraisal

An **appraisal** is an evaluation of what is happening between a person and the environment around them. Appraisals establish a person's feelings towards a situation and help determine the amount of stress involved. The **primary appraisal** is the first assessment of whether or not the situation is harmful to a person's well-being. The **secondary appraisal** follows the primary appraisal and is an evaluation of the options and resources available for coping with the situation. A person experiences stress when the available resources are not enough to completely manage or cope with the situation.

Different Types of Stressors

A **stressor** is an event that causes a person to experience feelings of stress. The three main types of stressors are cataclysmic events, personal stressors, and chronic stressors. **Cataclysmic events** occur suddenly and involve many people, such as earthquakes or mass transit accidents. **Personal stressors** are events that cause personal life changes, such as the loss of a job or death of a family member. These events usually cause an immediate, emotional reaction that tapers off over time. In some cases, however, a personal stressor may cause a person to experience post-traumatic stress disorder (PTSD), which has long-term effects, such as nightmares and flashbacks. **Chronic stressors** are events that occur often, sometimes daily, such as getting stuck in traffic or working long hours. These stressors are often small but can summate over time and negatively affect a person's well-being.

Effects of Stress on Psychological Functions

The ability to cope with stress is an important part of maintaining a person's state of good health. Stress can affect a person's immune system and increase one's susceptibility to illness. Chronic stress, coupled with a lack of effective coping mechanisms, can also affect a person's psychological state and lead to depression and anxiety. Chronic stressors persist over a long time and require a person's body to cope on a daily basis. The body's energy stores get depleted faster as well. These physiological effects impair a person's psychological state over time and do not allow them to function normally.

Stress Outcomes

Physiological

The physiological response of the body to stress is often referred to as a **fight-or-flight response**. The stress stimuli cause a chain of chemical and hormonal reactions in the body that will either prepare a person to fight the stressor or flee from the stressor to avoid any harm. The body increases production of both adrenaline and cortisol. **Adrenaline** keeps the body in a state of readiness; it increases a person's heart rate and causes some muscles to tighten. **Cortisol** helps the body return to a normal state after the stressful situation is over. It first helps to increase production of blood sugar to provide the body with extra energy and then helps the blood sugar level return to normal. Cortisol also regulates the acidic/alkaline balance of the body.

Emotional

When a person has appropriate coping resources, small amounts of stress can help motivate them to take action or make a change. The emotional response can be positive and stimulating. Prolonged stress, on the other hand, can take a toll on a person's emotional well-being. The body's hormonal and chemical response to stressors is very fast. When the response lasts too long or becomes too intense, the byproducts of the hormones and chemicals can become sedative-like and cause a person to feel fatigued. The feelings of low self-confidence can often become part of a pattern when the same stressors are encountered repeatedly, which can eventually lead to depression.

Behavioral

Stress affects a person's behavior in two stages: the short-term and the long-term. Following the idea that stressful stimuli cause the body to prepare itself for either fight or flight, in the short-term, the brain starts to automate some habitual behaviors. For example, while under stress, a person may take the milk out of the refrigerator several times after they have already poured themselves a glass. The brain focuses in on preparing the body for the stressful situation. In the long-term, the body may feel the effects of the overproduced stress hormones by being over-stimulated or under-stimulated. Over-stimulation may cause a person to be ill-tempered. It can cause people to grind their teeth or bite their nails and may affect appetite. Under-stimulation may cause a person to feel a loss of energy that inhibits motivation and daily functioning and may lead to a feeling of being burnt out.

Managing Stress

There are many things that people can do to manage the stress that they feel. First, it is important to identify the stressors. Acute stressors are often easier to identify than chronic stressors. Stress is a part of daily life and having appropriate coping mechanisms can help people maintain their healthy physical and emotional well-being. Exercising is a positive way to manage stress. Physical activity releases endorphins that make a person feel good and elevate mood. It helps to distract a person from the stress in their life and reduces tension and frustration. The maximum benefit comes from exercising for at least thirty minutes in order to feel the effects of the endorphins, elevate the heart rate, and relieve stress.

Stress also causes a person's muscles to tighten as part of the fight-or-flight response. Relaxation can help loosen the muscles and relieve stress. Stretching, massages, and getting a good night's sleep can all help to ease the tension in muscles. Deep breathing is also a quick way of relaxing the muscles and getting some relief from stress.

Spirituality is a broader form of stress relief. It includes the development of a personal value system, connecting with oneself, and searching for more meaning in life. While in many cases, spirituality is connected to a religion, it can also be found with a connection to nature, music, or art, among many other things. It helps a person feel a sense of purpose in their community and in the world, which helps can help relieve mental anxiety about smaller stressors in life.

Foundational Concept 7: Biological, psychological, and sociocultural factors influence behavior and behavior change.

Individual Influences on Behavior

Biological Basis of Behavior

As mentioned, the nervous and endocrine systems are the primary physiologic systems involved in behavior.

Neuronal Communication and its Influence on Behavior

Communication between neurons occurs through electrochemical processes and plays a major role in human behavior, as it is the structure of communication throughout the nervous system. This process begins when the dendrites at the end of one neuron receive neurotransmitters into receptor sites, causing the neuron to depolarize and send an electrical charge down the axon to the other end of the neuron. This is called the **action potential** and follows the **all-or-none** principle. A neuron either fires or does not fire; there can be no weak or partial action potential. Neurotransmitters, the chemical messengers of the brain, are then released from the synaptic vesicles within the axon terminal at the end of the neuron into the synaptic gap between the first neuron and the next one.

If enough neurotransmitters bind to receptor sites on the post-synaptic neuron, then the action potential will be set off again and the process will continue to the next neuron. Neuronal communication within the nervous system plays a major role in human behavior as it allows communication from the body to the brain, between different parts of the brain, and from the brain to the rest of the body. The primary way in which neural communication influences behavior is through mood fluctuations, which, in turn, influence a person's behaviors. Certain behaviors will also trigger the release of particular neurotransmitters, such as dopamine, leading to a pleasurable feeling which encouraging the repetition of those behaviors. Although neuronal communication influences behavior, it does not dictate behavior and is only one factor involved in how humans act.

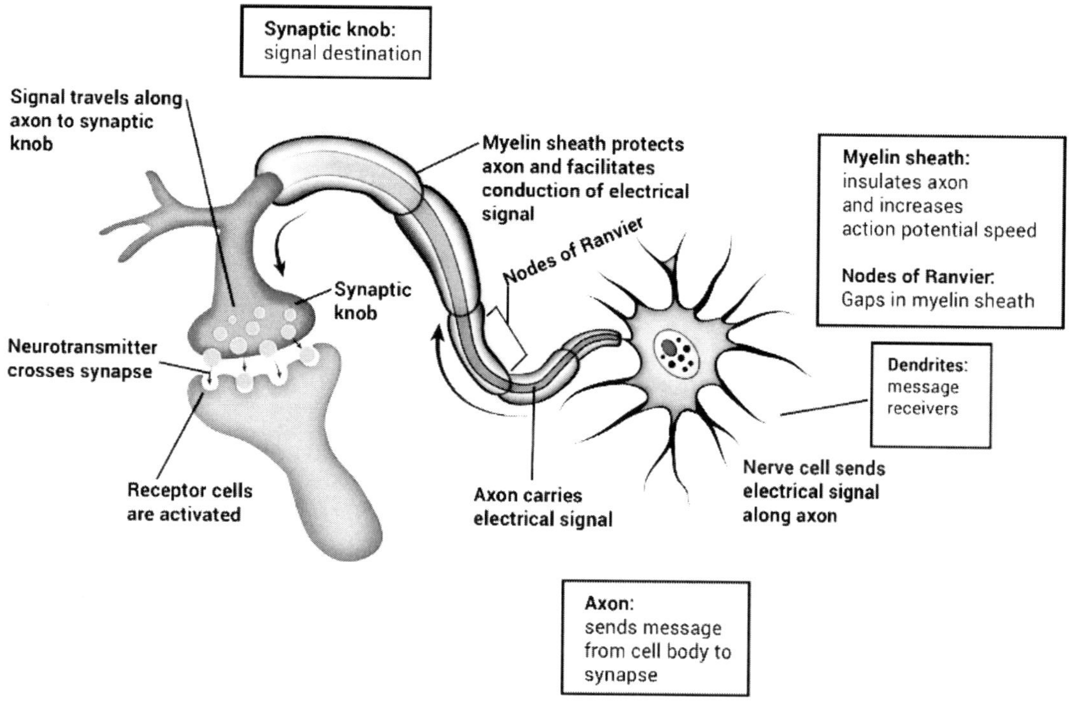

Influence of Neurotransmitters on Behavior

Neurotransmitters are active in the process of communication between neurons. Different types of neurotransmitters are released by various types of cells, and all have an impact on behavior in different ways. Some neurotransmitters, such as norepinephrine and serotonin, can directly impact one's mood. Others have a role in motor movement, such as acetylcholine. Endorphins are a natural painkiller and glutamate is involved in memory. Some neurotransmitters are considered **inhibitory** and others are **excitatory**. The release of more excitatory neurotransmitters is likely to lead to an action potential in the post-synaptic neuron, whereas the release of inhibitory neurotransmitters serves to prevent an action potential. Many mental health medications and treatments for other diseases function by mimicking, blocking, or changing the levels of certain neurotransmitters. Depression, schizophrenia, Alzheimer's, and Parkinson's are just a few examples of conditions or diseases that are directly connected to high or low levels of certain neurotransmitters. Recreational drugs have a similar effect to medications, often increasing or mimicking mood-enhancing neurotransmitters.

Behavioral Genetics

Behavioral genetics is the study of the interplay between environment and genes on human behavior.

Genes, Temperament, and Heredity

Genes, constructed of DNA, are the building blocks of **heredity**, which is the transmission of certain traits from parents to their offspring. Temperament, which consists of the basic and innate components of personality, has been shown to be highly genetic and individual variations can be viewed as early as infancy. A fully-developed personality is influenced by many factors, both genetic and environmental, but certain aspects of personality are inherited from parents.

Adaptive Value of Traits and Behaviors

Traits and behaviors can adapt to new situations or environments. This is true for species-wide traits, as the process of natural selection eliminates traits that are less useful for survival and promotes traits that are more advantageous. However, it can also be true for individuals who may learn new behavioral patterns when necessary for more effective functioning in a new environment.

The Interaction Between Heredity and Environmental Influences

The study of genetics seeks to understand the magnitude of the influence of nature versus nurture, or whether one's biological predispositions or one's environment have the greatest influence on behavior. Adoption and twin studies have been conducted as one way to determine the variations in individual behavior. Twins raised apart share common traits but also maintain certain differences, showing the impact of both heredity and environment. Heredity and environment can be viewed as two sides of the same coin, and always interact with each other in the development of individual differences.

Influence of Genetic and Environmental Factors on the Development of Behaviors

Experience and Behavior

Two people may share the same genetic makeup, such as identical twins, but still have varying personalities and display different behaviors. This is due to the environmental factors and the different experiences each of these people go through. A person's experiences, in addition to genetics, play a major role in shaping behavior.

Regulatory Genes and Behavior

Epigenetics refers to the changes that may occur in the expression or activation of genes, although the overall genetic sequence remains the same. **Gene regulation** is the process by which gene expression is regulated through the production of proteins or RNA. Gene expression can either decrease or increase through gene regulation, and these changes can be passed on to the next generation. These genetic adaptations, which are influenced by environment and individual behaviors, help the individual adjust to new environmental situations, but may also increase the risk of certain diseases or mental illnesses.

Genetically-Based Behavioral Variation in Natural Populations

Populations of both humans and animals share certain behavioral patterns that are a result of genetics. But within populations, there are genetically-based behavioral variations among individuals. These differences can be explained by differences in genetic makeup as well as the social and environmental context, which may cause the expression of certain genes.

Human Physiological Development

Indicators of Normal Physical Growth and Development

It is important to understand normal developmental milestones. While not all children progress at the same rate, one must know some benchmarks to determine if the child has any developmental delays that prevent him or her from reaching goals by a certain age.

Infancy Through Age 5

During the first year of life, abundant changes occur. The child learns basic, but important, skills. The child is learning to manipulate objects, hold their head without support, crawl, and pull up into a standing position. The toddler should be able walk without assistance by 18 months. By age two, the child should be running and able to climb steps one stair at a time. By age three, the child should be curious and full of questions about how the world works or why people behave in certain ways. The child should have the balance and coordination to climb stairs using only one foot per stair. By age four, the child is increasingly independent, demonstrating skills like attending to toilet needs and dressing with some adult assistance.

School Age to Adolescence

By age five, speech is becoming more fluent, and the ability to draw simple figures improves. Dressing without help is achieved. By age six, speech should be fluent and motor skills are strengthened. The youth is now able to navigate playground equipment and kick and throw a ball. Social skills, such as teamwork or friendship development, are evolving. The child must learn to deal with failure or frustration and find ways to be accepted by peers. They become more proficient in reading, math, and writing skills. Towards the end of this phase, around age 12, secondary sexual characteristics, such as darker body hair or breast development may occur.

Adolescence

This is a period of extraordinary change. The process of **individuation** is occurring. The teen views himself or herself as someone who will someday live independently. More time is spent with peers and less with family. Identity formation arises now, and the teen often experiments with different kinds of clothing, music, and hairstyles to see what feels comfortable and what supports their view of the world. Sexuality is explored, and determinations are being made about sexual preferences and orientation. Sexual experimentation is common, and some teens actually form long-term intimate relationships, although others are satisfied to make shorter-term intimate connections. There is sometimes a period of experimentation with drugs or alcohol. As the thinking process matures, there may be a questioning of rules and expectations of those in authority. Moodiness is common, and troubled teens are likely to "act out" their emotions, sometimes in harmful ways.

Human Genetics

The study of human genetics is important in a clinical setting. Many disorders, health problems, and various personality traits are passed from parent to child. Understanding the whole person is a necessary part of being a competent clinician. **Genes** are what carry the information that determines an individual's characteristics. It is well known that physical features, such as hair and eye color, are passed on genetically. Medical doctors know that illnesses, such as diabetes and high blood pressure, run in families.

It is also true that one's genetic background impacts one's psychological make-up. There is a strong genetic link to alcoholism and other addictions. Psychiatric disorders may also be passed on from generation to generation. Persons prone to depression and anxiety often have a parent, grandparent, or other relative who struggles with these issues. Scientific research has only scratched the surface in terms of understanding the role of genetics. It is important to recognize that although people are not enslaved by their genetic makeup, they are influenced by it and may have risk factors that should be considered.

Personality Theories

Sigmund Freud's Psychosexual Stages of Development

Sigmund Freud was an Austrian neurologist who is considered the father of psychoanalysis. Freud developed important concepts in Western psychology such as the id, ego, and superego, and wrote literature focusing on what he called the **unconscious** and the repression and expression that stems from it.

Freud also focused on human development, especially relating to sexuality. Freud theorized that each stage of human development is characterized by a sexual focus on a different bodily area (**erogenous zone**), which can serve as a source of either pleasure or frustration. He believed that **libido** (psychosexual energy) is the determinant of behavior during each of five fixed stages, and that if a developing child experiences frustration during one of these stages, a resulting **fixation** (or lingering focus) on that stage will occur.

To understand Freud's developmental stages fully, one must also understand his conceptualization of the human personality.

Freud describes three levels of the mind as follows:

- **Conscious:** the part of the mind that holds accessible and current thoughts
- **Pre-conscious:** the area that holds thoughts that can be accessed by memory
- **Unconscious:** where the mind motivates behaviors and contains thoughts, feelings, and impulses that are not easily accessible

Freud believed that the personality, or **psyche**, consists of three parts called the **Psychic Apparatus**, each of which develops at a different time.

Id

The **id** is the most basic and primitive part of the human psyche, based on instincts and all of the biological aspects of a person's being. An infant's personality consists only of the id, as the other aspects have not yet developed. The id is entirely unconscious and operates on the pleasure principle, seeking immediate gratification of every urge. It has two instincts: a death instinct called **thanatos** and a survival instinct called **eros**. The energy from eros is called the **libido.**

Ego

The **ego** is the second personality component that begins to develop over the first few years of life. The ego is responsible for meeting the needs of id in a socially-acceptable, realistic manner. Unlike the id, the ego operates on the reality principle, which allows it to consider pros and cons, to have awareness that other people have feelings, and to delay gratification when necessary.

Superego

The **superego** is the final personality component, developed by about age five. The superego is essentially a person's internal moral system or sense of right and wrong. The superego suppresses the instincts and urges of the id, but also attempts to convince the ego to act idealistically, rather than realistically.

In a healthy personality, there is balance between the three personality components. The individual has **ego strength**—the ability to function well in the world despite the conflicting pressures that the id and superego place upon the ego.

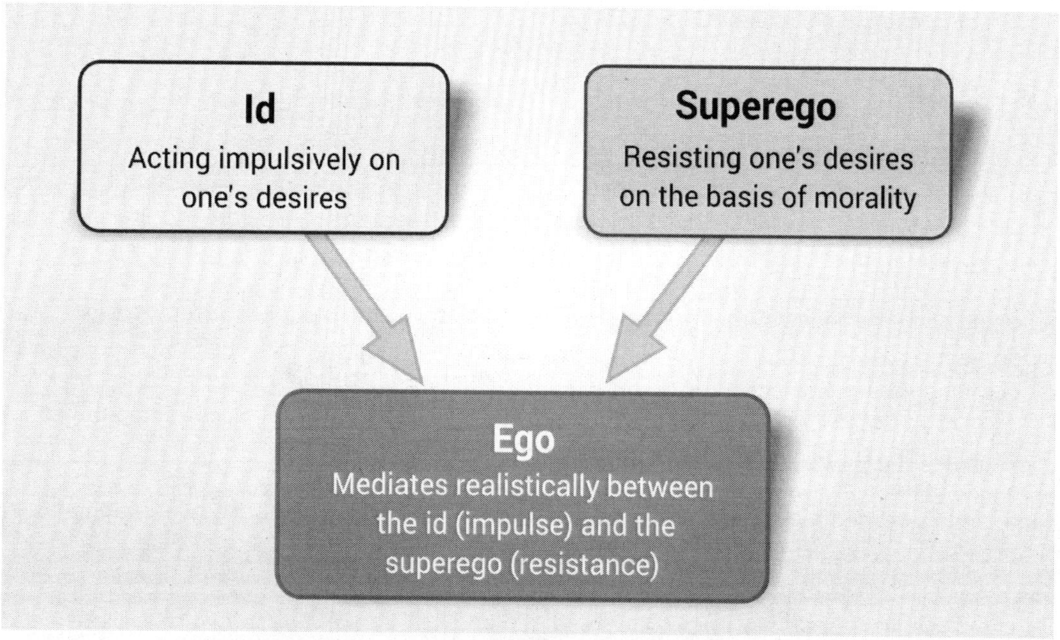

Five Stages of Psychosexual Development

Oral Stage (Birth to Eighteen Months): The infant satisfies its libido by feeding and by exploring the environment, primarily by putting objects in its mouth. The id dominates the oral stage of development, and every action an infant undertakes is guided by the pleasure principle. The key task of this phase is weaning from the breast, which also results in the infant's first experience of loss. Too much or too little focus on oral gratification at this stage was theorized to lead to an oral fixation and an immature personality. Examples of an oral fixation were believed to be excessive eating, drinking, or smoking.

Anal Stage (Eighteen Months to Three Years): The key task of this stage is toilet training, which causes a conflict between the id (which wants immediate gratification of the urge to eliminate waste) and the ego (which requires delay of gratification necessary to use the toilet). A positive experience with toilet training was believed to lead to a sense of competence that continues into adulthood. Anal-retentive personality results from overly-strict toilet training, characterized by rigid and obsessive thinking. Likewise, anal-expulsive personality results from a lax approach to toilet training, characterized by disorganization and messiness.

Phallic Stage (Three to Six Years): The libidinal focus during this stage is on the genital area, and it is during this stage that children learn to differentiate between males and females. The **Oedipus Complex** develops during this stage; Freud believed that a young boy views his father as a rival for his mother's attention and the boy may want to eliminate his father in order to take his place. Similar to the Oedipus Complex, the **Electra Complex** says that a young girl may view her mother as her rival. Freud also believed that girls experience penis envy. The key task of this stage is identification with the same-sex parent.

Latency (Six years to Puberty): During this period, libidinal energy is still present, but the child is able to direct that energy toward school, friendships, and activities.

Genital Stage (Puberty to Adulthood): The libidinal focus is once again on the genital area (as it is during the phallic stage), but at this point, the psyche is more developed. During the genital stage, an individual achieves sexual maturation, becomes independent of their parents, resolves any remaining conflict from the earlier stages, and is able to function as a responsible adult in terms of both work and relationships.

Carl Jung's Psychoanalytic Theory

Jung's theory is similar to Freud's psychoanalytic theory, with differences related to the purpose of the libido, the unconscious, and behavioral motives. Libido is a psychic energy that motivates individuals.

Jung theorized two parts to the unconscious:

- **Personal unconscious:** contains information not accessible to the conscious mind
- **Collective unconscious** (transpersonal): the memories from a person's ancestors that the individual has from birth

Jung identified this collective unconscious into four main archetypes.

- **Persona:** the artificial self that individuals show to the world to hide who they really are
- **Anima/Animas:** the masculine qualities that women express to society and the feminine qualities that men express to society
- **Shadow:** similar to Freud's id, signifies raw needs and desires
- **Self:** the unconscious and conscious mind come together to form a unified whole; occurs as a consequence of individuation

Object Relations Theory

Object Relations Theory was developed as an offshoot of Freud's theory. Melanie Klein is the person most closely associated with Object Relations Theory. In this theory, **object** typically refers to a person; thus, the theory is concerned with relationships between people, and it particularly emphasizes the relationship between the mother and child. A basic idea is that all people are driven to develop relationships with others, and failure in early interpersonal relationships causes later dysfunction.

- External object: a person, thing, or place
- Internal object: one's idea or mental representation of an actual object

Developmental Theories

Erikson's Psychosocial Stages of Development

Erikson proposed a lifespan theory of psychosocial development as an alternative to Freud's psychosexual stages. According to Erikson's epigenetic principle of maturation, human beings pass through eight developmental stages, each of which builds upon the preceding stages and sets the groundwork for the stages that follow.

Erikson's Psychosocial Stages of Development

Stage	Age	Psychosocial Crisis	Basic Virtue
1	Infancy (0 to 1½)	Trust vs. mistrust	Hope
2	Early Childhood (1½ to 3)	Autonomy vs. shame	Will
3	Play Age (3 to 5)	Initiative vs. guilt	Purpose
4	School Age (5 to 12)	Industry vs. inferiority	Competency
5	Adolescence (12 to 18)	Ego identity vs.role confusion	Fidelity
6	Young Adult (18 to 40)	Intimacy vs. isolation	Love
7	Adult hood (40 to 65)	Generativity vs. stagnation	Care
8	Maturity (65+)	Ego integrity vs. despair	Wisdom

All eight stages are present at birth, but remain latent until both an innate schedule and an individual's cultural upbringing cause a stage to begin to unfold.

An individual does not have to "master" a stage to proceed to the next stage, and the outcome of a particular stage may later be changed by an individual's life experiences. As with Freud's theory, Erikson proposed that each stage of development is characterized by a crisis; however, for Erikson, the crisis involves a conflict between the needs of the developing individual and the needs of society. Successfully mastering a stage and its psychosocial crisis leads to the development of a healthy personality and possession of basic virtues.

Erikson's theory centers around the development of ego, or a sense of self that is acquired by interacting with the social environment.

Psychosocial Stages

The first stage is **Trust vs. Mistrust**. This stage is centered in infancy (birth to eighteen months). An infant with consistent and stable care will develop a sense of trust that extends beyond the primary caregiver and is necessary for feeling secure in the world and in future relationships. An infant who does not develop trust becomes fearful and sees the world as an unsafe, unpredictable place. Mastery of this stage results in the virtue of **hope.**

The second stage is **Autonomy vs. Shame and Doubt**. This stage occurs during early childhood (eighteen months to three years). The focus of this stage is development of personal control, as the stage typically occurs when young children are beginning to gain motor control, explore the physical environment, and satisfy some of their own basic needs (e.g., by starting to dress themselves, eat independently, and use the toilet). Mastery results in a sense of autonomy; however, if a child's caregiver has expectations that are too high, restricts a toddler's independence, or belittles the child, shame and doubt may develop instead. The virtue acquired during this stage is **will**.

The third stage is **Initiative vs. Guilt.** This stage occurs in the preschool/play age (three to five years). Through play, being active, and planning activities, children in this stage begin taking risks and initiating tasks for specific reasons. Initiative is developed when adults support children's exploration and assist them in making good choices for themselves. Lack of support during this phase may instead cause the child to experience guilt related to their wants and needs. The virtue resulting from this stage is **purpose**.

The fourth stage is **Industry vs. Inferiority**. This stage occurs during childhood/school age (five to twelve years). During this stage, teachers and peers play a much larger role in a child's life and social interactions. As cognitive ability increases, children are able to understand more complex concepts, acquire skills such as reading and writing, and begin to form their own opinions and values. Per Erikson's theory, the early school years are essential to a child's sense of self-confidence. If children are encouraged and praised, they learn to take pride in accomplishments and to display industrious, goal-oriented behavior. If they experience discouragement, ridicule, or lack of opportunities for success, they may doubt their own abilities and develop feelings of inferiority. The virtue associated with this stage is **competence.**

The fifth stage is **Identity vs. Role Confusion** (or **Diffusion**). This stage occurs in adolescence (twelve to eighteen years). During the adolescent phase, as their bodies are rapidly maturing, children exert greater independence, often exhibit rebellious behavior, and begin to develop a sense of who they are as human beings. Establishment of ego is the crucial task of this developmental stage. If adolescents successfully navigate this stage, they emerge with a sense of self, an understanding of who they want to be, and comfort within their sex role. On the other hand, adolescents who are unable to find a solid sense of self and their place in the society around them may instead experience role confusion. The virtue associated with this stage is **fidelity** (being able to show one's true self to others and to relate to them in a genuine and sincere manner).

The sixth stage is **Intimacy vs. Isolation**. This stage occurs during young adulthood (eighteen to forty years). During this stage, young adults explore relationships and learn to commit to others beyond their immediate family. Erikson proposed that successful ego development during adolescence was crucial in order for adults to develop intimate relationships with others successfully during this subsequent stage. The virtue resulting from this stage is **love.**

The seventh stage is **Generativity vs. Stagnation**. This stage occurs in adulthood (forty to sixty-five years). During this stage, individuals turn their focus to family, careers, contributing to the world around them, and guiding the next generation. The virtue resulting from mastery of this stage is **care**.

The eighth stage is **Integrity vs. Despair**. This stage occurs during maturity (sixty-five years or older). Older adulthood is a time of existential reflection. Erikson proposed that looking back upon accomplishments and finding meaning in one's life results in satisfaction and ego integrity. Alternatively, those who are dissatisfied with their past may experience despair and regret. The virtue associated with this stage is **wisdom**.

Piaget's Theory of Cognitive Development

Piaget was the first to systematically study cognitive development. He believed children have a basic cognitive structure and continually restructure cognitive frameworks over time through maturation and experiences.

Key terms in this theory:

- **Schema:** introduced by Piaget, a concept or a mental framework that allows a person to understand and organize new information
- **Assimilation:** the way in which an individual understands and incorporates new information into their pre-existing cognitive framework (schema)
- **Accommodation:** in contrast to assimilation, involves altering one's pre-existing cognitive framework in order to adjust to new information
- **Equilibrium:** occurs when a child can successfully assimilate new information
- **Disequilibrium:** occurs when a child cannot successfully assimilate new information
- **Equilibration:** the mechanism that ensures equilibrium takes place

Piaget also recognized and defined the following *four stages of cognitive development*:

Stage 1: Sensorimotor Stage (birth to age 2)

- The infant becomes aware of being an entity separate from the environment.
- Object permanence occurs as the baby realizes that people or objects still exist, even if they are out of sight. Object permanence builds a sense of security as the baby learns that though mommy has left the room, she will still return. This reduces fear of abandonment and increases their confidence about the environment.

Stage 2: Pre-operational Stage (age 2 to age 7)

- The child moves from being barely verbal to using language to describe people, places, and things.
- The child remains egocentric and unable to clearly understand the viewpoint of others.
- The process of quantifying and qualifying emerges, and the child can sort, categorize, and analyze in a rough, unpolished form.

Stage 3: Concrete Operational Stage (age 7 to age 11)

- The ability to problem-solve and reach logical conclusions evolves.
- By age 10 or 11, children begin to doubt magical stories, such as the Tooth Fairy or the Easter Bunny.
- Previously-held beliefs are questioned.

Stage 4: Formal Operational Stage (age 12 through remaining lifetime)

- More complex processes can now be assimilated.
- Egocentrism diminishes.
- One assimilates and accommodates beliefs that others have needs and feelings too.

- New schemas are created.
- The individual seeks their niche in life in terms of talents, goals, and preferences.

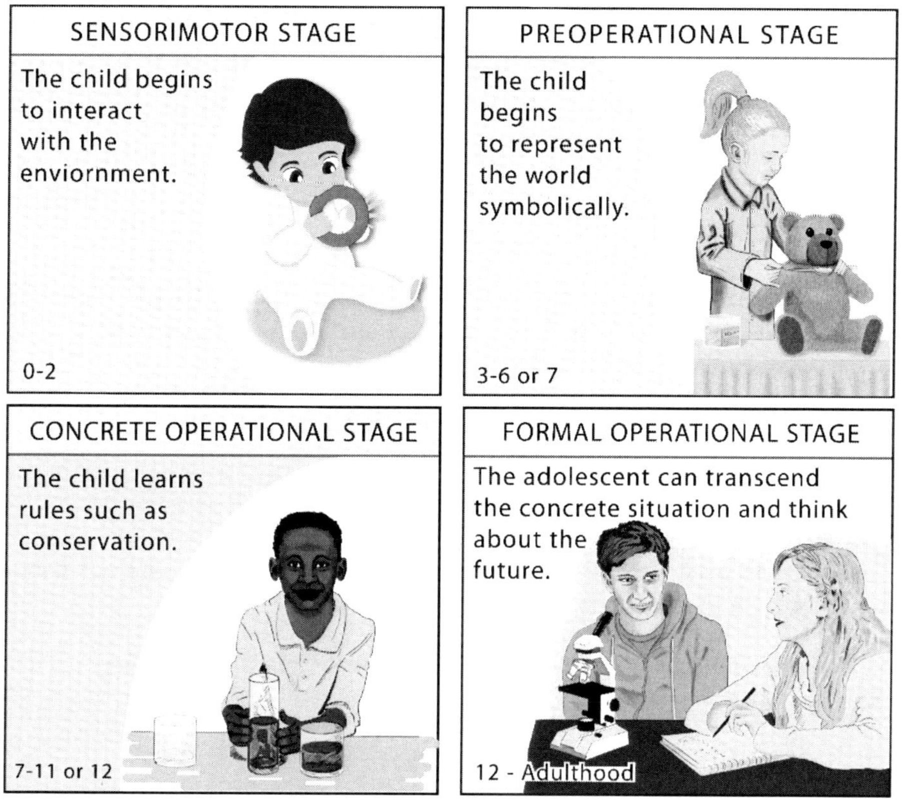

Gesell

American pediatrician and psychologist Arnold Gesell (1880–1961) conducted longitudinal observational studies over fifty years to produce several theories regarding human development. His **maturationist theory** states that beginning at the fetal stage, individuals will follow set, linear steps of physical and cognitive development. Gesell argued that human development is primarily governed by an individual's genetic makeup. External influences, such as society, parents, siblings, and teachers, are most effective when their actions support the physiological progress that will take place.

Personality Theories

There are several noted theories as to how personality is formed. In 400 B.C.E., Hippocrates attempted to identify personalities based on four temperaments. He called these **humors**, and these were associated with body fluid presence, such as phlegm or bile.

In the 1940s, William Sheldon came up with his body type theories that included the **endomorph**—an overweight individual, with an easy-going personality; the **mesomorph**—a muscular person, with an aggressive personality; and the **ectomorph**—a thin individual, with an artistic or intellectual personality.

Gordon Allport developed the trait theory of personality development. He believed that certain personalities were comprised of clusters of traits and that these traits could be categorized into cardinal, central, and secondary traits.

As mentioned, Freud believed the personality was composed of the id, the ego and superego. The **id** refers to a person's unconscious, with its suppressed desires and unresolved conflicts, whereas the **ego** and **superego** are more influenced by the conscious mind. He believed that these three components were often in conflict with one another and that how one resolved these conflicts determined personality. He also stressed the importance of childhood experience in personality development.

Carl Rogers was a proponent of the **humanistic theory** of personality development. This approach emphasized self-perception and a desire for striving to become the best person one can become. His theory was based on the basic goodness and potential of each person.

The behavioral theories of B.F. Skinner and others related to personality development imply that one's persona is developed as a result of classical or operant conditioning. Reinforcement and punishment guide behavioral choices.

Holland's Theory and Hexagon

Holland developed a theory in which personality was the basic factor in career choice. He created the **Vocational Preference Inventory** and **Self-Directed Search (SDS)** to assess traits and match them with specific occupations. He believed that individuals want careers with like-minded others of similar personalities. Most individuals fall into at least one of six personality types, depicted by a hexagon, which shows the correlation between jobs and personality traits.

Holland's Six Personality Types

Realistic types enjoy working with their hands: building, fixing, assembling, and operating tools and equipment. People with these personalities can enjoy working outdoors. Occupations of interest include engineer, mechanic, pilot, electrician, computer technologist, sportsperson, and park ranger.

Investigative types enjoy problem-solving, research, and discovery. People with these personalities like to observe, investigate, and experiment. Investigative individuals have excellent analytical, communication, and calculation skills. They can be best suited for careers in science, which include medical, health, and research occupations.

Artistic types express themselves through art, music, drama, and creative design. They enjoy performing, singing, dancing, planning, and presenting. Occupations of interest include artist, illustrator, fashion designer, photographer, and musician.

Social types like working with people. These personalities enjoy meeting new people, teaching, training, and coaching. They are skilled at treating others (as in a health setting) as well as providing care and support. Careers of interest can include athletic trainer, nurse, counselor, social worker, and dental hygienist.

Enterprising types like to meet people and enjoy working in business. They like talking, leading people, influencing, and encouraging others. People with these personalities are skilled at organizing, planning, developing, selling, promoting, and persuading. Careers of interest include lawyer, accountant, promoter, entrepreneur, manager, and business owner.

Conventional types like working with data and numbers. They enjoy accuracy, organization, and clear procedures. Conventional types are skilled at tasks that require orientation to detail. They excel at recordkeeping, handling money, working independently, and organization. Occupations of interest include librarian, office worker, bank clerk, and computer operator.

Psychological Disorders

Understanding Psychological Disorders

Psychological disorders can be difficult to define because they are based on determining what qualifies as normal or abnormal behavior. Psychological disorders are characterized by behaviors that are not only abnormal, but are maladaptive, distressing to the individual and disruptive to daily functioning.

Biomedical Versus Biopsychosocial Approaches

There are many theoretical approaches to viewing the etiology and treatment of psychological disorders. Some are more medically-focused, identifying psychological disorders as diseases that have physical causes and can be treated exclusively through medicine and in hospitals. The focus is on brain functioning, neurotransmitters, genetic factors, and other aspects of biology. Other approaches are more comprehensive, viewing psychological disorders as the combined result of biological, psychological, and social factors. These biopsychosocial approaches consider environmental factors, such as the influence of family and school, or psychological factors, such as a person's coping style.

Classifying Psychological Disorders

Psychological disorders are classified using the *Diagnostic and Statistical Manual of Mental Disorders, 5th Edition (DSM-V)*. Within this manual, the various disorders are listed, and the diagnostic criteria are provided. The DSM is periodically updated to integrate new research findings, and the newest edition was released in May, 2013. The DSM-5 includes several broad categories of psychological disorders, including mood disorders, dissociative disorders, anxiety disorders, and personality disorders.

Rates of Psychological Disorders

In the United States, approximately 20-25% of the adult population struggles with some type of mental disorder in a given year. The rate of serious psychological disorders is less, at roughly 4-8%. The United States has a high rate of mental disorders compared to other countries. Anxiety disorders are the most common type of psychological disorder, followed by mood disorders.

Types of Psychological Disorders

Anxiety Disorders

Anxiety disorders are characterized by persistent worry, anxiety, or fear. They may also include maladaptive patterns of behavior that are intended to reduce the fear or anxiety. This category of disorders includes generalized anxiety disorder, post-traumatic stress disorder (PTSD), specific phobias, panic disorder, and obsessive-compulsive disorder.

Obsessive–Compulsive Disorder

Obsessive-compulsive disorder is a specific type of anxiety disorder that consists of obsessive and recurring thoughts, and compulsive behaviors that are meant to reduce the stress related to the obsessive thoughts. For example, a person who has persistent thoughts related to cleanliness may engage in compulsive behaviors that would reduce the risk of germs, such as repetitive washing of hands.

Trauma- and Stressor-Related Disorders

Trauma related disorders, most notably PTSD, develop in reaction to stressful and traumatic experiences that a person has endured. For example, rape or a natural disaster can lead to a trauma-related disorder. These disorders involve fear responses to triggers, anxiety and depression, insomnia, hyper-arousal, etc.

Somatic Symptom and Related Disorders

Somatic symptom disorders are psychological disorders that manifest with physical symptoms even though there is no identifiable physical cause for the symptom. Conversion disorder and illness anxiety disorder (formerly **hypochondriasis**) are two examples of somatic symptom disorders.

Bipolar and Related Disorders

Bipolar disorder (formerly **manic-depressive disorder**) is considered a mood disorder and involves a mood that fluctuates between depression and mania or hypomania. The length and severity of the cycles of elevated mood and depressed mood vary from person to person. **Cyclothymia** is a related disorder in which a person experiences a fluctuation between minor depression (**dysthymia**) and mild mania (**hypomania**). Children who experience this fluctuating mood are diagnosed with disruptive mood dysregulation disorder rather than bipolar disorder.

Depressive Disorders

Major depressive disorder (MDD) is characterized by a depressed, sad, or hopeless mood. Some other symptoms are changes in sleep and appetite patterns, lethargy, decreased interest in previously-enjoyed activities, and suicidal ideation. These symptoms must persist for at least two weeks to receive a diagnosis of MDD. Persistent depressive disorder or dysthymia is another depressive disorder. It is a milder form of depression than MDD and persists for at least two years.

Schizophrenia

Schizophrenia is one of the more genetically-determined psychological disorders and usually involves psychotic symptoms such as hallucinations and delusions, in which a person loses touch with reality. Auditory or visual **hallucinations** are when a person perceives something that is not there. **Delusions** are false beliefs, such as a delusion of grandeur in which a person believes they are the president of the United States. Odd or disorganized speech and catatonia are other symptoms of schizophrenia.

Dissociative Disorders

Dissociative disorders are a controversial category of disorders, characterized by dissociation or detachment within a person's consciousness. The most well-known and debated dissociative disorder is **dissociative identity disorder** (formerly **multiple personality disorder**). A person with dissociative identity disorder (DID) can develop two or more distinct personalities. These personalities may have different names, genders, ages, and behaviors. Dissociative disorders also include a fugue state and depersonalization disorder.

Personality Disorders

Personality disorders are characterized by maladaptive and enduring patterns of social functioning and interactions, including manipulative or lying behaviors, social avoidance, or anti-social behavior. Some common personality disorders are narcissistic personality disorder, anti-social personality disorder, borderline personality disorder, and histrionic personality disorder.

Biological Bases of Nervous System Disorders

Schizophrenia

Schizophrenia has a strong genetic component, with a correlation between high levels of dopamine and schizophrenia. Anti-psychotic medications used in the treatment of schizophrenia serve to decrease the levels of dopamine, but also have the risk of causing tardive dyskinesia or Parkinson's disease, which are both associated with low levels of dopamine. Schizophrenia has also been shown to have a high genetic predisposition, with biological family members of those with schizophrenia being more likely to develop the disorder.

Depression

Mood disorders, including depression, are connected to levels of neurotransmitters in the brain. Specifically, serotonin, norepinephrine, and dopamine levels can affect a person's mood. Although not as strong as in schizophrenia, research indicates that there is a genetic predisposition to depression.

Alzheimer's Disease

Alzheimer's is the most common form of dementia and is associated with a deficit in the neurotransmitter acetylcholine. Alzheimer's is a progressive disease of the brain that is caused by the development of plaques and tangles, both parts of proteins, in and around nerve cells. Early-onset Alzheimer's is strongly genetic and inherited from parents. Late-onset Alzheimer's is most likely the result of a combination of genetic and environmental factors.

Parkinson's Disease

Parkinson's disease is associated with low levels of dopamine, so it is often treated with medications that will increase the levels of dopamine in the brain. However, an unfortunate side effect of these medications may be the development of some schizophrenia-related psychotic symptoms. There is also a genetic predisposition to Parkinson's.

Stem Cell-Based Therapy to Regenerate Neurons in the Central Nervous System

Stem cells have been discovered to have a reparative value within the nervous system because of their self-renewal properties. Much research has been conducted related to the implantation of stem cells within the brains of those suffering from different diseases in order to regenerate deteriorating cells. Stem cell-based therapy is used in treatment of degenerative diseases of the nervous system, such as Alzheimer's and Parkinson's disease.

Motivation

Factors that Influence Motivation

Motivation, a psychological construct, is the direction and intensity of an individual's effort. There are several forms of motivation including intrinsic and extrinsic motivation, achievement motivation, and motivation associated with skill development. It should be noted that individuals generally experience more than one type of motivation, and these can vary depending on the activity being performed, perceptions of competency, the level of importance the individual places on the activity, in addition to other factors.

Intrinsic Motivation

Intrinsic motivation is an individual's internal desire for their behavior to be competent and self-determined. It originates from the person's love and interest in the activity and personal satisfaction (i.e., inherent reward) in performing it. Intrinsic motivation is generally considered the best form of motivation. Intrinsic motivation can help one maintain focus on achieving short-term goals that require consistent effort.

Extrinsic Motivation

Extrinsic motivation, used extensively in sports and careers, comes from external sources (e.g., coaches, teammates, managers) in the form of individualized rewards such as praise from coaches and supervisors, bonuses or raises, social acceptance, avoidance of punishment, and the desire for positive reinforcement.

Achievement Motivation

Achievement motivation reflects an individual's effort to master a specific task, achieve excellence, perform better than others, and overcome obstacles. There are two types of achievement motivation. The **motive to achieve success** (MAS) is characterized by a desire to challenge and evaluate one's ability and be proud of accomplishments. People with greater MAS like challenging situations, where the likelihood of success or failure is approximately the same. The **motive to avoid failure** (MAF) is characterized by the desire to avoid being perceived as a failure, preserve one's ego and self-confidence, and minimize shame. People with greater MAF prefer either easy situations where they will likely succeed and avoid shame or difficult situations where success is unlikely and feelings of shame are minimized. In the athletic arena, athletes with high levels of achievement motivation are more competitive and generally perform better than athletes with lower levels of achievement motivation.

Theories that Explain How Motivation Affects Human Behavior

Abraham Maslow is the most notable researcher in the area of basic human needs. **Maslow's Hierarchy of Needs** (1943, "A Theory of Human Motivation") is a theory typically depicted as a pyramid, with the most fundamental needs forming the base. Maslow proposed that people are motivated to meet their most basic needs before turning their attention to the fulfillment of more advanced needs.

Maslow theorized that human needs could be described in the form of a pyramid, with the base of the pyramid representing the most basic needs and the higher layers representing loftier goals and needs. Unless the basic needs are met, a person cannot move on to higher needs. For example, a homeless woman living under a bridge will need food, shelter, and safety before she can consider dealing with her alcoholism. The foundational layer in Maslow's hierarchy is physiological needs, and the final layer at the pinnacle of the pyramid is self-transcendence.

Maslow's Hierarchy of Needs

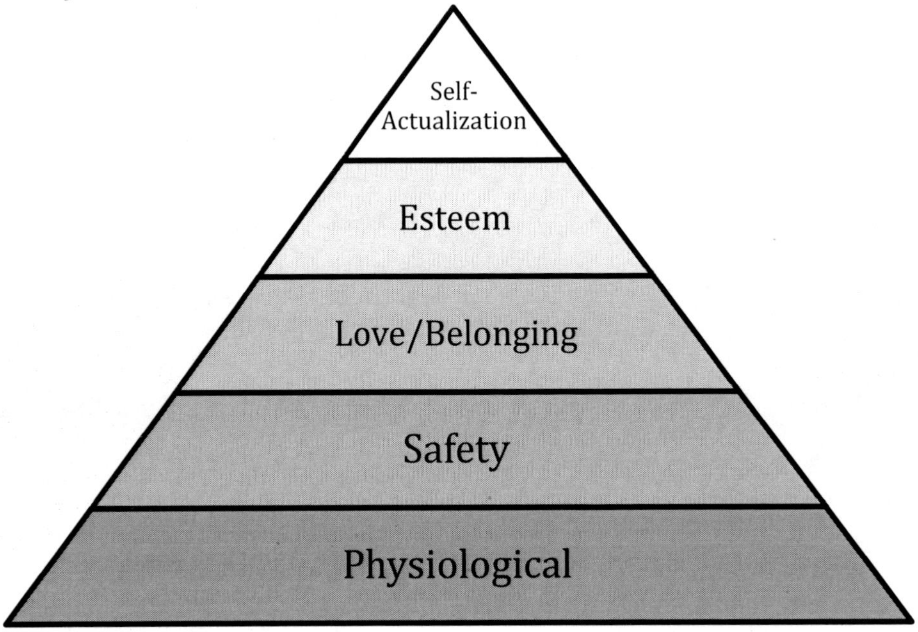

Physiological Needs: These needs must be met first and pertain to what humans need to survive. These include basics, such as food, water, clothing, and housing.

Safety Needs: Once primary needs are met, the person may now focus on safety issues, including safety from abuse and neglect, natural disaster, or war.

Love and Belonging: Once the first levels of needs have been satisfied, people are next driven to find a sense of acceptance and belonging within social groups, such as family, community, or religious organizations. Maslow suggests that humans have a basic need for love, affection, and sexual intimacy. Failure to achieve this level can lead to difficulty in forming and maintaining close relationships with others.

Esteem: The need for esteem is driven by a desire for recognition, respect, and acceptance within a social context.

Self-Actualization: The U.S. Army slogan, "Be All You Can Be," expresses this layer of need. Reaching one's highest potential is the focus. According to Maslow, this cannot be achieved until all the other needs are mastered.

Self-Transcendence: This level was devised by Maslow in his later years because he felt that self-actualization did not completely satisfy his image of a person reaching their highest potential. To achieve self-transcendence, one must commit to a goal that is outside of oneself, such as practicing altruism or finding a deeper level of spirituality.

Biological and Sociocultural Motivators that Regulate Behavior

Some human motivators are more biologically based and others are more strongly influenced by sociocultural factors, although biology and environment play a role in both. Biological factors involved in hunger motivation include the lateral and ventromedial areas of the hypothalamus, metabolic rate, and glucose levels. However, hunger is also influenced by social factors such as body perception and cultural customs around food. Sex drive, though powerfully influenced by the biology of hormones such as testosterone and progesterone, is also motivated by social constructs and social norms for sexual behavior. Substance addiction includes both biological and sociocultural motivation, as it impacts a person physically, psychologically, and socially.

Attitudes

Components of Attitudes

Cognition refers to a person's thought patterns, beliefs, and ideas. The affective component has to do with feelings or emotions. The behavioral element relates to a person's actions, which are usually the direct result of one's attitude. The three components of attitude are interconnected and influence each other.

The Link Between Attitudes and Behavior

Processes by Which Behavior Influences Attitudes

The **foot-in-door phenomenon** refers to when someone influences another person to do a greater behavior or action, by first getting them to agree to a small step. If someone has loaned a friend $5, the loaner may later be willing to increase the loan to $20. The first action, though small, leads to an attitude that allows for a greater action. Role-playing is another behavior that can powerfully influence attitudes. Philip Zimbardo's prison experiment, in which students were asked to role-play guards and prisoners, is a classic example of the power of role-playing. The participants' attitudes were so influenced by their roles that they began to act in dangerous and extreme ways.

Processes by Which Attitudes Influence Behavior

The attitudes people have toward other people, situations, or things will strongly influence their behaviors. Attribution theory asserts that people attribute someone's behavior either to their disposition or their situation. This will then influence actions toward that person. Icek Ajzen's **theory of planned behavior** (TPB) states that a combination of perceived behavioral control, attitudes, and normative beliefs work together to influence behavior.

Cognitive Dissonance Theory

Cognitive dissonance theory states that when a person holds two conflicting beliefs, or acts in a way that is inconsistent with their beliefs, the person will experience tension or dissonance. In an effort to reduce this tension, the person will act to reduce this tension by changing their attitudes or actions.

Social Processes that Influence Human Behavior

How the Presence of Others Affects Individual Behavior

There are many ways in which a social context can influence individual behavior, either positively or negatively. **Social psychology** looks at the person-environment interaction and explores the many ways the social setting influences a person's attitudes and actions.

Attitudes toward, and influenced by, those around play a major role in a person's behaviors. **Attribution theory** has to do with how one views the behavior of others, whether attributing their behaviors to disposition or situation. If one wrongly attributes someone's negative action to their disposition—the **fundamental attribution error**—then one may think more negatively about others than is deserved.

The concept of **conformity**—the tendency for a person to conform personal behaviors to the behaviors of those around him or her—helps explain everything from style trends to mass genocide. Solomon Asch performed a study which showed that people tend to conform to the people around them, even if it means giving an answer that they know is false. The phenomenon of conformity stems from the idea that people act in a way to get approval from others and to avoid disapproval, called **normative social influence**. Another impact of the social sphere that people live in is **deindividuation**, in which a person loses a sense of personal responsibility or individualism. This may happen in crowds at a concert or sports event, or a riot, leading people to behave in ways they would not normally behave if they did not feel anonymous and emotionally-charged by the social setting.

People tend to automatically form groups, often developing the in-group and out-group. The **in-group** consists of those who are part of the group, who share its identity and unifying characteristics. The **out-group** consists of those outside the group, particularly those who may be in opposition or share opposite beliefs to those in the in-group. This in-group and out-group concept may lead to patriotism or working together towards a common goal, but it may also lead to prejudice and discrimination.

Some other key concepts related to the effects of social context on behavior are social loafing and social facilitation. **Social loafing** happens in a context of shared responsibility for a task. In this case, there is a tendency for some people to abdicate responsibility, assuming that others will fulfill the obligations of the work. **Social facilitation**, on the other hand, is when having an audience inspires people to perform tasks they do well even better. Alternatively, it can also cause them to do worse in tasks they find more difficult or challenging.

Group Decision-Making Processes

Group Polarization

Group polarization refers to the phenomenon that when a people gather with others who hold similar beliefs, they will become stronger in their shared beliefs. When the majority of the group either opposes or supports a particular idea, they are more likely to make a more extreme decision than they would do as an individual.

Groupthink

Groupthink occurs when people in a group are unwilling to express ideas in opposition to everyone else, due to a desire to maintain harmony. This results in the group making a unanimous decision even though some people may secretly disagree. Negatively, groupthink can prevent all the options from being fully and reasonably explored which may lead to poor decision-making.

Normative and Non-Normative Behavior

Social Norms

Social norms are the unspoken expectations of behavior in a culture or society. Norms may be established through formal laws and regulations but are often unofficially assumed. Social norms are the underlying structure of every society and are necessary to the smooth and cohesive functioning of a group of people.

Sanctions

Sanctions are a form of behavioral reinforcement used to encourage conformity to social norms. They can be mild or severe, depending on how norms have been violated. Many sanctions are informal, whether verbal praise of a particular behavior or shaming when someone does not conform. But formal legal sanctions may also be used in extreme cases where there is a deviation from social norms. Formal and informal sanctions may be implemented by peers, parents, police, teachers, or others.

Folkways, Mores, and Taboos

Folkways are simply everyday customs that are common to a particular population or society. They are the daily habits and behaviors of a culture, such as shaking someone's hand upon being introduced to them. **Mores**, by nature, have a moral emphasis behind them; these behaviors are considered either right or wrong and are often established through religion. Lying or cheating, for example, are considered morally unacceptable in many cultures. Those who engage in mores will usually receive informal sanctions from others, being shamed or ostracized in some way. **Taboos** are actions that are so strongly forbidden by the culture that a person is universally rejected or ostracized from the group because of the behavior. An example of this may be incest or pedophilia.

Anomie

Emile Durkheim developed the term **anomie**, which refers to a mismatch between individual needs, norms or morals, and the expectations of the society. When there is a breakdown of values or norms, there is a de-integration of individuals and the social structure. This can result when social norms fail to evolve and grow with the changing population and the needs of the individual people. Social norms then serve to frustrate or hinder people from reaching their goals. People, instead of being led by appropriate and moral norms of society are left to create and pursue their own norms, which can result in individualism and isolation.

Deviance Perspectives

Deviance is a behavior that violates or dramatically departs from social norms. Some behavior is considered deviant in a particular context while being perfectly normal in another setting or group. The **differential association** perspective of deviance states that deviant behavior is learned and that people who engage in deviance have adopted it through observing others. **Labeling theory** looks at the power of labels and how those with social power or influence can assign the label of deviant to certain behaviors. Those who are labeled in a certain way may either change their behaviors in order to conform to social norms or they may embrace those behaviors more fully as their identity. Finally, the **strain theory** puts the blame on the social system or structure. One major way this plays out is when society has certain expected goals of individuals but does not provide the means by which people can achieve those goals. As a result of this strain, people may resort to deviant behavior, such as criminal activity.

Aspects of Collective Behavior

Collective behavior occurs when groups of people share in the same activity under special circumstances. One obvious example of collective behavior is **fads**, which are short-lived popular trends in behavior, speech, or clothing. **Mass hysteria** results when something happens that causes a widespread and irrational fear among people. The universal panic can result in mass responses that can be as dangerous as the threat that caused the hysteria. **Riots** are when a group of people engage in a spontaneous emotional reaction, often involving violence. Riots are very often in protest of something perceived as negative, but they can also occur spontaneously in joyful reaction to a positive outcome or event.

Socialization

Agents of Socialization

Social development begins right from birth as a child learns to attach to their mother and other caregivers. During adolescence, social development focuses on peer relationships and self-identity. In adulthood, social relationships are also important, but the goal is to establish secure and long-term relationships with family and friends.

Another important contributor to social development, are social institutions, such as family, church, and school, which assist people in realizing their full potential. Lev Vygotsky was a pioneer in this field with his concept of cultural mediation. This theory emphasizes that one's feelings, thoughts, and behaviors are significantly influenced by those in their environment.

Attitude and Behavior Change

Habituation and Dishabituation

When a person or animal shows a decreased response to a stimulus over time, it is considered habituation. Something that may at first provoke a response will, after time and repeated exposure to the stimulus, cease to yield the same response. A person who moves to a new city with lots of traffic may at first have trouble sleeping but will after time adjust to the new stimulus and resume old patterns of sleep. **Dishabituation** occurs when there is again an increase in responsiveness to the same stimulus as prior to the habituation. This happens when a similar and stronger stimulus is presented and then the old stimulus is presented again. A person who has adjusted to the noise of traffic in a new house may experience dishabituation if one night many emergency vehicles with sirens drive by. The sound of normal traffic again may then disrupt sleep patterns.

Associative Learning

Ivan Pavlov (Classical Conditioning)

Another important concept of development has to do with learning and the way in which humans learn new behaviors. A famous psychologist, Ivan Pavlov, conducted research with dogs that proved to be ground-breaking in the field of classical conditioning. In his experiment, a ringing bell was paired with the presentation of food, which produced salivation in the dog. The ringing sound eventually produced salivation from the dog even in the absence of food. Salivation then became the conditioned response to hearing a bell, and thus, the theory of classical conditioning was developed. The important finding of this research is that humans learn by association.

B.F. Skinner (Operant Conditioning)

Skinner also did important research in the field of learning, specifically **operant conditioning**. Operant conditioning theory focuses on behavioral changes that can be seen or measured. The basic concept is that behavior that is reinforced will increase and behavior that is punished will decrease. There are several key concepts integral to an understanding of this form of learning:

- **Positive Reinforcement:** Anything that serves as a form of reward, including food, money, praise, or attention
- **Negative reinforcement:** An unpleasant stimulus that is removed when behavior is elicited, such as a man finally cutting the grass to stop his wife from nagging him about it
- **Punishment:** An unpleasant response from the environment—e.g., a slap, an unkind word, or a speeding ticket—that, when encountered, increases the likelihood that a behavior will cease. Two problems arise with using punishment. Once the negative stimulus is removed, the behavior is likely to continue. Punishment can also cause humiliation, anger, resentment, and aggression.
- **Superstition:** An incorrect perception that one stimulus is connected to another. Skinner found that when teaching a rat to press a lever for food, if the rat chases its tail before pressing the lever, it will mistakenly believe that the tail chase is required and will do both behaviors each time it wants food.
- **Shaping:** The process of changing behavior gradually by rewarding approximations of the desired behavior (for example, first rewarding a rat for moving closer to the lever).

Skinner found that there are different schedules of reinforcement and that some work better than others. These include the following:

- **Continuous rate:** Person or animal is rewarded every time a behavior is demonstrated
- **Fixed ratio:** Reward is given after a fixed number of attempts
- **Variable ratio:** Reward is forthcoming at unpredictable rates, like a slot machine
- **Fixed interval:** Reward is given only after a specific length of time has passed
- **Variable interval:** Reward is given after an unpredictable amount of time has passed
- **Extinction:** Occurs when a behavior disappears or is extinguished because it is no longer being reinforced. To stop tantrum behavior in toddlers, ignoring the behavior will decrease or stop the tantrum if the desired reward is parental attention or parental aggravation.

Observational Learning

Observational learning takes place when someone's behaviors are adjusted or changed in response to watching someone else.

Modeling

Modeling happens when behaviors are displayed by one person and imitated by another. This most powerfully shows itself in the case of children, who emulate the behaviors of adults or their peers. Modeling was clearly displayed in Albert Bandura's Bobo Doll Experiment. Children who observed adults acting violently toward a blow-up doll were more likely to act violently in the same way.

Biological Processes that Affect Observational Learning

Mirror Neurons

Mirror neurons are a specific type of neuron in the frontal and parietal lobes of the brain that are involved in imitating the behavior of others and in feeling what others are feeling. First observed in monkeys, mirror neurons fire both when observing someone else perform a behavior and when engaging in that behavior oneself. These neurons help explain observational learning and the capacity for imitation, as well as the phenomenon of empathy.

Role of the Brain in Experiencing Vicarious Emotions

Vicarious emotions are an aspect of empathy, in which people feel the same emotions another person is experiencing. When one observes someone else in a particular situation, it stimulates the parts of the brain that would activate the emotions that a person would feel if they were in that situation themselves.

Applications of Observational Learning to Explain Individual Behavior

Children, in particular, learn to adopt the behaviors that they observe around them. Thus, the modeling set by parents and others will impact how they speak and act toward others, their work ethic, their levels of aggression, and countless other areas. Observational learning also impacts the individual behaviors of adults. For example, the kinds of television programs and movies that people watch will influence their behaviors.

Theories of Attitude and Behavior Change

Elaboration Likelihood Model

The **elaboration likelihood model** seeks to explain attitude changes that lead to behavioral changes and decision-making. These changes happen primarily through persuasion. A person engaged in the central route to persuasion will assess the true characteristics of a thing or the actual issues being debated. The peripheral route to persuasion, on the other hand, relies on secondary and superficial means rather than the actual issues. For example, someone may be persuaded to purchase a particular item because it was advertised by a famous or attractive person, rather than because on the quality of the item itself. When there is high cognitive engagement, or elaboration, there is a higher chance that the central route to persuasion will be utilized, which typically leads to more long-term and enduring changes in attitude.

Social Cognitive Theory

The **social cognitive theory**, popularized by Albert Bandura, looks at the interaction between the person, environment, and behaviors. The 'person' refers to individual characteristics and traits, especially cognition or thinking processes. Although they are not constantly equal in influence, each of the three are all continually present and have an impact on each other, which Bandura referred to as **reciprocal determinism**. This theory plays out in an aspect of observational learning that proposes that people not only learn through their own behaviors but from watching other people's actions and observing the consequences they face.

Factors that Affect Attitude Change

Just as attitude can influence behavior, behavioral change can influence attitude change. For instance, the action of smiling can encourage the feeling of happiness. The action of role playing can create attitudes in line with the role being played. Secondly, when those presenting a particular message are considered more attractive, knowledgeable in their field, or trustworthy, it is more likely that the listener will accept the speaker's message and change their attitude. Finally, social factors can affect attitude change. Attitudes are formed and altered by observing others and people tend to conform to the beliefs of their peers and society.

Foundational Concept 8: Psychological, sociocultural, and biological factors influence the way we think about ourselves and others, as well as how we interact with others.

Self-identity

Self-Concept, Self-identity, and Social Identity

The Role of Self-esteem, Self-efficacy, and Locus of Control in Self-concept and Self-identity

Self-esteem is the feeling of personal value or worth, and **self-efficacy** is an individual's feeling of competence in accomplishing a task. Someone who has strong self-esteem and self-efficacy will be proactive and confident, both socially and vocationally. Having an internal locus of control vs. external locus of control also plays a role in one's identity. An **internal locus of control** is when someone has the perception that he or she has control over their environment. An **external locus of control** is when someone believes that their future and life are controlled by factors outside of himself or herself. Those with an internal locus of control have a stronger self-concept and self-identity, leading to superior achievement, greater emotional stability, and more individual responsibility for behaviors.

Different Types of Identities

Identity is best understood as a person's view of self, which may include the many different aspects of race, gender, age, sexual orientation, and class. **Race** typically denotes distinctive physical characteristics, such as skin color, while **ethnicity** encompasses all of a person's cultural traditions and background. **Gender** refers to a person's subjective experience of being male or female. **Sexual orientation** has to do with sexual attraction, and includes those who identify as homosexual, heterosexual, asexual, or bisexual. Chronological and felt age, as well as economic class, can contribute significantly to one's identity. All aspects of identity are influenced by social factors and issues of discrimination and prejudice based on specific identity characteristics.

The Impact of Culture, Race, and Ethnicity on Self-image

Culture, race, and ethnicity can greatly impact one's self-image, whether one is part of a privileged population or of a minority or disenfranchised population. One's ethnic and racial background provides a sense of belonging and identity. Depending on a country's treatment of a particular group, self-image can be negatively impacted through racism and discrimination. Non-whites are more likely to be arrested than whites and often receive harsher sentences for similar offenses. Racial jokes and racial slurs are common. Stereotypes abound, and some people judge entire racial groups based on the behavior of a few. Such treatment consistently impacts the self-esteem of those in minority groups. As children become aware of the environment and the culture in which they live, they inevitably notice a lack of prominent non-white politicians, entertainers, CEOs, and multi-millionaires. Non-white Americans who grew up in the fifties or earlier were denied access to restaurants, theaters, high schools, professions, universities, and recreational activities. Even within the last fifty to sixty years, African Americans who had achieved great status in the fields of music, sports, and entertainment were still denied access to certain clubs, hotels, or restaurants.

Every person must explore and come to terms with their own culture, ethnicity, and race. Sometimes, this even means rejecting cultural aspects with which he or she disagrees and embracing new and evolving cultural norms. This is a significant part of self-identity development for teenagers and young adults, as they are part of a new generation that may be culturally different from their parents. Those that have more exposure to other cultures and backgrounds likely will have a more open perspective and will be better able to evaluate their own culture and ethnicity objectively.

Cultural, Racial, and Ethnic Identity Development

Race refers to biologically distinct populations within the human species. **Ethnicity** is a cultural term referring to the common customs, language, and heritage of a category of people. **Ethnic identity** is the identification with a particular group of people who share one's culture and heritage.

William Cross's Stages of Identity Development

The following lists William Cross's Stages of Identity Development for people of color:

Pre-Encounter

Unless prompted to do so, children do not critically evaluate the race-related messages that they receive from the world around them.

Encounter

Often experienced in early adolescence, the individual has one or more experiences that are related to race. Although it is possible for the experiences to be positive, this is often when an individual first experiences racism or discrimination and begins to understand the personal impact of their race.

Immersion-Emersion

After experiencing a race-related incident, the individual strongly identifies with their racial group and may seek out information about history and culture.

Internalization

Racial identity is solidified, and the individual experiences a sense of security in identifying with their race.

Internalization-Commitment

Racial identity is taken one step further into activism pertaining to issues related to the experiences of the individual's racial group.

Sue & Sue's Stages of Racial/Cultural Identity Development

The following lists Stages of Racial/Cultural Identity Development:

Conformity

The individual displays a distinct preference for the dominant culture and holds negative views of their own racial and/or cultural groups. He or she may also experience shame or embarrassment.

Dissonance

The individual undergoes a period of re-thinking or challenging their beliefs. For the first time, the individual examines and appreciates positive aspects of their own racial/cultural group.

Resistance and Immersion

The individual shows preference for minority views and actively rejects the views of the dominant culture, experiencing pride about and connection to their racial or cultural group.

Introspection

The individual becomes aware of the negative impact of the resistance and immersion stage and may realize that he or she does not actually disagree with all majority views or endorse all minority views.

Integrative Awareness

The individual is able to appreciate both their own culture and differing cultures.

Gender

Gender identity is a person's understanding of their own gender, especially as it relates to being male or female. **Sexual orientation** is a more complex concept as it refers to the sexual attraction one feels toward others.

Types of Gender Identity

- **Bi-gender:** An individual who fluctuates between the self-image of traditionally male and female stereotypes and identifies with both genders.
- **Transgender:** A generalized term referring to a variety of sexual identities that do not fit under more traditional categories; a person who feels to be of a different gender than the one he or she is born with.
- **Transsexual:** A person who identifies emotionally and psychologically, and sometimes physically, with the gender other than that assigned at birth; lives as a person of the opposite gender

Those who are transgender or transsexual may be homosexual, heterosexual, or asexual. Sexual identity and sexual attraction are independent.

Impact of Sexual Orientation and/or Gender on Self-Image

Self-Image corresponds to how one views one's self based upon reactions from others. Everyone goes through a process of determining their own identity and figuring out who they are, a process that can be more complicated for those who are not heterosexual. The impact of sexual orientation depends greatly upon one's cultural experiences. **Coming out**—sharing one's sexual orientation with others—can be gratifying or demoralizing. Everything depends on the importance of the relationship and response from those who are given this information. When a person is embraced by loved ones following the disclosure, this can positively impact self-image. If the opposite occurs, the impact is generally negative. There are multiple factors involved in the process of coming out.

Here are some example situations that may negatively impact self-image:

- Location: It is often easier to "come out" to friends and family in San Francisco, for example, than in a small town in Kentucky.
- Religious Issues: If friends and family members belong to a highly conservative religious organization, there may be negative impact on self-image, depending on the extent to which that group embraces diversity and equality.
- Peers: There may be a negative impact on self-image from one's peer group, especially in adolescence, depending on the group's ability to embrace the individual and their sexual orientation.

- Family Values: A narrow-minded and judgmental family can have a negative impact on self-image, as opposed to a positive impact from an open and accepting family dynamic.
- Setting: A university campus in Berkley, California will likely be more supportive than a small religious college in the Deep South.

Other factors include the individual's access to people who have a similar sexual preference and are comfortable with their sexuality. Sometimes rejection by parents or other significant persons can be counterbalanced with the support of like-minded individuals who can provide understanding, guidance, and acceptance. When the individual feels that their lifestyle is seen as a viable one, self-image will be enhanced. When the person feels unloved or judged, self-image will likely be negative.

Formation of Identity

Identity Development

Identity includes **self-concept** and **self-esteem**. Self-concept is the beliefs one holds about one's self. Self-esteem is how one feels about one's self-concept.

The physical changes of adolescence can have a strong influence on an adolescent's self-esteem. Adolescents also incorporate comments from others, particularly parents and friends, into their identity.

Adolescents also undergo important emotional development and begin to hone the skills that are necessary for stress management and effective relationships with others. Some of the skills necessary for stress management are recognizing and managing one's own emotions, developing empathy for others, learning appropriate and constructive methods of managing conflict, and learning to work cooperatively rather than competitively.

A normal part of adolescence is a yearning for independence. Health professionals can help parents understand that the desire for independence is healthy and age-appropriate. They can educate both parents and adolescents about the importance of positive peer relationships during this time. Peer groups help adolescents learn about the world outside of their families and identify how they differ from their parents. Adolescents who are accepted by their peers and who have positive peer relationships may have better psychosocial outcomes in both adolescence and adulthood.

An increase in conflict with parents is normal during adolescence and seems to be most prevalent between girls and mothers. Parents may need reassurance that this conflict does not represent rejection, but rather a normal striving for independence.

Some theories seek to explain the prevalence of risk-taking behaviors among adolescents. One theory of risk-taking behavior explains that the need for excitement and sensation-seeking outweighs any potential dangers that may come from sensation-seeking. Another theory says that risk-taking often occurs within groups as a way to gain status and acceptance among peers. Additionally, adolescents who engage in risk-taking behavior may be modeling adult behavior that has been romanticized.

There are many ways in which professionals and guardians can provide guidance to young people with regard to their risk-taking behavior. They should become comfortable discussing uncomfortable topics, so that adolescents can safely talk about their decision-making and peer pressure. Additionally, it is wise to steer adolescents toward healthy outlets that channel their talents or get them involved in positive activities.

Adolescent resilience and positive outcomes are associated with these factors:

- Having a stable and positive relationship with at least one involved and caring adult (e.g., parent, coach, teacher, family member, community member)
- Developing a sense of self-meaning, often through a church or spiritual outlet

- Attending a school that has high, but realistic, expectations and supports its students
- Living in a warm and nurturing home
- Having adequate ability to manage stress

Social Thinking

Attributing Behavior to Persons or Situations

Attributional Processes

Attribution theory states that people attribute the behavior they observe in others either to their situation or their disposition, or unchanging qualities. The fundamental attribution error happens when someone mistakenly attributes observed behavior to someone's disposition rather than their situation. There are also cultural variations when it comes to attribution styles. Western cultures that are more individualistic tend to attribute behaviors to a person's disposition. On the other hand, some collectivist Asian cultures are more likely to consider situational factors in behavior attribution.

How Self-Perception Shapes the Perception of Others

Self-perception shapes the way people view others and interpret their behaviors. Individuals tend to believe that other people are more similar to them than they are in reality. Additionally, if someone has a weak perception of self or low self-esteem, he or she may perceive others to be more attractive or more successful.

How Perceptions of the Environment Shapes Perceptions of Others

Environment and social context shape perceptions of how someone acts, speaks, or dresses. Something that would be perceived as normal and appropriate in a particular environment may not be perceived in the same way in a different environment, such as wearing a bathing suit to the grocery store. Additionally, a positive or comfortable environment may cause others to be viewed more positively, whereas a negative environment may have the opposite effect.

Prejudice and Bias

Prejudice and Various "-isms"

Prejudice—the perceived opinions and beliefs that cause someone to feel or act in a negative manner toward a particular group—can present itself in several forms:

- **Anti-Semitism:** prejudice against the Jewish religion and culture
- **Racism:** prejudice against a particular race
- **Sexism:** prejudice against one or the other sex
- **Ageism:** prejudice against someone based on age, either young or old
- **Classism:** prejudice against someone based on their socio-economic class
- **Ableism:** prejudice against someone with disabilities or handicaps
- **Homophobia:** prejudice against the gay and lesbian community
- **Transphobia:** prejudice against the transgender community
- **Nationalism:** prejudice against non-natives in a specific country

Prejudice may also present itself as discrimination against someone due to immigration status, national origin, religion, or weight.

Processes that Contribute to Prejudice

Prejudice is most often a negative belief about others that is based on pre-judging with limited information and faulty assumptions. Unfortunately, prejudice can, and is, shown toward people due to their race, gender, sexual orientation, religion, and many other factors.

Power, Prestige, and Class

Some common contributors to prejudice have to do with a person's position, reputation, or economic status. Those with more political or personal **power** may be prejudiced against those who are perceived as weaker. **Prestige** has to do with a person's position or job, which can contribute to prejudice against those in less prestigious positions. Finally, a person's **class** or socioeconomic status can serve as a trigger for prejudice against those in lower socioeconomic positions.

The Role of Emotion in Prejudice

People tend to show prejudice toward those whom they feel certain emotions, such as disgust, pity, or envy. These emotions are felt toward those who are part of various outgroups, whereas positive emotions are felt toward those who are in the same group or category as oneself.

The Role of Cognition in Prejudice

The human brain, in processing and retrieving memories, tends to categorize information about others. These mental groupings can lead to oversimplified categorizations and reduce complex human beings to specific labels or characteristics. **Belief perseverance**—the tendency to persist in one's beliefs no matter what the contrary evidence may be—can lead people to hold onto the faulty ideas they have developed about certain groups or types of people.

Stereotypes

Stereotypes are the labeling or categorizing of people based on fixed ideas about the group to which they belong, thus leading to assumptions about others based solely on their group membership. These generalizations can lead to prejudice and discrimination.

Stigma

Stigma has the connotation of a mark or blot, and is a strong societal aversion to someone, or disapproval of them, based on a particular characteristic or circumstance. Those who are stigmatized will feel shame and disgrace because of the social censure they experience. Those suffering from mental illness and those who identify as homosexual are two groups that have historically been stigmatized, although many other examples exist.

Ethnocentrism vs. Cultural Relativism

Ethnocentrism is the tendency to view one's own ethnicity more positively than other ethnicities, and to view everything about one's own culture as better than other cultures. On the other hand, **cultural relativism** views each culture as being equally valid and good, although different from each other.

Processes Related to Stereotypes

Self-Fulfilling Prophecy

Self-fulfilling prophecies are beliefs or expectations someone has about a person, which cause them to act in a certain way toward that person, thus eliciting the very behavior they expect of them. This has been clearly observed in experiments conducted with school teachers and children, where the teachers were given faulty expectations about students, either that they were more or less intelligent than they actually were. The students' performances reflected the expectations of their teachers, because the teachers treated the students according to the expectations they had of them.

Stereotype Threat

A **stereotype threat** occurs when there is a negative stereotype against a particular group, and a member of that group experiences anxiety about fulfilling the stereotype. Their performance will suffer, due to the anxiety of conforming to the stereotype, even though there is no legitimate reason for a poorer performance.

Social Interactions

Elements of Social Interaction

Status

Status is the position that someone has within a group or society and how they fit into the social structure. **Achieved status**, good or bad, covers everything that a person earns or acquires in their life through their own efforts and choices, whether financial, vocational, or educational positions. **Ascribed status** is what a person obtains by no individual choice or effort, including race or socioeconomic status inherited at birth.

Role

Roles usually play out within a status, as a person who has a particular status is expected to play a certain role. **Social role theory** emphasizes the fact that people's behaviors are motivated by the role that person has in society. The societal expectations for that particular role have a strong influence on how someone carries out the responsibilities of the role.

Role Conflict and Role Strain

Each person plays multiple roles and there can either be strain within one role or conflict between the responsibilities of different roles. There may be a conflict between the parenting role and professional role if a working parent wants to attend a child's school performance but needs to be at the office. A nurse might struggle with role strain if he or she wants to spend quality time with each patient, but in order to meet the needs of everyone on their caseload, the nurse is forced to decrease individual time with patients.

Role Exit

Role exit occurs when someone leaves a role that has been central to their identity, in order to take on a new role or identity. Many students at the end of college will leave that role to move on to a new role in the work force.

Groups

Primary and Secondary Groups

Everyone is a part of many groups, which simply consist of two or more people who join together for a specific purpose or because of a shared characteristic. **Primary groups** are the relationships that are long-lasting, personal, and close-knit, such as family or friends. **Secondary groups** are temporary and built on more superficial reasons. These may be study or work groups that get together to accomplish a particular task and then disperse after the task is accomplished.

In-Group and Out-Group

Those considered to be part of the in-group are the ones who share a common identity that joins them. Anyone without the same shared characteristics (such as race or religion) as those in the in-group is considered different and part of the out-group.

Group Size

Social groups can be any size, as long as there are at least two people. **Dyads** are groups made up of only two people, such as a marriage or a pair of study partners. Adding another person to the group creates a **triad**, a group of three. Group size strongly impacts the dynamics of the group, whether there are two people or more than one hundred.

Networks

Networks consist of people or organizations that are connected or tied to each other. They differ in size, strength, and purpose.

Organizations

Formal Organizations

Formal organizations are professional social structures that aim to provide a particular service or achieve a certain goal. The relationships of those connected through formal organizations are not usually personal or long-term.

Bureaucracy

A **bureaucracy** is a group of people that make decisions in government but are not elected representatives.

Characteristics of an Ideal Bureaucracy

Max Weber is known for developing a set of ideal principles for a bureaucracy, with an emphasis on efficiency and rationalism. First, the ideal bureaucracy has a clear, well-defined distribution of labor. There is also a hierarchy, with those higher up making decisions and supervising those directly below them. Formal selection of participants is used to ensure that people are selected and promoted based on objective qualifications, rather than on preference or personality.

Perspectives on Bureaucracy

McDonaldization is a term used to refer to a society that has taken on the characteristics of a fast food restaurant, like efficiency and predictability. McDonaldization in a society can also have side effects, like substituting quantity for quality. The iron law of oligarchy states that all governments and organizations will inevitably shift in the direction of an oligarchy, where a government or group is controlled by a small group of powerful or elite people.

Self-Presentation and Interactions with Others

Expressing and Detecting Emotion

The Role of Gender in the Expression and Detection of Emotion

Several studies that have been conducted related to gender and emotion have found that women are better at reading emotions, consider themselves more open to emotions, experience more empathy, and interpret emotional events with more brain activity than men. Anger is the only emotion that people assume to be more masculine. The notion that women express and detect emotion more than men may be influenced by societal expectations around men and women.

The Role of Culture in the Expression and Detection of Emotion

At least six emotions are universally, cross-culturally recognized—anger, fear, surprise, happiness, disgust, and sadness. However, other more complex emotions, such as pride or jealousy, are less universally-detected. There are significant cultural variations in how these more complex emotions reveal themselves, as well as how freely people express emotions and what causes certain emotions.

Presentation of Self

Impression Management

Impression management is the way people shape how others perceive them or their priorities. Impression management involves verbal communication as well as clothing choices and actions conducted in front of others.

Front Stage vs. Back Stage Self

According to the **dramaturgical approach**, human behavior and social interactions are viewed as actors performing on a stage. Front stage self involves the behavior that is intended for public display, or for an audience. Back stage behavior is what a person engages in when they have no audience.

Verbal and Nonverbal Communication

Verbal communication consists of the words that people use when interacting with others. Nonverbal communication includes body language, gestures, tone of voice, and facial expressions. It is usually possible for people to understand the emotions and feelings of other expressed through nonverbal cues.

Animal Signals and Communication

Communication between animals takes place through a variety of verbal, tactile, auditory, and even chemical signals. The signals can serve as warnings to other animals, play a role in courtship, or signal bonding and affection. For example, the bark of a dog, scent of a skunk, raised fur of a cat, or grooming behavior of monkeys all send different messages.

Social Behavior

Attraction

Attraction occurs when someone is drawn toward others for friendship or romantic love. Familiarity, which often comes through close proximity, contributes to attraction, since people tend to like the things with which they are familiar. Similarity is another determiner of attraction; those who are more alike tend to be drawn to each other and have a liking that lasts. Finally, physical attractiveness, often influenced by social or cultural norms, plays a role in the attraction people feel toward each other.

Aggression

Aggression can be verbal or physical and is intended to harm or destroy someone or something. Many factors contribute to aggressive behavior. Biologically, high levels of testosterone are associated with aggressive behaviors, and aggression is more common in men. Environmental contributors include modeling and observational learning, as illustrated in the Bobo Doll experiment. Another contributor is the frustration-aggression principle that posits that people will act out in anger and aggression if they are thwarted in achieving a goal.

Attachment

Attachment is an emotional bond that a child develops with a primary caregiver and is crucially important during the early months or years of life. If a child establishes an avoidant, disorganized, or anxious attachment rather than a secure attachment with the caregiver, it will impact the child's emotional stability and function, as well as future relationships.

Altruism

Altruism refers to the social phenomenon of people showing an unselfish care or concern for the needs of others. There is conflict about whether pure altruism actually exists among humans, as there is nearly always some type of subtle or intrinsic reward that comes from seemingly selfless behaviors. Either way, acting on behalf of others at the risk or inconvenience to oneself has a positive impact on a person emotionally and physically.

Social Support

Having social support is important for people of all ages and contributes to greater overall health and happiness. Social support can consist of family or friends, and includes the financial, physical, emotional, and psychological care they provide.

Biological Explanations of Social Behavior in Animals

Foraging Behavior

Although sometimes foraging for food is done as a solitary activity, at other times, animals will do this in groups to obtain the greatest amount of energy for the least effort.

Mating Behavior and Mate Choice

Mating among animal partners for the purpose of reproduction may be an uncomplicated event or involve exotic mating rituals. Sometimes there is competition among those of the same sex to gain the rights to sexually reproduce with the chosen mate. Mating behavior among animals may be polygamous or monogamous, short-term or long-term.

Applying Game Theory

Game theory views animals as different players in a game, making strategic decisions based on a cost-benefit analysis. This means that sometimes animals will choose strategies other than competition, such as cooperation or altruism, if it ultimately assists survival.

Altruism

Altruism, acting to help another even at risk to oneself, will be chosen by animals over competition if it is seen to have the greater benefit. For example, an altruistic act toward one member of the species may be done if it contributes toward the greater strength of the group, thus ultimately benefiting the individual who is a member of that group.

Inclusive Fitness

Related to altruism is **inclusive fitness**, which proposes that organisms in different species will not only seek their own benefit directly, but also the benefit of those with whom they share similar genes. This promotes successful reproduction and the passing on of common traits.

Discrimination

Individual vs. Institutional Discrimination

Discrimination is the unfair or unequal treatment of a person or group based upon a characteristic, such as race, ethnicity, religion, age, sex, or sexual orientation. There are several forms of discrimination:

Direct discrimination refers to unfair treatment based on someone's characteristics. An example would be refusing to hire someone because of their ethnicity.

Indirect discrimination refers to situations in which a policy applies the same to everyone, but a person or group of people are negatively impacted due to certain characteristics. For example, a company might require that everyone help unload shipments that come to the office. The policy is the same for everyone, but it's discriminatory towards any disabled employees. In a workplace environment, indirect discrimination can sometimes be allowed if there's a compelling reason for the requirement. For example, firefighters have to meet certain physical criteria due to the nature of their work.

Another form of discrimination is **harassment**. This involves unwanted bullying or humiliation intentionally directed to a person of minority status. **Secondary victimization** refers to the unfair treatment received when a person reports discrimination and is not supported by authorities.

Effects on the individual:

- Depression, anxiety, and other mental health issues
- Medical/health-related problems caused by lack of access to health resources

Effects on society:

- Diminished resources (e.g., employment, educational opportunities, healthcare)
- A culture characterized by fear, anger, or apathy

Systemic (Institutionalized) Discrimination

Systemic (institutionalized) discrimination refers to discrimination taking place within a society or other institution (e.g., a religion or educational system).

- Such discrimination can be either intentional or unintentional and results from the majority of people within the institution holding stereotypical beliefs and engaging in discriminatory practices.
- Systemic discrimination is often reflected in the laws, policies, or practices of the institution.
- Systemic discrimination creates or maintains a disadvantage to a group of people by way of patterns of behavior; it can have wide-reaching effects within a region, profession, or specific institution.

Examples:

- Hiring practices that create barriers or result in lower wages for certain groups
- U.S. Supreme Court case, Plessy vs. Ferguson (1896) – "separate but equal" public facilities for African-Americans
- Oppression of women in certain countries (e.g., being unable to vote, obtain education, or hold jobs)

The Effects of Discrimination Based on Sexual Orientation and/or Gender

While more individuals feel it is safe to come out to family, friends, and employers, there are still vocations in which gays and lesbians choose not to disclose their sexuality, fearing that doing so will invite discrimination in some form. These include professions such as teaching, childcare, politics, and medicine.

Within the lesbian-gay-bisexual-transgender (LGBT) community, discrimination is common, with this group reporting ten times more discrimination based on sexual orientation than heterosexuals. One of the most detrimental forms of discrimination is parental rejection of teenagers. One study reported that 30% of LGBT teens experience a physical abuse from parents when they come out to them and 26% report being kicked out of their house. This explains, in part, why 40% of homeless youth are members of the LGBT community.

In addition, LGBT youth have a higher incidence of being bullied at school, with 85% of these teens reporting at least one incident of peer harassment within the last school year. Almost 20% of these youths have been victims of assault while at school. Gay adults in the workforce often experience discrimination. In one study, researchers sent out two identical resumes with one exception: one indicated college participation in a neutral organization and the other indicated participation in an LGBT advocacy program. Those with affiliations to a LGBT group were 40% less likely to be called for an interview.

Discrimination based upon gender has existed for centuries and can be seen in multiple cultures across the world. In many nations, women—either by law or religious custom—are relegated as subordinates. This is clearly exemplified in those cultures where women are forbidden to drive, choose their own attire, or file for divorce. In China, where, until recently, laws mandated that couples raise only one child, infant girls have been killed or left on orphanage steps.

In more developed countries, such as the U.S., women continue to experience discrimination. Women are more likely to experience sexual harassment in the workplace, and women continue to struggle to secure or maintain jobs if they are pregnant, despite laws to protect them. Outside of the workplace, women are far more likely to be sexually assaulted or become the victims of domestic violence than men. Girls and young women are also at far greater risk of sexual trafficking than are males. One form of gender discrimination experienced by males is related to child custody. Women have a greater chance of receiving custody in legal battles over children than men, even if the father is as responsible and upstanding as the mother.

These multiple forms of discrimination lead to depression, anxiety, anger, and poor self-esteem. When these emotions are experienced, there may be an increased use of drugs, alcohol, or other addictive behaviors. Additionally, there is a higher rate of attempted suicide amongst the LGBT population than those who are heterosexual. For LGBT adults who have experienced family rejection, the likelihood of a depressive disorder is six times greater than those not rejected by family. This group is also eight times more likely to attempt suicide than persons who have not experienced family rejection. Lastly, being the victim of a violent hate crime has a greater impact on self-image and mood than being victimized for similar crimes that are not based on sexual orientation or other differences. LGBT victims of hate crimes report a sense of depression, anxiety, and anger that lingers for an average of four years longer than those harmed for other reasons.

The Effects of Discrimination Based on Age or Disability

Age discrimination refers to a process of differential treatment of older adults based on age-related stereotypes. People sometimes assume that an older person is incompetent, inflexible, and unable to assume the same responsibilities of younger persons. Age bias can cause older persons to feel depressed, anxious, or unworthy. This may, in turn, exacerbate the symptoms of physical illness that the elderly person already endures. Economic problems may emerge if the older person is refused interviews or promotions in the workplace. Overall, these victims of ageism have a discouraged attitude. They may lack the desire to pursue romantic relationships, climb economic ladders, or identify themselves as being able to positively contribute to society.

Discrimination against the physically and/or mentally disabled members of society is common. The physically disabled face many obstacles. They are frequently bullied, have difficulty finding gratifying or decent paying employment, and have limited choices regarding accessible housing and public transportation. There are still many buildings that have not been made handicap accessible. Numerous physically disabled persons feel that they are misunderstood and that others judge them as intellectually impaired, when, in fact, they are not.

The mentally ill and developmentally-delayed populations also face a myriad of barriers. These persons are often the brunt of jokes or harassment. This group is sometimes viewed as violent or unpredictable, and although some violent crimes are committed by members of this group, these individuals are far more likely to be the victims of violence rather than perpetrators.

Foundational Concept 9: Cultural and social differences influence well-being.

Understanding Social Structure

Theoretical Approaches

Microsociology vs. Macrosociology

Many sociological perspectives differ in their scope of analysis. Functionalists and conflict theorists, for instance, gravitate toward a more macro-level orientation in their analyses: these sociologists tend to examine large-scale social patterns with a broad focus on the ways in which specific social structures affect the whole (and vice versa). Symbolic interactionists, however, gravitate toward a micro-level orientation in their analyses: instead of focusing on the "big picture," they tend to focus on a "street level," studying the individual, household, or neighborhood. These micro-level sociologists are interested in everyday interactions.

Functionalism

Functionalism is a framework of sociological analysis based on the premise that society is a whole unit is comprised of a variety of interrelated parts, each with their own function that work together. Functional analysis, the study of society's function's, became relevant in sociology when two pioneering sociologists, August Comte (1798-1857) and Herbert Spencer (1820-1903), began labeling society as a sort of "living organism" that has certain interrelated "organs" that function together much like in the body of a human or an animal.

According to Emile Durkheim (1858-1917), an heir to Comte and Spencer's sociological perspectives, "To love society is to love something beyond us and something in ourselves." In other words, society is both an external set of functions that shape humanity and an internalized expression of society's functions that, in turn, reshape societal expressions and motivations. Robert K. Merton (1910-2003) also implemented functional analysis in his work, noting that society is also in direct interaction with human dysfunctions, which bring about unintended negative consequences. All of these sociologists, from Comte to Merton, adhered to a functionalist perspective—a broader system of thinking that encouraged global citizens to examine the ways in which smaller functions harmoniously interact with superstructural frameworks.

Conflict Theory

Karl Marx (1818-1833) departed from the aforementioned functionalist perspective by declaring that society's functions are not predisposed to collaborative harmony with the whole, but rather, are predisposed to competition over resources. Growing up in the Industrial Revolution, Marx developed a conflict theory that stressed class conflict (i.e., the struggle between certain socioeconomic brackets in society) instead of cooperative alliances. Initially, conflict theory remained tied to Marxist notions of class struggle (i.e., the struggle between the working class and the capitalists), but in the 20th and 21st centuries, many sociologists extended conflict theory to include societal clashes regarding race and gender. For instance, feminist conflict theory, which developed in the 1960s, emphasizes the conflict between patriarchy and femininity rather than the conflict between the proletariat (working class) and the bourgeoisie (capitalists).

Symbolic Interactionism

Symbolic interactionism is often attributed to German sociologist Max Weber (1864-1920), author of *The Protestant Work Ethic and the Spirit of Capitalism* (1905). A symbolic-interaction approach emphasizes the everyday interactions of individuals at a "street level." Unlike functionalists and conflict theorists, symbolic interactionists tend to see society as a reality defined by individualized identities and micro-level orientations. Weber's work, for instance, emphasizes individual "point of views" over superstructural shifts. Weber and his followers concerned themselves not with the macro-level changes, but rather, with what people do when they are in a certain context or within the presence of another person.

Social Constructionism

Social constructionism refers to the use of individual and proximal biases, worldviews, information, and life experiences to define and understand reality. In this sense, humanity's sense of reality is both collectively learned and individually analyzed. In either case, society—and reality at large—is **constructed;** that is, human beings inherit and create reality through a subjective process of understanding. Society and reality, therefore, are constructed products of human belief and ingenuity.

Exchange-Rational Choice

"Exchange-rational choice" is used to describe the coalescence of two major sociological theories—social exchange theory and rational choice theory. Developed by scholars such as George Homans (1910-1989) and Peter Blau (1918-2002), social exchange theory states that all social interactions and all social changes or stabilities are guided and negotiated by a subjective cost-benefit analysis by all human beings and parties involved in the exchange. Social interaction, in this sense, is guided and negotiated by what one seeks to gain or lose from others. Likewise, rational choice theory explains that all parties involved in an exchange will possess individual preferences, filtered through their particular brand of rationale, when it comes to the cost-benefit choices in exchange. **Exchange-rational choice** is thus an overarching sociological term used to describe the motivations and cost-benefits for social interactions.

Feminist Theory

Feminist theory aims to understand the nature of gender constructs and inequality in society by deconstructing and reconstruction the role of feminism (and, by extension, masculinity and patriarchy) in history, sociology, art, literature, education, and all other academic categories. Feminist theory is not a singular lens of study, but rather, a wide range of diverse (and often competing and contradicting) lenses of critical gender analysis. Feminist theory is a direct product of **feminism**, which traditionally has opposed patriarchy and sexism in advocacy for socioeconomic equality for women. All feminist theory critically analyzes the personal experiences of women, men, and transgender persons, taking a close look at the ways in which gender identity, gender roles, and gender stratification shapes society and vice versa. Although there are various types of feminist theories (i.e., liberal feminist theory, socialist feminist theory, radical feminist theory, etc.), almost all strains of feminist theory support five general principles:

1. Eliminating gender stratification
2. Working to increase gender and socioeconomic equality
3. Expanding human choice (especially with concern to gender roles)
4. Promoting sexual freedom
5. Ending sexual violence.

Each type of feminist theory may approach these general principles in different ways, but almost all types of feminist theory at least interact with these broad categories.

Social Institutions

Education

Hidden Curriculum

Scholars of education, such as John Dewey (1859-1952), Paulo Freire (1921-1997), and Jean Anyon (1941-2013), employed the term **hidden curriculum** to describe the implicit, unwritten rules of behavior embedded within formal curricula in schools across the globe. According to many conflict theorists, global educational systems employ various forms of hidden curricula to reinforce socioeconomic stratification and racial segregation. For instance, in *Social Class and the Hidden Curriculum of Work* (1981), author Jean Anyon explains that working-class students are often exposed to implicit curricular biases that emphasize work ethic over intellectual curiosity. In contrast, according to Anyon (1981), middle-class students are often exposed to implicit curricular biases that emphasize inquiry-based learning over social compliance. According to conflict theorists, these differing social classes rarely "mingle" within national and international school systems because their implicit curricular biases reinforce competition and stratification rather than collaboration and unification.

Teacher Expectancy

Teacher expectancy refers to a symbolic interactionist theory that states that social interactions between teachers and students help develop a set of expectations that have profound consequences in terms of student performance and student behavior. According to this theory, a teacher's expectations, in particular, will dramatically affect student grades and test results. If a teacher has low expectations of their students, then the students are more likely to internalize these low expectations as truth and seek other forums for personal expression and positive feedback. Likewise, if a teacher maintains high expectations for students, then their students are more likely to internalize those high expectations as truth and live up to their potential.

Educational Segregation and Stratification

Throughout the history of the United States, racial segregation and socioeconomic segregation have long encouraged educational segregation and stratification. Poor and minority communities have historically been forced into struggling, segregated public schooling districts. Resources are limited within these school districts, making it difficult for teachers and students to remain competitive within the global economy. Court decisions such as *Brown vs. Board of Education* (1954) have limited legal educational segregation in the United States, yet educational segregation continues in countless neighborhoods in the 21st century as a result of political engineering and illegal housing policies.

Family

The Effects of Family Dynamics on Individuals

There are many ways in which the family influences the individual socially, emotionally, and psychologically. All family systems have their own unique characteristics, with both good and bad functional tendencies. The family interactions are among the earliest and most formative relationships that a person has, so they define the relational patterns that the individual develops and utilizes with all subsequent relationships. Parenting styles, conflict resolution methods, beliefs and values, and coping mechanisms are just a few things that a person learns from their family of origin. It is also within the family that a person first develops an image of self and identity, often having to do with the role that he or she is given within the family system and the messages communicated by parents. If a child has a secure and healthy relationship with the family members, it will likely lead to favorable overall well-being and emotional stability as an adult.

When it comes to physical or mental illness, the role that the family plays is critical in lowering risk factors and minimizing symptoms. A strongly supportive family will help a person function at the highest level possible. Oftentimes, family members can serve as caregivers or play less formal—but still critical—roles in supporting a person's health.

Dysfunctional Family Dynamics

Dysfunction within families comes in different forms. It may be in the form of physical, verbal, emotional, or sexual abuse, or in the form of neglect. On the other hand, it may be ongoing conflict, unrealistic expectations, and poor communication patterns that lead to stressful relationships and situations. Alcoholism or mental health issues can also create dysfunctional family patterns, as individuals struggling with these things will be unable to function as healthy members of the family. There may be unequal treatment of children in the family, such as treating one child as the favorite, or one as the **scapegoat**, and blaming him or her for things for which he or she is not responsible. Whatever the dysfunction may be, it can affect the various individuals in the family in negative ways. In families where there are dysfunctional dynamics, there is a failure to affirm the uniqueness and value of each individual.

The impact of family dysfunction, though not deterministic, is very influential when it comes to the long-term health and well-being of family members. Negative family relationship patterns, whether abuse, neglect, or high levels of conflict, have a greater likelihood of leading to later mental health issues. These early family experiences may also result in poor health, insecurity, and an inability to cope with life stressors as an adult. Even if separated from the family later in life, the person has learned to view himself or herself and the world through the lens of personal childhood experiences. If a person does have ongoing contact with family members, there may be a constant re-affirmation of the dysfunctional habits, promoting low self-image, poor communication, or even abusive behaviors.

The Impact of Physical Illness on Family Dynamics

When a family member is diagnosed with a serious physical illness, it can have a significant impact on family dynamics. Not only will that person's role within the family change, as he or she will probably have to give up some of the responsibilities he or she had before, but the roles of other members will change as well. Family members may have to share the responsibilities that the sick person had, in addition to the added responsibilities of caring for that person. This could include frequent doctor's visits, medication management, or helping the patient with tasks that he or she can no longer accomplish independently.

It may even be that a family member must take on the role of full-time caregiver, which adds new stress and complications to the relationship. It can also impact the family financially, if either the sick person or the caregiver was previously one of the primary financial providers for the family. There may be feelings of guilt, as well as re-evaluation of identity on the part of the sick person. If it is a parent who is sick, there may be a reversal of the parent-child relationship. If it is a child who is sick, there may be confusion or even resentment on the part of other siblings because of the attention that child is taking from the parents.

No matter who is diagnosed with the illness, it will certainly put a strain on the family dynamics and make it more difficult to ensure that each family member's needs are being met adequately. The family's ability to cope also depends on the level of functioning that the family had before the illness occurred. If there were already strained relationships or patterns of conflict, these will be exacerbated by the diagnosis. If the family had a high level of emotional and relational functionality, it is more likely that they will be resilient and better able to cope with the changes.

Religion

Religiosity

Most sources agree that the sociological term **religiosity** is somewhat difficult to define, and it may be used differently in various situations. The most common usage of religiosity is in reference to piety or the degree to which someone's religious beliefs and involvement affect their life. In this sense, it deals with one's devoutness toward their faith.

Types of Religious Organizations

Sects are typically formed when a faction has broken away from the "parent" or larger, initial religious organization or denomination, often because of some degree of conflict or disagreement about some of the values and norms of that religion that are or are not being practiced by the denomination. Usually, the members of the sect feel that important tenants and original views of the religion have been lost in the current practice of the parent organization and they seek to restore focus on these areas. Because sects are sort of "side groups," they are relatively small, and they often lack the bureaucracy and formally-trained clergy of a denomination. They often have a large focus outside of services on proselytizing—recruiting new members and growing the sect. However, ultimately, as membership grows, so does the bureaucratic nature of the sect. Therefore, much of what was initially desired when the sect was formed is lost as the sect grows into a more formalized denomination

Cults are small religious organizations that usually originate on their own, rather than by breaking off of a mainstream religion, as in the case of sects. Another difference from sects is that cults tend to be more secretive and receive all of their leadership from one highly charismatic leader.

In sociology, a **church** is a religious organization that tends to be integrated into the surrounding society. There are two types of these bureaucratically-organized institutions: an ecclesia and a denomination. An ecclesia is the state or national religion, meaning it is a recognized as a formal part of the state and its membership body includes most or all citizens of the state. Rather than members "joining" an ecclesia, they are automatically anointed members at birth. There is very little separation between church and state in an ecclesiastic society. A denomination is still integrated into society, but it is not a formal constituent of the state, and nations can have numerous coexistent denominations. Members usually self-select to join the denomination or join because their parents are members.

Religion and Social Change

Religions, like all other social institutions, evolve with time. Currently, sociologists study three major categories of change when it comes to religious evolution: modernization, secularization, and fundamentalism. Many scholars, including Max Weber, have concluded that religion can be both a product and a driving force for modernization (i.e., the transition from antiquity to modernity and/or the transition from traditional society to industrial/technological society).

In the 19th and 20th centuries, for instance, religion is believed to have been a major driving force of the Industrial Revolution and the global shift toward capitalist society. Max Weber argues in *The Protestant Ethic and the Spirit of Capitalism* (1905) that Christian Protestantism helped create a work ethic that drove the so-called "spirit of capitalism" as Western society shifted toward modernity. Likewise, the tides of modernity seemed to have shape the Protestant religion as much as the work day: the Industrial Revolution of the 19th and 20th centuries paved the way to the construction of hundreds of thousands of Protestant churches in the United States of America. Although Weber's arguments have been criticized as being Protestant-centric, they still shed light on an important aspect of the interrelated forces of modernization and religiosity – any historical transformation or technological progress has the potential to (re)shape humanity's relationship with theology.

Another historical force studied by many sociologists is secularization. **Secularization** is a term used to describe the process of gradual decline in the importance of spiritual matters in society. Secularization is a force of modernization – it is a modern phenomenon that has replaced otherworldly concerns with a focus on world affairs. Trends indicate that citizens of the United States are becoming increasingly secularized in their beliefs, becoming less influenced by religion and more influenced by a 20th- and 21st- brand of secular morality. Religion is not "dead," so to speak, but it is in decline in Western nations such as the United States.

In the Middle East, and even in the United States, however, there appears to be a rise and/or reemergence of religious fundamentalism. Many religious devotees across the globe are adhering to fundamentalist, conservative doctrines of belief that are in direct conflict with the forces of modernization and secularization. These religious fundamentalists favor the restoration of traditional, literal analyses of sacred texts and oppose the tides of secular humanism. In the Middle East and the United States, many Muslim believers have warned against the excesses of secular modernity, condemning Western culture and its frivolous excesses. The emergence of ISIS in the Middle East, for example, illustrates that even an era of increased secularization, many people rely on fundamental religiosities as a means of understand life and the afterlife.

Government and Economy

Politics is the process of governance, typically exercised through the enactment and enforcement of laws, over a community, or most commonly, a state. Political theory involves the study of politics, especially concerning the efficacy and legitimacy of those responsible for governance. The major concepts in political theory include power and authority. The concepts of power and authority are closely related but possess certain significant distinctions.

Power is the ability of a ruling body or political entity to influence the actions, behavior, and attitude of a person or group of people; in short, power implies a degree of control over a human community. In order to possess **authority**, the ruling body or political entity must be recognized as having the right and justification to exercise power. This is commonly referred to as *legitimacy*. In representative governments, authority is garnered from the citizens through democratic processes, but in more autocratic regimes, influential elites grant that authority. In some cases, a ruling body or political entity may possess authority recognized by its citizens or influential elites but lack the power to influence those citizens and political entities or effect change within the system of governance. When power and authority are not properly aligned, governments are extremely weak, often deadlocked, and at risk of collapse or revolution.

Government is the result of the decisions made by a society during the political process and is a physical manifestation of the political entity or ruling body. The government determines and enforces the power of the state. A government includes the formal institutions of a society with the power and authority to enact, enforce, and interpret laws. The many different forms of government are determined based on this delegation of power between those institutions. Government encompasses the functions of law, order, and justice and is responsible for maintaining the society.

Sovereignty refers to a political entity's right and power to self-govern, including enacting and enforcing its own taxes and laws without interference from external forces. A political entity may possess varying degrees of sovereignty, as some sovereign states may still be subject to influence by outside political entities. For example, the members of the European Union cede some sovereignty in order to enjoy membership. A state's sovereignty is legitimate when outside political entities recognize the right of the state to self-govern. Both sovereignty and legitimacy are requirements to form a state.

The terms **nation** and **state** are often used interchangeably, but in political theory, they are two very distinct concepts. Nation refers to a people's cultural identity, while state refers to a territory's political organization and government.

Unlike states, there are no definitive requirements to be a nation; the nation just needs to include a group that is bound together by some shared defining characteristics such as the following:

- Language
- Culture and traditions
- Beliefs and religion
- Homeland
- Ethnicity
- History
- Mythology

The term **state** is commonly used to reference a nation-state, especially in regard to its government. There are four requirements for a political entity to be recognized as a state:

1. **Territory:** a clearly defined geographic area with distinct borders

2. **Population:** citizens and non-citizens living within the borders of the territory with some degree of permanence

3. **Legitimacy:** legal authority to rule that is recognized by the citizens of the state and by other states

4. **Sovereignty:** a political entity's right and power to self-govern without interference from external forces

Nation-state is the term used to describe a political entity with both a clearly defined nation and state. In a nation-state, the majority population of the state is a nation that identifies the territory as their homeland and shares a common history and culture. It is also possible to have several nations in the same nation-state. For example, there are Canadians in Canada and nations of Aboriginal peoples. The presence of multiple nations raises issues related to sovereignty.

Example of a nation: Sikhs in India

Example of a state: Vatican City

Example of a nation-state: Germany

Modern Political Parties

Franklin D. Roosevelt, a Democrat, was elected president in 1933. Roosevelt instituted the New Deal, which included many social policies that built an expansive social welfare program to provide financial support to citizens during the Great Depression. The Republican Party opposed this interference by the government, and the two parties became more strongly divided. The political landscape again shifted during the Civil Rights Movement, as Southern Democrats fled to the Republican Party over their opposition to enforcing federal civil rights onto states. This strengthened the modern coalition between economic conservatives and social conservatives.

Today, the Democrats and Republicans are still the two major parties, although many third parties have emerged. The Republicans and Democrats hold opposing views on the degree of state intervention into private business, taxation, states' rights, and government assistance. The ideals of these parties include:

Republican (or the Grand Old Party [GOP])

- Founded by abolitionists
- Support capitalism, free enterprise, and a policy of noninterference by the government
- Support strong national defense
- Support deregulation and restrictions of labor unions
- Advocate for states' rights
- Oppose abortion
- Support traditional values, often based on Judeo-Christian foundations

Democrat

- Founded by anti-Federalists and rooted in classical Liberalism
- Promote civil rights, equal opportunity, and protection under the law, and social justice
- Support government-instituted social programs and safety nets
- Support environmental issues
- Support government intervention and regulation, and advocate for labor unions
- Support universal healthcare

Some prominent third parties include:

- **Reform Party:** support political reform of the two-party system
- **Green Party:** support environmental causes
- **Libertarian Party:** support a radical policy of nonintervention and small, localized government

Interest Groups

An **interest group** is an organization with members who share similar social concerns or political interests. Members of political interest groups work together to influence policy decisions that benefit a particular segment of society or cause. Interest groups might include:

- Activist groups, like the NAACP, American Civil Liberties Union (ACLU), or People for the Ethical Treatment of Animals (PETA)
- Corporations, like pharmaceutical companies or banks
- Small-business advocates
- Religious groups, like the Muslim Public Affairs Council and the Concerned Women PAC
- Unions, such as the Association of Teacher Educators and International Brotherhood of Electrical Workers

Health and Medicine

Medicalization

Medicalization is a sociological term used to describe a social process by which human issues are described in medical terms. An example of medicalization is when society attempts to describe any kind of social deviance as a medical matter that demands the attention of the public or medical profession. Often people who deviate from social norms are mislabeled as "mentally ill." This is a form of medicalization because not all forms of social deviance are directly rooted in mental illness. Some controversial scholars, such as Thomas Szasz (1920-2012), actually believe the emergence of attention-deficit disorder (ADD) is actually a historic example of the ways in which behavioral deviance can be medicalized. Additionally, homelessness is a form of social deviance that is often described as a medical matter when it is not always directly rooted in disease.

The Sick Role

According to the pivotal 1951 study by Talcott Parsons, society affords people a pattern of behavior deemed appropriate for illness. According to Parsons, this pattern of acceptable behavior is called a "**sick role**." According to this sick role, society strategizes to keep its members healthy, by allowing ill citizens the opportunity to be released from their normal civic duties, such as work and schooling. Parsons consequently links illness and medical practices to societal orientations and dispositions, claiming that members of society are often forced to "look the part" when it comes illness. In other words, they are asked to assume a "sick role" in society and seek the expertise of a medical professional. Parsons' theory indicates that both illness and treatment are social constructions, just like any other facet of social interaction.

Delivery of Healthcare

Healthcare is also a social construction much like illness and treatment. Access to and the delivery of healthcare is shaped by the social orientations and dispositions of a particular culture. For instance, in the United States, despite attempts in recent years to introduce changes to health insurance, access to and the delivery of healthcare remains inequitable due to the nation's historic aversion to universal healthcare. In other countries, access to and the delivery of healthcare is a universal right. Still in other countries, normal citizens do not have any access to healthcare due to infrastructural deficiencies. In many capitalist countries, such as the United States, there is a profit motive when it comes to healthcare access and delivery. Conflict theorists continue to lambast the pharmaceutical industry for placing profit over equity. In this sense, medicine and healthcare remain tied to the political economy and the tides of social norms and (supra)national politics.

Illness Experience

In medical sociology, illness differs from disease in that illness refers to a person's subjective relationship to health issues while disease refers to professional or objective definitions of health issues. Illness experience is therefore a "lay" experience – it emphasizes the ways in which people define and orient themselves in relationship to their perceived health concerns. Since illness experience emphasizes personal perception over professional diagnosis, it is, therefore, theoretically possible for a person to experience illness without being medically diagnosed with a disease.

Social Epidemiology

Social epidemiology is the study of how illness, health, and medical practice is distributed across society. Social epidemiologists analyze the intersection between nationality, race, ethnicity, age, and gender; they examine the connections between health, illness, politics, social interaction, and geography. Social epidemiologists often study the cultural patterns that define health, the cultural standards that change health over time, the technological advances that affect health, and the social inequalities that stratify health standards

Culture

Elements of Culture

Cultures differ throughout society, but they maintain some similar elements. These elements include: beliefs, language, rituals, symbols, and values. **Beliefs** are particular ideas or statements that people hold to be true or false. **Language** is any system of symbols or speech that allows human beings to communicate with one another. **Rituals** are certain rites, practices, or programmatic traditions that human beings participate in as a means to convey their individual or collective beliefs, symbols, or values. Rituals are typically tied to religion (i.e., baptisms, rites of passage, etc.), but human beings can also participate in secular or popular rituals. **Values** define the parameters of social living for cultural participants; these values determine what is morally good, socially desirable, or aesthetically pleasing. All of these elements of culture are subjective; they differ from one community to the next as a result of contextual and individual variables.

Material vs. Symbolic Culture

Material culture refers to the material objects—technology, computers, machines, buildings, weapons, infrastructure, clothing, hairstyles, utensils, jewelry, etc.—that distinguish a group of people or a specific sector of society. Material culture is not "natural," so to speak; rather, it is the material manifestation of human beliefs and practices. Symbolic cultures, sometimes referred to as immaterial or non-material culture, refers to a specific group or sector's beliefs, values, and assumptions about the world. Symbolic culture includes a central set of symbols such as language, gestures, folkways, mores, religiosity, norms, rules, and sanctions. Symbolic culture is not driven by the material world but can be influenced by humanity's relationship to the material world.

Culture Lag

Cultural lag, a term coined by sociologist William Ogburn (1886-1959), refers to the theory that many cultural changes are unevenly adopted, implemented, or absorbed throughout a particular culture or institution. According to Ogburn, a group's material culture (things) is more likely to be formed more rapidly than a group's immaterial culture (ideas or beliefs). Ogburn observed that, in particular, technology transforms the world's culture of things at a fast pace while customs and beliefs surrounding these things are typically delayed in their adoption, implementation, or absorption. The rapidity and efficiency of technology, therefore, has humanity constantly trying to "catch up" to technological transformation. This cultural lag creates a gap in the relationship between technological use and human custom.

Culture Shock

Culture shock refers to the kind of personal uneasiness or disorientation that is experienced when a person interacts with an unfamiliar way of life. Travelers, foreign ambassadors, and international students often feel culture shock when they are either thrust into a new environment or return to a familiar environment after a long-term experience with an unfamiliar culture. Nevertheless, culture shock is not just a global phenomenon, but rather, it can occur within a domestic context. For instance, a first-generation, low-income Mexican-American student may experience may experience culture shock when she or he is thrust into the culture of a primarily white institution (PWI). Additionally, a white, middle-class teacher may experience culture shock when providing a public service to a dilapidated urban neighborhood. Culture shock is an important facet of sociological analysis because it illustrates that there is no "natural" or "uniform" way of life, but rather both micro- and macro-level environments display a diversity of cultural orientations.

Assimilation

Assimilation is a term used to describe the process by which certain ethnic, racial, or religious minorities slowly adopt the beliefs, practices, and institutions of the majority culture. Assimilation is often referred to when discussing the immigrant experience in the United States and the ways in which immigrant minority groups adopt majority norms and values. Assimilation is often the product of oppression, colonization, or coercion, but it can also be the result of self-determination or collective choice. The process is usually followed by shifts in customs, eating habits, political and religious values, and clothing.

Multiculturalism

Multiculturalism is a socio-intellectual platform for recognizing cultural diversity and advocating for an equality of cultural traditions. Instead of promoting monolithic cultural homogeneity, multiculturalism recognizes, celebrates, and advocates for a diverse range of coexisting cultures. Rather than downplaying cultural diversity for the sake of national or cultural centrism, multiculturalism warns against the dangers of Eurocentrism or Americentric perspectives that negate the cultures and histories of certain groups and subgroups of society. Multiculturalism is, therefore, in direct opposition to assimilationist policies that disregard the cultural values of certain racial, religious, or ethnic groups.

Subcultures and Countercultures

Subculture refers to cultural groups, patterns, or values that reside outside or within a subcategory of the subjective parameters of mainstream culture. Subcultural groups can form around any collective interest or personal activity. Memberships within these subcultural groups are not awarded easily and are often the result of intensified rites of passage and selective processes. Subcultures do not necessarily have to conjure up negative connotations; however, many people are often inaccurately placed within certain subcultures in order to oppress or disenfranchise their existence. Some subcultures are looked down upon by the mainstream culture while other subcultures are in direct opposition with the broader culture. Subcultures that are in direct opposition to mainstream values are called **countercultures.**

Mass Media and Popular Culture

Mass media is defined by an efficient delivery of impersonal communications to a popular audience. **Popular culture**—culture that is both consumed and displayed by the popular masses—is greatly shaped by the images, symbols, and messages distributed by mass media. Televisions, newspapers, magazines, and social media shape society's social norms as well as social constructs concerning race, gender, sexuality, and socioeconomic status. Historically, mass media has been centered on white, middle-class, male norms, making the mass media a beacon of racism, sexism, and class-based prejudice.

Transmission and Diffusion

Transmission is the process by which cultural elements are passed from one generation to the next. Language is a crucial component of cultural transmission. **Diffusion** refers to the spread of cultural elements from one society to another. Language and trade are crucial components of cultural diffusion.

Demographic Characteristics and Processes

Demographic Structure of Society

Demography, or the study of human populations, involves a variety of closely related stimuli. First, as has been previously addressed, economic factors play a significant role in the movement of people, as do climate, natural disasters, or internal unrest. For example, in recent years, millions of immigrants from the war-torn country of Syria, have moved as far as possible from danger. Many even risked their own lives in rickety boats on their way across the Mediterranean Sea. Although people are constantly moving, some consistencies remain throughout the world.

First, people tend to live near reliable sources of food and water, which is why the first human civilizations sprung up in river valleys like the Indus River Valley in India, the Nile River Valley in Egypt, and the Yellow River Valley in Asia. Second, extreme temperatures tend to push people away, which is why the high latitudinal regions near the North and South Poles have such few inhabitants. Third, the vast majority of people tend to live in the Northern Hemisphere, due to the simple fact that more land lies in that part of the Earth. In keeping with these factors, human populations tend to be greater where human necessities are easily accessible, or at least are more readily available. In other words, such areas have a greater chance of having a higher population density than places without such characteristics.

Demographic patterns on Earth are not always stagnant. In contrast, people move and will continue to move as both push and pull factors fluctuate along with the flow of time. For example, in the 1940s, thousands of Europeans fled their homelands due to the impact of the Second World War. Today, thousands of migrants arrive on European shores each month due to conflicts in the Levant and difficult economic conditions in Northern Africa. Furthermore, as previously discussed, people tend to migrate to places with a greater economic benefit for themselves and their families. As a result, developed nations such as the United States, Germany, Canada, and Australia, have a net gain of migrants, while developing nations such as Somalia, Zambia, and Cambodia generally tend to see thousands of their citizens seek better lives elsewhere.

It is important to understand the key variables in changes regarding human population and its composition worldwide. Religion and religious conflict play a role in where people choose to live. For example, the Nation of Israel won its independence in 1948 and has since attracted thousands of people of Jewish descent from all over the world. Additionally, the United States has long attracted people from all over the world, due to its promise of religious freedom inherent within its own Constitution. In contrast, nations like Saudi Arabia and Iran do not typically tolerate different religions, resulting in a decidedly uniform religious (and oftentimes ethnic) composition. Other factors such as economic opportunity, social unrest, and cost of living also play a vital role in demographic composition.

The Influences of Age and/or Disability

There are many influencers on how happy and satisfactory old age can be. Physically, a person's independence and health depend on many things, including genetics, nutrition, exercise, and bad habits, such as smoking or drinking. Those who have lived unhealthy lifestyles are likely to suffer from more severe and earlier onset disease and disability. Psychosocially, according to Erik Erikson, those who are aging face the crisis of integrity vs. despair. At this stage, people are looking back on their lives and evaluating what they have done and how they have lived. Those who can look back with integrity and satisfaction will have a happier, more fulfilling old age than those who feel guilt or dissatisfaction regarding their past. Socially, a person who has family and a strong social support and community will do better in old age.

Living successfully with disability is also influenced by many different factors. First and foremost, it is important to have access to resources, whether familial, educational, social, or physical, that will assist the disabled person in living at a high level of function. Those persons who have an optimistic outlook and have a desire to take charge of their own lives will do better. Optimism has to do with many things, including family support, an internal locus of control, one's positive perception of the future and the world, and the severity of the disability.

The Impact of Age and/or Disability on Self-Image

Aging is an inevitable phase of human development, and the impact is physical, psychological, social, and economic. Self-image is the perception of oneself, but the perception is influenced by societal values. Some cultures revere the elderly and look to them for wisdom and strength. These cultures include the Native Americans, Chinese, Koreans, and Indians, among others. In the United States, there is a different perception of aging. Many elderly Americans feel less valuable or important once they enter retirement. At the same time, they are coping with undesirable body changes and learning to accept that, physically, they can no longer do what they once did. In the U.S., youth and physical attractiveness are highly valued. The elderly are seldom seen as important social figures. They are also less connected with families today, with only 3.7% of homes reporting multigenerational households, per U.S. Census Bureau reports. Currently, family support and family contact are less available. However, for some segments of the population, technology has allowed relatives to visit regularly with grandchildren and even participate in family meals or get-togethers.

Disabilities impact self-image regardless of age; however, an individual who is born with a disability tends to fare better than one who acquires one later in life. Responses vary based upon severity of impairments. Some later-life medical conditions cause the individual to give up independence as the person is forced to retire the car keys or move to an institutional setting. Less severe acquired disabilities that still allow the person to maintain much of their previous lifestyle are painful but easier to accept. An individual's personality make-up and resilience to coping with change are also important factors. It is not uncommon for older adults to lapse into depression. This is often generated by a combination of losses. As one enters the later stages of life, loss of friends and family members is common. There may be declines in status, earning capacity, or physical abilities, all of which contribute to depression and negatively impact self-image.

Social Significance of Aging

Ages, and, more specifically, the process of aging, are now believed to be social constructions much like race and gender. Attitudes toward ages and aging are very much rooted in cultural values and differ from culture to culture. Ageism is the act of being prejudicial due to subjective notions of age and aging. The so-called "life course perspective of age cohorts" plays on the notions of social constructivism, noting that human beings can choose their own journeys in life and they can choose to subjectively analyze aging and the meaning of aging according to their own goals and values. The life course perspective on age cohorts helps to further diversify perspectives on aging and offers individualized and culture-specific alternatives.

The Social Construction of Gender

"The social construction of gender" refers to the concept that the philosophical and sociological notion of gender is actually a subjective creation of humanity rather than an objective reality. According to this constructionist view, people are assigned gender roles by society, and these gender roles force human beings into frivolous categories that demand certain prescribed behaviors or values. Gender theorists have moved beyond the tradition male-female dichotomy, noting alternatives such as being agender, transgender, and gender fluid.

Gender Segregation

One consequence of the social construction of gender has been centuries of gender segregation. **Gender segregation** is the categorization and separation of human beings by gender. One of the most obvious modern examples is bathroom designations, which has come under fire by gender theorists recently. Traditionally, bathrooms have been separated into male and female quarters. However, as more people move beyond this gender dichotomy, many consumer spaces and public places have chosen to not be gender-specific in their designations. Throughout history, however, there have been much more severe forms of gender segregation such as the separation of schools by gender.

Race and Ethnicity

Racialization

Racialization refers to the process of categorizing and separating people in society based on race, or physical characteristics that distinguish them from other groups. Race is both a reality and a myth/construct. By nature of the diversity of humanity, certain groups are distinguished by their unique skin tones or physical features. However, race is mostly a myth/construct, historically used to endow superiority and/or inferiority to certain groups. Racialization, therefore, occurs not only when people are categorized or separated by race, but also when the spatial distribution of society is also categorized or separated by race. The most extreme form of spatial racialization, therefore, is racial segregation.

Racial Formation

Developed by sociologists such as Howard Winant (b. 1946), **racial formation** an analytical framework in sociology used to describe the process by which race is socially constructed by individuals. Racial formation focuses on the relationship between race and identity, and the manifestation of racial formation is dependent upon many variables, including social context, economic disposition, and political forces. According to the theory, race is formed (and reformed) dynamically throughout history in relationship to the contexts and identities of individuals and groups. Race, in this sense, is not a fixed set of categories, but rather, an ever-changing sense of self. Although race is a constructed myth, it can become an intense reality for persons or groups who analyze and categorize the world in racialized terms.

Immigration Status

Immigration status describes the citizenship and/or resident status of an immigrant or immigrant family. Types of immigrant statuses differ according to the laws of the state. In some countries, immigrants may obtain work visas, asylum, or deferred action with regards to their resident/citizenship status. Conversely, some immigrants maintain an "undocumented status," meaning they unlawfully immigrated to a nation without going through the proper channels to obtain work visas, asylum, deferred action, or citizenship. Currently, in the United States of America, there is an ongoing debate regarding the status of millions of undocumented persons residing on U.S. soil.

Patterns of Immigration

Migration is governed by two primary causes: **push factors**, which are reasons causing someone to leave an area, and **pull factors**, which are factors luring someone to a particular place. These two factors often work in concert with one another. For example, the United States of America has experienced significant **internal migration** from the industrial states in the Northeast (such as New York, New Jersey, Connecticut) to the Southern and Western states. This massive migration, which continues into the present-day, is due to high rents in the northeast, dreadfully cold winters, and lack of adequate retirement housing, all of which are push factors. These push factors lead to migration to the **sunbelt**, a term geographers use to describe states with warm climates and less intense winters.

In addition to internal migrations within nations or regions, international migration also takes place between countries, continents, and other regions. The United States has long been the world's leading nation in regard to **immigration**, the process of having people come into a nation's boundaries. Conversely, developing nations that suffer from high levels of poverty, pollution, warfare, and other violence all have significant push factors, which cause people to leave and move elsewhere. This process, known as **emigration**, is when people in a particular area leave in order to seek a better life in a different—usually better—location.

Patterns of migration are generally economically motivated. For example, the United States underwent a significant population shift from 1916-1930 due to its entrance into the First World War. Because of the war, thousands of factories opened and needed workers to produce munitions for the war effort. Answering the call of opportunity, thousands of African Americans, who had lived on farms since the cessation of the Civil War, packed up their belongings and moved to cities like Detroit, Los Angeles, Milwaukee, and Cleveland. This mass internal migration, which historians termed the **Great Migration**, is an excellent example of how economic forces work to stimulate human migration, thus drastically altering a nation's demographic patterns.

Demographic Shifts and Social Change

Demographic shifts—the apparent changes in the size, distribution, composition, and growth of a population—inevitably catalyze social changes as micro- and macro-communities expand disperse, shift, and contract. Demographic shifts influence human beings to respond in different ways. Demographic shifts can be the root of war, immigration, genocide, famine, and panic. Additionally, they can be the root of harmony, peace, stability, and social justice. Demography and sociology are so integrally linked that it is hard to disassociate the two fields.

Theories of Demographic Change

In sociology, there are two major theories of demographic change: the Malthusian theory and the demographic transition theory. Created by English economist Thomas Malthus (1766-1834), **Malthusian theory** argues that if births and population increases burgeon in an unchecked fashion, then a national, regional, or global community will outstrip its food supply. According to Mathus, who authored a book entitled *An Essay on the Principle of Population* (1789), food supplies increase arithmetically or linearly (1, 2, 3, 4, etc.) while population increase geometrically (2, 4, 8, 16, etc.). Inheritors of the Malthusian theory, frequently referred to as the New Malthusians, later developed the exponential growth curve, which states that population growth tends to double at near-equal intervals.

Detractors of Malthusian theory, traditionally called Anti-Malthusians, gravitate toward the so-called **demographic transition theory**. Demographic transition refers to a three-stage historical process of population growth: 1) high birth rates/high death rates, 2) high birth rates/low death rates, 3) low birth rates/low death rates. Some inheritors of this theory add a fourth stage: 4) deaths outnumber births.

Population Growth and Decline

The availability of resources affects the human population. Humans require basic resources such as food and water for survival, as well as additional resources for healthy lifestyles. Therefore, access to these resources helps determine the survival rate of humans. For much of human existence, economies have had limited ability to extract resources from the natural world, which restricted the growth rate of populations.

However, the development of new technologies, combined with increasing demand for certain products, has pushed resource use to a new level. On the one hand, this led to higher living standards that ensured that fewer people would die. However, this has also brought mass population growth. Admittedly, countries with higher standards of living often have lower birthrates. Even so, the increasing exploitation of resources has sharply increased the world's population as a whole to unsustainable levels. The rising population leads, in turn, to more demand for resources that cannot be met. This creates poverty, reduced living conditions, and higher death rates. As a result, economics can significantly influence local and world population levels.

Technology is also intricately related to population, resources, and economics. The role of demand within economies has incentivized people to innovate new technologies that enable societies to have a higher quality of life and greater access to resources. Entrepreneurs expand technologies by finding ways to create new products for the market. The Industrial Revolution, in particular, illustrates the relationship between economics and technology because the ambitions of businessmen led to new infrastructure that enabled more efficient and sophisticated use of resources. Many of these inventions reduced the amount of work necessary for individuals and allowed the development of leisure activities, which, in turn, created new economic markets.

However, economic systems can also limit the growth of technology. In the case of monopolies, the lack of alternative suppliers reduces the incentive to meet and exceed consumer expectations. Moreover, as demonstrated by the effects of economics on resources, technology's increasing ability to extract resources can lead to their depletion and create significant issues that need to be addressed.

Population Growth and Decline

A population's size can grow or decline based on fluctuating birth rates, death rates, immigration, and emigration. The **birth rate** is defined as the total number of live births per 1,000 individuals in a defined population in a year. The **death rate**, or **mortality rate**, is defined as the total number of deaths per 1,000 individuals in a defined population in a year. **Immigration** refers to a person or organism coming from another population to the one currently being examined, and **emigration** refers a person or organism leaving that population to settle elsewhere. Because these are the chief factors affecting a population's size, the rate of its growth can be determined from them.

Other variables such as food availability, adequate shelter, and water supply can also affect population. These resources are finite and help determine the carrying capacity of a particular geographic area. **Carrying capacity** is defined as the maximum number of individuals that can be sustained indefinitely in a particular habitat. As a population of humans grows, other factors such as government, education, economics, healthcare, and cultural values will also begin to influence the population.

As time goes on, certain countries may experience population growth while others experience its decline. Population growth, especially if unchecked, can be troubling when a community grows to a point that exceeds its carrying capacity. Ultimately, levels of emigration may rise as individuals leave in search of more favorable conditions. Conversely, population decline can also be threatening due to the diminished pools of individuals available for labor and reproduction. Ultimately, rising levels of immigration will be needed to remedy this stress on the population.

Demographic Transition Model

The **Demographic Transition Model** (DTM) explains changes in two key areas, birth rate and death rate, and their effect on the total population of a country as it undergoes economic and industrial development. This model was introduced in 1929. Birth rate is defined as the number of live births per 1,000 individuals in a population over the course of an entire year, while death rate is defined as the total number of deaths per 1,000 individuals in a population over the course of an entire year.

As a general rule, a country will progress through stages as it undergoes economic and industrial development. Very few countries are in stage 1 of the model. Most of the developing countries are grouped in stage 2 or 3 of the model, while most of the industrialized countries are categorized in stage 3 or 4 of the model.

The Demographic Transition Model has the following stages:

- **Stage 1—High Stationary:** Both a high birth and a high death rate characterize stage 1 of the DTM. These factors combine to produce a constant, relatively low total population. High birth rates may be accounted for by factors such as poor family planning, high infant and child death rates, and child labor requirements for farming and manufacturing. High death rates may be accounted for by factors such as famine, poor sanitation, poor healthcare, and disease epidemics. Before the Industrial Revolution, most of the world's countries were categorized as stage 1. Today, only the least economically developed countries would be classified as this stage.
- **Stage 2—Early Expanding:** A high birth rate and a rapidly decreasing death rate characterize stage 2 of the DTM. These factors converge to produce a rapid increase in the total population. Rapidly decreasing death rates may be explained by falling infant and child death rates, improved sanitation, improvements in healthcare, and better nutrition. Today, the African countries of Ethiopia, Kenya, and Egypt are examples of countries classified in this stage.
- **Stage 3—Late Expanding:** A decreasing birth rate along with a continued falling (but less rapid) death rate characterizes stage 3 of the DTM. These factors continue to produce an increase in total population, but at a slower rate than seen in stage 2. Child welfare laws, a desire for smaller families, and the changing role of women in the workplace may explain the effect of falling birth rates on the total population. Current examples of countries grouped in this stage are Brazil, South Korea, and India.
- **Stage 4—Low Stationary:** Both a low birth rate and death rate characterize stage 4 of the DTM. As a result, the factors combine to have a stabilizing effect on total population. Current examples of countries classified in this stage are the United States, Canada, and Great Britain.

Factors Influencing Birth and Fertility Rates

Fertility rate is defined as the average number of children a woman will bear over her lifetime for a given population. By convention, the reproductive lifetime of a woman ranges from about 15 to 45 years old. The fertility rate is an artificial measure, and does not represent the real fertility rate of any particular group of women, nor does it consider child mortality. Fertility rate is not the same as **birth rate**, and it is, instead, defined as the total number of live births per 1,000 individuals in a defined population in a year.

Key factors influencing birth and fertility rates of a particular country include:

- Urbanization: Rates are lower amongst individuals living in urban areas because they tend to have smaller families than those living in rural areas.
- Child labor: Rates are lower in developed countries because fewer children are required to work at a young age and help cultivate the land.
- Education costs: Rates are lower in developed countries because these costs are higher due to the fact children enter the work force in their late teens to early twenties.

- Women labor: Rates are lower in developed countries because women have access to education and paid employment outside of the household.
- Infant mortality: Rates are lower in locales with low infant mortality rates because individuals tend to have fewer children if those children don't die at an early age.
- Age of marriage: Rates are lower in countries where the average age at which women marry or have their first child is greater than 25. Women who marry or have children later in life tend to have fewer children.
- Pension systems: Rates are lower in developed countries as pensions and social security eliminate the burden of children providing for aging parents.
- Abortions: Rates are lower in countries where women have access to legal elective abortions.
- Contraception: Rates are lower in developed countries, because individuals have access to reliable birth control methods.
- Cultural norms and religious beliefs: Rates are lower in countries that don't hold particular norms and beliefs that strongly oppose abortion or birth control.
- Fertility and Mortality Rates

Two major demographic variables are fertility and mortality rates. **Fertility rates** convey the average number of children an average woman bears within a particular town, city, state, region, or nation. **Fecundity**, a term often associated with fertility rates, conveys the number of children women are capable of bearing. **Crude birth rates** illustrate the annual number of births per every 1,000 people. **Total birth rates** illustrate the net number of annual births. **Age-specific birth rates** illustrate the number of births per age group in a particular town, city, state, region, or nation.

Mortality rates, on the other hand, convey the average number of annual deaths within a particular town, city, state, region, or nation. **Crude death rates** illustrate the annual number of deaths per every 1,000 people. **Total death rates** illustrate the net number of annual deaths. **Age-specific death rates** present the number of births per age group in a particular town, city, state, region, or nation.

Patterns in Fertility and Mortality

In order to discover patterns in fertility and mortality, one must also consider migration as an additional variable. The net migration rate will illustrate the difference in the total number of emigrants and immigrants per every 1,000 people. This net migration rate is crucial for understanding broader patterns in fertility and mortality. These broader patterns can be discovered by using the basic demographic equation (births – deaths + net migration) to find an approximate growth rate. The growth rate allows sociologists to discover patterns in fertility and mortality by adding births, subtracting deaths, and then adding/subtracting the net migration rate. In some cases, a country may experience "zero population growth," which indicates that the women of that particular town, city, state, region, or nation can bear only enough children to maintain the population. Global fertility and mortality patterns indicate the Middle Africa has one of the highest growth rates, while Southern Europe has one of the lowest growth rates.

Social Movements

Social movements can be looked at as a group of people getting together to organize themselves to advocate for social or political change. Members of social movements engage in actions like political campaigns, rallies, petitions, and meetings. Typically, people who feel marginalized or oppressed, or sympathize with those they view as such, join social movements. Representative historical social movements include abolitionists, suffragists, civil-rights advocates, and women's rights advocates. In the U.S. today, there are gay-rights advocates on the left and Tea Party patriots on the right.

Political and social scientists categorize social movements in the following ways:

- **Reform movements** are social movements with the goal to change social and political norms. Examples include the movements to abolish capital punishment and abortion.
- **Radical movements** are social movements with the goal to change the fundamental values and trajectory of a society. Examples include the Black Panther Party and Polish solidarity movements.
- **Innovation movements** are social movements with the goal of implementing new solutions to old problems. Examples include the promotion of electric cars and artificial intelligence.
- **Conservative movements** are social movements with the goal of generally preserving tradition, or the political status quo. Examples include groups opposed to transgender people using common public bathrooms and groups supportive of unrestricted gun rights.
- **Group-focused movements** are social movements with the goal of changing a particular group. Examples include political parties and smaller factions.
- **Individual-focused movements** are social movements with the goal of advancing personal change. Examples include self-help groups that focus on individual self-improvement and change.
- **Peaceful movements** are social movements with the goal of using nonviolent methods to achieve some social goal. Examples include the civil-rights movement in the U.S. and the anti-Apartheid movement in South Africa.
- **Violent movements** are social movements who use violence to achieve their political ends. Examples include the Ku Klux Klan (KKK) and the Islamic State in Iraq and Syria (ISIS).
- **Old movements** are social movements that typically started in the twentieth century or earlier. Examples include the labor movement and the National Association for the Advancement of Colored People (NAACP).
- **New movements** are social movements that started after 1950. Example groups include feminists, right to life advocates, and environmentalists.
- **Global movements** are social movements that mobilize activists from around the globe to address a particular cause or issue. Examples include the International AIDS Society, the Save Darfur Campaign, and Nigeria's #BringBackOurGirls movement.
- **Local movements** are social movements with the goal of making changes at the community or local level. Examples include people who advocate for school reform, clean water, and jobs.
- **Multi-level movements** are social movements that work on local, regional, national, and international levels. Examples include human rights and environmental groups.

Relative Deprivation

Relative deprivation theory indicates that people are more likely to join social movements as a result of what they *think* they are deprived of and what they *think* they should have in relativity to others rather than any semblance of actual, concrete deprivation. According to this theory, the human desire for better conditions fuels social change, even if a person is not absolutely deprived of their own quality conditions.

Organization of Social Movements

Social movements are sociological phenomena that bring large numbers of people together to promote or resist social shifts. There are five stages to consider when studying the organization and growth of social movements: initial agitation, resource mobilization, organization, institutionalization, and decline and death. **Initial agitation** emerges when a charismatic leader or group of people verbalize their unrest. **Resource mobilization** forces a social movement to bring together financial and human capital. **Organization** allows for a division of labor to efficiently utilize financial and human capital. **Institutionalization** occurs when organization is efficiently bureaucratized. **Decline and death** occur only when the movement withers away as a result of political shifts or defunding. Some sociologists also entertain a sixth stage: resurgence. During this stage, after years of death or decline, a social movement may be reinvigorated by a breath of fresh air.

Movement Strategies and Tactics

Depending on their scope and intent, social movements can rely on rioting, rumors, panics, mass hysteria, fads, and mass media to convey their messages. Almost all social movements develop some sort of propaganda—persuasive, one-sided forms of advertisement and communication used to influence people's beliefs and public opinion. Propaganda can be dispersed by—or can lead to—rioting, rumors, panics, mass hysteria, and fads. Typically, propaganda is disseminated through the mass media. In the 21st century, propaganda has also been disseminated on social media, spawning many contemporary social movements and political revolutions such as Black Lives Matter and the Arab Spring.

Globalization

Globalization is the process that occurs when businesses and governments sign trade agreements, establish tariffs or quotas, or exchange information. In effect, it is the integration and internationalization of trade, communication, and people-to-people engagement. The speed and ease of globalization is increasing due to gains in information technology, the seeming ubiquity of the English language, the ease of global travel, the growth of truly global multinational corporations, the growth of regional and international trade, and the creation of the World Trade Organization.

Globalization has detractors in the West and across the globe. Critics cite problems with the concentration of wealth and power in the hands of rich multinational corporations, regional trade agreements being made in secret, the loss of jobs in the West, the exploitation of cheap labor in the global south, poor environmental policies, low human-rights standards, among other issues. Political opportunists across the globe are making populist – and sometimes nativist – appeals, designed to protect local economies and advance their political interests.

Fragmentation, Interlinked Economies, Global Culture, and Regionalism

Operationally, **fragmentation** is defined as weakening in the ties that bind members of the global community. In some instances, fragmentation can be massively disruptive as countries, economies, regional organizations, and industries have been known to dissolve. Due to globalization, economies across the globe are interlinked. As such, a crisis in one country can have political and economic repercussions in other countries. Over time, a global culture has emerged that appeals to many in the middle and upper class around the globe. This process has helped to produce loyalties beyond the state, as publics identify with regional organizations like the EU. Conversely, **regionalism** is defined as the allegiance that one has to a particular part of a country and not the country at large.

Factors Contributing to Globalization

Globalization—the historical process of breaking down national boundaries in order to create an increasingly interconnected world culture and economy—has been catalyzed by revolutions in corporate capitalism, communication technology, trade, and travel. The so-called "globalization of corporate capitalism"—the process by which corporate capitalism has become the dominant economic system of the entire globe—has spawned economic interdependence in the increasingly interconnected world economy. Communication and technological revolutions have made this advancement possible. In particular, the advent of computer technology, the Internet, and social media has brought disparate global economies closer together under the umbrella of corporate capitalism. Computers allow nations and supranational businesses to maintain 24/7 operations, uniting producers and consumers across the globe. Travel and trade advancements have also assisted this process. Thanks to technological advancements in shipping and travel, people can now access different global economic sectors at a much more regular and efficient rate.

Perspectives on Globalization

Some scholars and activists hail the "progress" made by globalization. They point to the increased communication and understanding between disparate persons, groups, and nations. Other scholars and activists deride globalization and the destruction it has wrought on local communities and the environment. Specifically, many scholars and activists point to the ways in which globalization has catalyzed domestic deindustrialization in countries such as the United States, while simultaneously increasing economic exploitation in at-risk underdeveloped nations. Environmental justice warriors note that globalization has come at an ecological cost. The growing need for resources has inaugurated an age of unsustainable farming, animal slaughtering, and mining.

Social Changes in Globalization

Many sociologists note the direct correlation between globalization, civil unrest, and global terrorism. As more supranational businesses and elite countries compete for limited global resources, more communities are placed at risk of war, terrorism, and genocide. Civil unrest, in this sense, has emerged in this globalized era of human history because many global residents are fighting the forces of economic interdependence and resource competition. Terrorism, specifically Islamic terrorism, has emerged as a strategic response to the growing influence of the West in the globalized economy.

Urbanization

Urbanization is the process by which there is a mass migration to city centers and/or populated regions that results in a rapid population expansion. These urban sectors can expand to become metropolises, a series of interconnected cities or a large central city surrounded by smaller cities. In some cases, urbanization even allows metropolises to expand to the point in which several metropolises conjoin to form a megalopolis. Likewise, urbanization may increase the population of a particular city to over 10 million, which may result in that urban center being rebranded as a "megacity." Urbanization, therefore, not only affects local statistics, but also global economics and politics—the process of urbanization has become so influential in the postindustrial era that cities continue to expand as epicenters of globalization.

Industrialization and Urban Growth

In its nascent stages, urbanization is typically shadowed by **industrialization**, a process by which labor-based sectors expand to offer more working-class jobs to residents. The process of industrialization, brought on by a broader, global Industrial Revolution, has significantly helped developing countries expand through the 19th, 20th, and 21st centuries. Many developing countries, such as Brazil and Mexico, continue to industrialize in the 21st century, making them epicenters of population growth, while many older industrial hubs such as the United States and the United Kingdom have entered multi-decade eras of deindustrialization.

Suburbanization and Urban Decline

Suburbanization is the process by which city residents and surrounding regions come together in a mass exodus to the outskirts (i.e., suburbs) of a particular city. Suburbanization affected the Industrial North pervasively in the 1950-1980s in response to deindustrialization and globalization. As a result, many urban centers entered several decades of **urban decline** in which the "inner city" became synonymous with deindustrialized dilapidation, poverty, drug use, and higher crime rates.

Gentrification and Urban Renewal

Gentrification is the process by which middle-class residents move or return to an urban environment, reinvigorating local real estate prices and local economies. Gentrification is one approach to **urban renewal**—the process of revitalizing rundown sectors of a city. Gentrification, however, remains a controversial approach to urban renewal because it typically displaces and disenfranchises lower-income residents and contributes to the suburbanization of poverty.

Foundational Concept 10: Social stratification and access to resources influence well-being.

Social Inequality

Spatial Inequality

Residential Segregation

Residential segregation occurs when certain groups within society live in neighborhoods that are separated along racial-, ethnic-, socioeconomic-, religious-, or gender-based lines. Some religious sects, such as the Amish of Lancaster, Pennsylvania, choose to segregate themselves from the rest of the world in order to maintain their traditions. Nevertheless, most historical instances of residential segregation have occurred as a result of social engineering techniques by majority populations. In the United States, for instance, racial segregation was made legal in the late 19th and early 20th centuries through Jim Crow laws in the South. Even after these Jim Crow laws diminished as a result of the Civil Rights Movement in the 1960s, residential segregation continues in the United States, due to illegal housing practices.

Neighborhood Safety and Violence

Neighborhood safety and violence is socially engineered within communities. Spatial inequalities place marginalized minority populations at a greater risk of violence while protecting the safety of those with power, privilege, and prestige. Racially and socioeconomically segregated neighborhoods are especially at risk of violence due to lack of adequate policing and resources.

Environmental Justice (Location and Exposure to Health Risks)

Environmental justice, and, conversely, environmental injustice, refers to the ways in which minority statuses, human segregation, and location can directly affect the health of certain marginalized communities. For instance, in Flint, Michigan, the minority status of the city residents led to a form of infrastructural political neglect and environmental injustice. Residents of Flint are still exposed to high amounts of lead in their drinking water due to environmental and infrastructural neglect. Environmental justice warriors are currently battling these wrongdoings, encouraging local, state, and national politicians to end the injustices in Flint, Michigan.

Social Class

Social class and culture influence each other. Class standing influences socioeconomic status, worldview, and personal values. Consequently, these affect the opportunities that might be available to someone in a particular class. Together, all of these aspects create variable cultures across social class strata.

Lower social classes may have restricted access to education, healthcare, or transportation so there may be more emphasis placed on getting a job for financial security as soon as possible, rather than paying money to attend college. Lower social class members may experience or instigate violence to procure resources. They may find more support in one another and have closer-knit communities if resources aren't available, such as trusting neighbors to watch children while at work, rather than paying for childcare. Some studies have reported that members of lower-class neighborhoods tend to be more giving, but usually have poorer overall health outcomes. All of these factors describe the culture often found within lower socio-economic classes.

Higher socio-economic classes may have more access to education, healthcare, and transportation, and usually, they do not have to rely on other people to meet their basic needs. With financial security, these members can focus on their needs and wants first. Their attitudes and beliefs tend to be somewhat entitled and less altruistic, and they are usually able to leverage their wealth to manage problems. Thus, the availability of resources to a particular socio-economic class shapes their worldview. Collectively, this becomes the socio-economic group's culture.

Living in a poor neighborhood causes a domino effect of difficulties. In such areas, there is less access to good healthcare, good educational institutions, and fewer resources for enrichment activities such as tutoring programs, summer camps, or other opportunities for cultural or social development. Residents of poor neighborhoods may engage in risky or maladaptive behaviors to achieve financial security or to express anger at others. There is a greater likelihood that a non-white person will be remanded to prison as opposed to being placed on probation. Research indicates that non-white individuals tend to receive harsher sentences and will spend more time in prison than Caucasians.

Mental health issues and poverty, which are often co-existent in minority cultures, correlate to higher rates of depression, anxiety, and PTSD. There is greater exposure to violence, contributing to feelings of fear, poor self-esteem, and grief. Exclusion and rejection contribute to anxiety and depression. Other minorities struggle with similar issues in the United States. Children of immigrants are often mistreated or bullied because they have not yet learned the language or customs. Clearly, being a nonwhite person in the U.S. can be a disadvantage on a myriad of levels, and the effects of discrimination are widespread and pervasive.

Non-white Americans are far more likely to live in impoverished neighborhoods. For example, young black citizens between the ages of 13 and 28 are ten times more likely to reside in a poor neighborhood than young Caucasians. In addition, there is the concept of **cumulative discrimination**, meaning that the discrimination has been ongoing for generations. Only 7% of white families remain in an impoverished neighborhood for two or more generations, while 48% of African Americans remain in poor neighborhoods for two generations. This indicates that upward mobility is less likely for African Americans.

Aspects of Social Stratification

Class Consciousness and False Consciousness

Within Marxist theory, **class consciousness** refers to a shared awareness and common identity based upon one's socioeconomic position within society. Marx believed class consciousness was necessary for catalyzing a working-class revolution. **False consciousness**, however, occurs when a lower-class citizen mistakenly identifies himself or herself as a member of the elite, capitalist class.

Cultural Capital and Social Capital

Coined by sociologist Pierre Bourdieu (1930-2002), **cultural capital** refers to the financial prowess that one gains from being a member of a certain social group or institution. **Cultural capital**, also coined by Pierre Bourdieu, refers to the non-economic resources (i.e., skills, leisure activities, knowledge, education) that are inherited or earned and consequently affect or enable social mobility.

Social Reproduction

Stemming from Marxist theory, **social reproduction** refers to the privileges and inequalities that are passed on from one generation to the next. People born into privilege are more likely to maintain privilege, while people born into inequality are more likely to inherit inequality.

Power, Privilege, and Prestige

According to intersectionality theory, power, privilege, and prestige often coalesce within a particular identity or group, leading to various displays of social control and coercion. **Power** manifests itself within an identity or group when one can get their way regardless of resistance or opposition. **Privilege** refers to both earned and inherited traits of cultural superiority; these traits can be manifested in reality or myth but are almost always displayed through social control or status reinforcement. **Prestige** refers to the inherited or earned cultural capital that symbolically conveys a sense of superiority or empowerment in the political economy. While power, privilege, and prestige can be used for the social good, the terms are often used pejoratively to describe various abuses of authority.

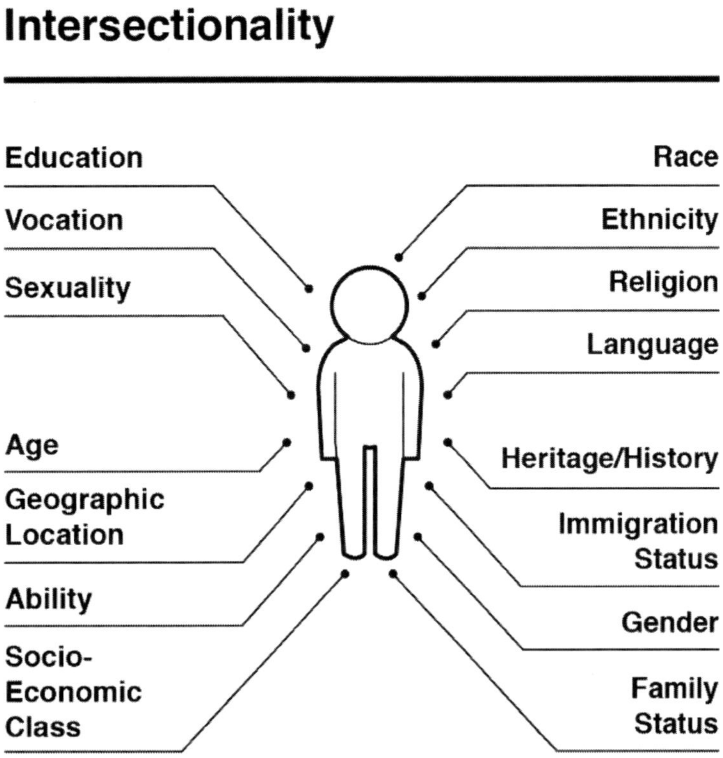

Intersectionality

Intersectionality theory indicates that within every identity there is a unique interplay of sociological variables such race, class, age, and gender. According to intersectionality theory, the interplay of these variables often results in multiple dimensions of oppression and disadvantage. On the flip side, the interplay of these variables may reinforce the power, privilege, and prestige of a particular group or individual.

Socioeconomic Gradient in Health

The **socioeconomic gradient** in health refers to the fact that a population's health status is directly correlated with its socioeconomic status in society. Due to global stratifications, many lower-income groups and sectors are more at-risk in terms of their health because they are denied access to proper healthcare as a result of inadequate resources and spatial inequalities.

Global Inequalities

Much in the way that inequalities exist among neighborhoods in a city, they also exist within the global community. Certain nations or groups are deemed second-class global citizens, and they are therefore denied the healthcare, infrastructure, and resources necessary to thrive in the political economy at large. Developed nations, for instance, tend to have better healthcare systems, infrastructures, and resources than developing or underdeveloped nations.

Patterns of Social Mobility

Intergenerational and Intragenerational Mobility

In the fields of sociology and history, scholars tend to differentiate between short-term and long-term changes in person's social and/or economic disposition. Sociologists and historians try to distinguish between intergenerational and intragenerational social mobility. **Intragenerational mobility** is a term used to describe social and/or economic changes that affect a person during their lifetime; it reveals short-term changes within a particular generation. **Intergenerational mobility** is a term used to describe the vertical mobility of children in relationship to their parents or an entire younger generation in relationship to an older generation; it reveals long-term changes in history, highlighting broad-sweeping superstructural shifts such as industrialization, urbanization, gentrification, and/or suburbanization.

Vertical and Horizontal Mobility

In sociology, **vertical mobility** refers to any kind of social or economic mobility that may increase or decrease the general standing of living for a person or family. Upward vertical mobility may occur when a person or family's social and/or economic standing increases as a result of personal entrepreneurship, marriage, college graduation, or a job promotion. Downward vertical mobility may occur from dropping out of school, loss of a job, inability to earn a college degree, health issues, or even divorce. These notions of upward and downward mobility are often skewed by one's historical context. In fact, most cases of vertical mobility (upward and downward) are actually a product of societal change rather than personal achievement. For example, the Internet tech boom dramatically pushed up the standards of living for millions of United States citizens in the 1990s.

Additionally, superstructural events like the Industrial Revolution positively affected the economies of the United States and Great Britain in the 18th and 19th centuries. Many scholars have, therefore, accepted the term "structural social mobility" to describe upward and downward mobility directly related to broader socioeconomic shifts. For instance, in the recent Great Recession, many global citizens had to cope with downward socioeconomic turns that had nothing to do with their personal merit and everything to do with the superstructural setbacks of a struggling world economy.

Horizontal mobility refers to a change of occupation that moves an employee to a position in a similar income level. These types of lateral shifts, which are common, may provide a worker with the opportunity to transition from blue collar work to white collar work (or vice versa), but they do not provide a significant amount of financial gain (or loss).

Meritocracy

Meritocracy is an academic term that refers to any form of social stratification or social mobility that appears to be dependent upon personal merit. In a pure meritocracy, every individual's position in society would be a direct product of their effort or ability. This, however, is an unrealistic perception. Most industrial and postindustrial societies maintain caste-like systems that limit vertical and horizontal mobility. Moreover, in many industrial and postindustrial societies, wealth is often inherited rather than achieved. This has led many scholars, such as H. Richard Milner, author of *Start Where You Are, But Don't Stay There: Understanding Diversity, Opportunity Gaps, and Teaching in Today's Classrooms* (2010), to point to a so-called "myth of meritocracy." According to scholars like H. Richard Milner, meritocracy is less of a social reality and more of an ideological myth that has been created to reinforce rampant inequality in both capitalist and communist nations.

In the United States, the notion of the "American Dream"—the idea that any American can pull themselves up by their bootstraps—is a notion traditionally based upon meritocratic ideals. In industrial and postindustrial nations such as the United States, many citizens are taught to embrace inequality as a natural byproduct of inherent differences in work ethic or ability. Nevertheless, this worldview ignores the fact that often one's socioeconomic condition is often actually a byproduct of their circumstances or context rather than that person's work ethic or ability. Poverty, like wealth, is often passed on from generation to generation.

Poverty

Poverty is the sociological term used to subjectively describe a certain person or group of people's socioeconomic condition and/or disposition. Within the field of sociology, the creation of a so-called "poverty line" assists sociologists in exploring and assessing global stratification.

Relative and Absolute Poverty

Absolute poverty refers to a lack of resources that may prove to be deadly for a person or group of people. Human beings residing in absolute poverty lack the resources and infrastructure that is necessary to thrive in the global economy. People suffering from absolute poverty often suffer from nutritional and health issues that threaten long-term survival. This means people experience absolute poverty are at high risk of death at a young age. In the United States of America, most citizens do not experience absolute poverty. Most people affected by poverty in the US are affected by **relative poverty**, which means they merely lack some resources that are taken for granted by their fellow U.S. citizens. Relative poverty is more pervasive than absolute poverty in the U.S. because very few poor people residing in the United States are affected by life-threatening situations. The United States has the infrastructure and social welfare institutions to limit the impact of poverty, while other lower-income countries have nearly one-third or more of their populace affected by absolute poverty.

Social Exclusion (Segregation and Isolation)

Poor communities throughout the world remain segregated by class. Poor people (including homeless populations) are typically forced into isolation and social exclusion by the power and privilege of their wealthier peers. In both rural and urban sectors throughout the world, communities remain extremely stratified and segregated along class lines. In the United States, for instance, poverty, once believed to be an "inner-city" phenomenon, is now suburbanizing in many cities at a rapid rate since gentrification is overtaking many of the nation's previously-dilapidated urban cores. In both cases—inner-city or suburban—impoverished communities remain segregated from wealthier ones. Despite many local and national efforts to incentivize cohabitation between the classes, cities across the United States and the world remain highly divided by class lines.

Health Disparities

There are measures that can determine the level of inclusiveness to women in a society. Figures that measure access to quality reproductive health, indices of empowerment, and the participation of women in the labor market are all good indicators of how well a society is achieving gender equality.

The **General Inequality Index** (GII) measures three broad areas: access to healthcare (specifically reproductive health), the empowerment of women in a society, and the amount of women participating in the labor market. Access to quality reproductive healthcare is a key area for women's equality. The GII measures a maternal mortality ratio and adolescent birth rates. The maternal mortality rate is the number of women who die from any type of pregnancy or childbirth complication. It is measured as a ratio of the number of deaths per 100,000 live births. The lower the maternal mortality rate is, the more access women have to quality reproductive healthcare. The adolescent birth rate is defined as the number of births by women aged 15-19. It is normally stated as the number of births per 1,000 women in that same age group. In general, a higher adolescent birth rate means that more young women have limited economic opportunities in a society. Young mothers tend to have less opportunity for education assuming that the society has education available. They also tend to have lower incomes than women of the same age who do not have children.

The second component of the GII seeks to measure the empowerment of women in a society. The empowerment component is a combination of the percentage of women who hold office in the nation's parliament and the proportion of adult women age 25 and older who have some secondary education. The term **secondary education** is used differently in different countries, but in general, it refers to a more advanced education beyond the primary level of education that focuses just on basic reading, writing, and math skills. In the United States, for example, secondary education refers to high school.

The final component of the General Inequality Index is the labor participation rate by women in an economy. The **labor participation rate** is defined as the number of women who are working or looking for work. It does not include any women who are not looking for work because they are either stay-at-home mothers or have just given up trying to find work because of limited opportunity. The participation rate is a good measure of inequality in two ways. First, it can be compared to the labor participation rate among men. A truly equal society would have equal male and female labor participation rates. The greater the difference between the male and female participation rates, the greater the inequality in the economy. Because the participation rate does not include those who have given up looking for work, a falling participation rate among women could be an indicator that a society has become less equal and there are fewer economic opportunities for women.

Human Development Index (HDI)

The **Gender Development Index** (GDI), created by the United Nations in 1995, attempts to measure inequality differences between men and women in three areas of life: health, knowledge, and standard of living. For the healthy life component of the index, the figures for life expectancy are used. A more developed society will have a higher life expectancy rate. The difference between the rate for males and the rate for females is calculated. It is interesting to note that the life expectancy for women in the United States is currently a few years longer than the rate for males. That is not the situation in many less developed nations with greater gender inequality.

The knowledge component measures the number of years of education that a person has. The mean number of years of schooling is assessed for both males and females. That number is then compared to the expected number of years of schooling. The comparison can yield two revealing figures. First, it can provide information about the degree of inequality between the genders. Second, it can give an overall evaluation of how well the society is educating the younger generation because the "mean vs. expected" figure is measured. How well a society is doing in terms of education is determined by the difference between those two figures. The "standard of living" component is measured by using the **Gross National Income** (GNI) per capita. The higher the GNI per capita, the higher the income that a person earns. That higher income allows the person to be able to purchase goods and services that are needed for a better quality of life.

The **Human Development Index** (HDI) was created by economists in the early 1990s to add a human dimension to the standard national income accounting use of GDP and GNI. The HDI attempts to measure more than just how much a nation produces by looking at how well the people in that nation are living. The HDI uses the same three components as the Gender Development Index (GDI). In fact, the GDI was developed after the HDI and was done so with the purpose of making the HDI more focused on gender inequality issues. Each year, the United Nations ranks the nations of the world based on their Human Development Index in an attempt to focus the world's attention on the human aspect of development rather than just the economic development.

Critical Analysis and Reasoning Skills

The Critical Analysis and Reasoning Skills section of the MCAT provides a passage to read and asks test takers to answer questions relating to the passage after they've read it. There are 53 questions in this section and all are passage-based, following complex passages that are roughly 500-600 words in length. The purpose of the Critical Analysis and Reasoning Skills section is to test a student's ability to retain complex text information with the ability to analyze and/or synthesize it, given a certain set of questions. The questions assess *Foundations of Comprehension, Reasoning Within the Text,* and *Reasoning Beyond the Text.* Medical students and physicians are constantly confronted with difficult texts that require tedious analysis, so this section is important for test takers to learn.

The passages and questions encountered on the MCAT will be drawn roughly equally from the social sciences and humanities. While the excepts used may be taken from a variety of books and journals, the social sciences passages are typically more objective and factual, while humanities passages may be more opinionated or conversational, with a focus on relationships of ideas and changes over time. The disciplines from which the content pulls include the arts, various global cultures, ethics, philosophy, literature, religion, architecture, and popular culture, among others. While not an exhaustive list, social sciences passages are typically drawn from education, anthropology, sociology, psychology, public health, linguistics, economics, geography, history, political science, and archeology. The sections below are a comprehensive list of characteristics you will encounter in the passages. Some of the sections, such as *Main Idea* or *Words Used in Context*, should be familiar to you. However, other sections, such as *Principles that Function in the Selection* or *The Impact of New Information*, are subjects that may be unfamiliar to new MCAT test takers.

It's important to remember that it is not necessary to have outside knowledge of the passage information before entering the test. Every question relies on the universe of the passage; therefore, it's important to read the whole passage first and at least designate what the primary purpose or main idea of the passage is. If test takers delve straight into the questions, they may not have a sense of the passage's entirety, and thus will waste time reading answers that have no meaning to them.

Main Idea or Primary Purpose

On the MCAT, some questions may ask test takers to identify the **main idea** or **primary purpose** of the passage. The main idea is what the writer wants to say about that topic. A writer may make the point that global warming is a growing problem that must be addressed in order to save the planet. Therefore, the topic is global warming, and the main idea is that *it's a serious problem needing to be addressed*. The topic can be expressed in a word or two, but the main idea should be a complete thought.

In order to illustrate the main idea, a writer will use **supporting details**—the details that provide evidence or examples to help make a point. Supporting details are typically found in nonfiction texts that seek to inform or persuade the reader.

For example, in the example of global warming, the author's main idea is to show the seriousness of this growing problem and the need for change. The use of supporting details in this piece would be critical in effectively making that point. Supporting details used here might include statistics on an increase in global temperatures and studies showing the impact of global warming on the planet. The author could also include projections for future climate change to illustrate potential lasting effects of global warming.

Some questions may also ask test takers to select the best title for the passage. Going back to the *topic*, for these questions it's important that test takers give a narrower answer that still encompasses the main idea of the passage. Asking for the appropriate title for passages is rare, but it's best to be prepared for anything.

Finally, the MCAT may ask test takers to summarize the passage they've read. Giving a **summary** is different than pointing out the main idea; in a summary, test takers should expect to choose a more comprehensive answer on the passage, one that includes the most important points. In the example of global warming, the summary might be the main idea merged with the most important supporting details. Reading the passage in its entirety before approaching the questions is key to getting a comprehensive look at what the most important aspects of the text will be.

Information that is Explicitly Stated

Readers want to draw a conclusion about what the author has presented. Drawing a conclusion will help the reader to understand what the writer intended as well as whether he or she agrees with what the author has said. There are a few ways to determine the logical conclusion, but careful reading is the most important. The passage should be read a few times, and readers should highlight or take notes on the details that they deem important to the meaning of the piece. Readers may draw a conclusion that is different than what the writer intended, or they may draw more than one conclusion. Readers should look carefully at the details to see if their conclusion matches up with what the writer has presented and intended for readers to understand. Of course, test takers may not have time to take notes or compare on the test itself. However, it may be helpful for test takers to practice this to make sure their comprehension skills are strong.

Textual evidence can help readers to draw a conclusion about a passage. Textual evidence refers to information such as facts and examples that support the main point; it will likely come from outside sources and can be in the form of quoted or paraphrased material. Readers should look to this evidence and its credibility and validity in relation to the main idea to draw a conclusion about the writing.

The author may state the conclusion directly in the passage. Inferring the author's conclusion is useful, especially when it is not overtly stated, but inferences should not outweigh the information that is directly stated. Alternatively, when readers are trying to draw a conclusion about a text, it may not always be directly stated.

As mentioned before, summary is another effective way to draw a conclusion from a passage. Summary is a shortened version of the original text, written in one's own words. It should focus on the main points of the original text, including only the relevant details. It's important to be brief but thorough in a summary. While the summary should always be shorter than the original passage, it should still retain the meaning of the original source.

Like summary, **paraphrasing** can also help a reader to fully understand a part of a reading. Paraphrase calls for the reader to take a small part of the passage and to say it in their own words. Paraphrase is more than rewording the original passage, though. It should be written in one's own way, while still retaining the meaning of the original source. When a reader's goal is to write something in their own words, deeper understanding of the original source is required. Again, applying summary and paraphrase to the passages during the test may not be the most efficient use of the test taker's time. However, these tools should be considered when one is practicing comprehending passages. Test takers who are familiar with carefully selecting important aspects of the passage will benefit from this experience on test day.

The Purpose of Words or Phrases as Used in Context

Knowledge of synonyms and antonyms is crucial for writing and identifying a good paraphrase, and it also helps readers expand their mental vocabulary network. Another useful vocabulary skill is being able to understand meaning in context. A word's **context** refers to all the other words and information surrounding it, and the context of a word can have an impact on how readers interpret that word's meaning. Of course, many words have more than one definition. For example, consider the meaning of the word *engaged*. The first definition that comes to mind might be "promised to be married," but consider the following sentences:

A. The two armies engaged in a conflict that lasted all night.
B. The three-hour lecture flew by because students were so engaged in the material.
C. The busy executive engaged a new assistant to help with his workload.

As you can see, *engaged* has a variety of other meanings. In these sentences, respectively, it can mean: "battled," "interested or involved," and "appointed or employed." With so many possible definitions, readers may wonder how to decide which one to apply in a given sentence. The appropriate meaning is prioritized based on context. For example, sentence *C* mentions "executive," "assistant," and "workload," so readers can assume that *engaged* has something to do with work—in which case, "appointed or employed" would be the best definition for this context. Context clues can also be found in sentence *A*. Words like "armies" and "conflicts" show that this sentence is about a military situation (and not about marriage or the office), so in this context, *engaged* is closest in meaning to "battled." By using context clues—the surrounding words in the sentence—readers can easily select the most appropriate definition for the word in question.

In addition to helping readers select the best meaning for a word with many definitions, context clues can also help readers when they don't know any meanings for a certain word. Test writers will deliberately ask about vocabulary that test takers are probably unfamiliar with in order to measure their ability to use context to make an educated guess about a word's meaning.

Which of the following is the closest in meaning to the word *loquacious* in the following sentence?
The loquacious professor was notorious for always taking too long to finish his lectures.

a. Knowledgeable
b. Enthusiastic
c. Approachable
d. Talkative

Even if the word *loquacious* seems completely new, it is still possible to utilize context to make a good guess about the word's meaning. Grammatically, it is apparent that *loquacious* is an adjective that modifies the noun "professor"—so l*oquacious* must be some kind of quality or characteristic. A clue in this sentence is "taking too long to finish his lectures." Readers should then brainstorm qualities that might cause a professor to be late. Perhaps he is "disorganized," "slow," or "talkative"—all words that might still make sense in this sentence. After brainstorming some ideas for the word's definition, take a look at the choices for the question. Choice *D* matches one word from the brainstorming session, and it is a logical choice for this sentence—the professor talks too much, so his lectures run late. In fact, *loquacious* means "talkative" or "wordy."

One way that readers can use context clues is to think of potential replacement words before considering the answer choices given in the question. However, if it is truly a struggle to come up with any possibilities, readers should turn to the answer choices first and try to replace each of them in the sentence to see if the sentence is still logical and retains the same meaning.

Which of the following is the closest in meaning to the word *dogma* in the following sentence?
Martin Luther was a revolutionary religious figure because he argued against Catholic dogma and encouraged a new interpretation of Christianity.

a. Punishments
b. Doctrines
c. Leadership
d. Procedures

Based on context, this sentence has something to do with religious conflict and interpretations of Christian faith. The only word related to religious belief is Choice *B*, *doctrines*, which is in fact the best synonym for *dogma*.

Yet another way to use context clues is to consider clues in the word itself. Most students are probably familiar with prefixes, suffixes, and root words—the building blocks of many English words. A little knowledge goes a long way when it comes to these components of English vocabulary, and they can point readers in the right direction when they need help finding an appropriate definition.

Which of the following is the closest in meaning to the word *antipathy* in the following sentence?
A strong antipathy existed between Margaret and her new neighbor, Susan.

a. Enmity
b. Resemblance
c. Relationship
d. Alliance

In this case, the sentence does not provide much context for the word *antipathy*. However, the word itself gives some useful clues. The prefix *anti-* means "opposite or against," so *antipathy* probably has a negative meaning. Also, if readers already know words like "sympathy" or "empathy," they might guess that the root word "path" is related to emotions. So, *antipathy* must be a feeling *against* something. *Alliance* is a positive connection, *relationship* is too neutral, and *resemblance* means two things are similar to each other. The only word that shows a negative or opposite feeling is Choice *A*, *enmity* (the feeling of being enemies). In this way, even an unfamiliar word contains clues that can indicate its meaning.

Author's Attitude in the Tone of a Passage

Style, tone, and mood are often thought to be the same thing. Although they're closely related, there are important differences to keep in mind. The easiest way to do this is to remember that style creates and affects tone and mood. More specifically, **style** is *how the writer uses words* to create the desired tone and mood for their writing.

Style

Style can include any number of technical writing choices, and some may have to be analyzed on the test. A few examples of style choices include:

- Sentence Construction: When presenting facts, does the writer use shorter sentences to create a quicker sense of the supporting evidence, or do they use longer sentences to elaborate and explain the information?
- Technical Language: Does the writer use jargon to demonstrate their expertise in the subject, or do they use ordinary language to help the reader understand things in simple terms?
- Formal Language: Does the writer refrain from using contractions such as *won't* or *can't* to create a more formal tone, or do they use a colloquial, conversational style to connect with the reader?
- Formatting: Does the writer use a series of shorter paragraphs to help the reader follow a line of argument, or do they use longer paragraphs to examine an issue in great detail and demonstrate their knowledge of the topic?

On the exam, test takers should examine the writer's style and how the author's writing choices affect the way that the text comes across.

Tone

Tone refers to the writer's attitude toward the subject matter. For example, the tone conveys how the writer feels about the topic he or she is writing about. A lot of nonfiction writing has a neutral tone, which is an important tone for the writer to take. A neutral tone demonstrates that the writer is presenting a topic impartially and letting the information speak for itself. On the other hand, nonfiction writing can be just as effective and appropriate if the tone isn't neutral. For instance, take this example:

> Seat belts save more lives than any other automobile safety feature. Many studies show that airbags save lives as well; however, not all cars have airbags. For instance, some older cars don't. Furthermore, air bags aren't entirely reliable. For example, studies show that in 15% of accidents airbags don't deploy as designed, but, on the other hand, seat belt malfunctions are extremely rare. The number of highway fatalities has plummeted since laws requiring seat belt usage were enacted.

In this passage, the writer mostly chooses to retain a neutral tone when presenting information. If the writer would instead include their own personal experience of losing a friend or family member in a car accident, the tone would change dramatically. The tone would no longer be neutral and would show that the writer has a personal stake in the content, allowing them to interpret the information in a different way. When analyzing tone, test takers should consider what the writer is trying to achieve in the text and how they *create* the tone using style.

Mood

Mood refers to the feelings and atmosphere that the writer's words create for the reader. Like tone, many nonfiction texts can have a neutral mood. To return to the previous example, if the writer would choose to include information about a person they know being killed in a car accident, the text would suddenly carry an emotional component that is absent in the previous example. Depending on how the writer presents the information, he or she can create a sad, angry, or even hopeful mood. When analyzing the mood, test takers should consider what the writer wants to accomplish and whether the best choice was made to achieve that end.

Types of Appeals

In nonfiction writing, authors employ argumentative techniques to present their opinion to readers in the most convincing way. Persuasive writing usually includes at least one type of appeal: an appeal to logic (**logos**), emotion (**pathos**), or credibility and trustworthiness (**ethos**). When writers appeal to logic, they are asking readers to agree with them based on research, evidence, and an established line of reasoning. An author's argument might also appeal to readers' emotions, perhaps by including personal stories and **anecdotes** (a short narrative of a specific event). A final type of appeal, appeal to authority, asks the reader to agree with the author's argument on the basis of their expertise or credentials. Consider three different approaches to arguing the same opinion:

Logic (Logos)

Below is an example of an appeal to logic. The author uses evidence to disprove the logic of the school's rule (the rule was supposed to reduce discipline problems, but the number of problems has not been reduced; therefore, the rule is not working) and call for its repeal.

> Our school should abolish its current ban on campus cell phone use. The ban was adopted last year as an attempt to reduce class disruptions and help students focus more on their lessons. However, since the rule was enacted, there has been no change in the number of disciplinary problems in class. Therefore, the rule is ineffective and should be done away with.

Emotion (Pathos)

An author's argument might also appeal to readers' emotions, perhaps by including personal stories and anecdotes. The next example presents an appeal to emotion. By sharing the personal anecdote of one student and speaking about emotional topics like family relationships, the author invokes the reader's empathy in asking them to reconsider the school rule.

> Our school should abolish its current ban on campus cell phone use. If students aren't able to use their phones during the school day, many of them feel isolated from their loved ones. For example, last semester, one student's grandmother had a heart attack in the morning. However, because he couldn't use his cell phone, the student didn't know about his grandmother's accident until the end of the day—when she had already passed away, and it was too late to say goodbye. By preventing students from contacting their friends and family, our school is placing undue stress and anxiety on students.

Credibility (Ethos)

Finally, an appeal to authority includes a statement from a relevant expert. In this case, the author uses a doctor in the field of education to support the argument. All three examples begin from the same opinion—the school's phone ban needs to change—but rely on different argumentative styles to persuade the reader.

> Our school should abolish its current ban on campus cell phone use. According to Dr. Bartholomew Everett, a leading educational expert, "Research studies show that cell phone usage has no real impact on student attentiveness. Rather, phones provide a valuable technological resource for learning. Schools need to learn how to integrate this new technology into their curriculum." Rather than banning phones altogether, our school should follow the advice of experts and allow students to use phones as part of their learning.

Rhetorical Questions

Another commonly used argumentative technique is asking **rhetorical questions**—questions that do not actually require an answer but that push the reader to consider the topic further.

> I wholly disagree with the proposal to ban restaurants from serving foods with high sugar and sodium contents. Do we really want to live in a world where the government can control what we eat? I prefer to make my own food choices.

Here, the author's rhetorical question prompts readers to put themselves in a hypothetical situation and imagine how they would feel about it.

The Organization or Structure

Good writing is not merely a random collection of sentences. No matter how well written, sentences must relate and coordinate appropriately to one another. If not, the writing seems random, haphazard, and disorganized. Therefore, good writing must be organized, where each sentence fits a larger context and relates to the sentences around it.

Text Structures

Depending on what the author is attempting to accomplish, certain formats or text structures work better than others. For example, a sequence structure might work for narration but not for identifying similarities and differences between concepts. Similarly, a comparison-contrast structure is not useful for narration. It's the author's job to put the right information in the correct format.

Readers should be familiar with the five main literary structures:

Sequence Structure

Sequence structure, sometimes referred to as the **order structure**, is when the order of events proceeds in a predictable order. In many cases, this means the text goes through the plot elements: exposition, rising action, climax, falling action, and resolution. Readers are introduced to the characters, setting, and conflict in the

exposition. In the **rising action**, there's an increase in tension and suspense. The **climax** is the height of tension and the point of no return. Tension decreases during the **falling action**. In the **resolution**, any conflicts presented in the exposition are resolved, and the story concludes. An informative text that is structured sequentially will often go in order from one step to the next.

Problem-Solution

In the **problem-solution structure**, authors identify a potential problem and suggest a solution. This form of writing is usually divided into two paragraphs and can be found in informational texts. For example, cellphone, cable, and satellite providers use this structure in manuals to help customers troubleshoot or identify problems with services or products.

Comparison-Contrast

When authors want to discuss similarities and differences between separate concepts, they arrange thoughts in a **comparison-contrast** paragraph structure. Venn diagrams are an effective graphic organizer for comparison-contrast structures because they feature two overlapping circles that can be used to organize similarities and differences. A comparison-contrast essay organizes one paragraph based on similarities and another based on differences. A comparison-contrast essay can also be arranged with the similarities and differences of individual traits addressed within individual paragraphs. Words such as *however*, *but*, and *nevertheless* help signal a contrast in ideas.

Descriptive

Descriptive writing structure is designed to appeal to the reader's senses. Much like an artist who constructs a painting, good descriptive writing builds an image in the reader's mind by appealing to the five senses: sight, hearing, taste, touch, and smell. However, overly descriptive writing can become tedious; likewise, sparse descriptions can make settings and characters seem flat. Good authors strike a balance by applying descriptions only to facts that are integral to the passage.

Cause and Effect

Passages that use the **cause and effect** structure are simply asking *why* by demonstrating some type of connection between ideas. Words such as *if*, *since*, *because*, *then*, or *consequently* indicate this relationship. By switching the order of a complex sentence, the writer can rearrange the emphasis on different clauses. Saying, *If Sheryl is late, we'll miss the dance*, is different from saying *We'll miss the dance if Sheryl is late*. The first example emphasizes Sheryl's tardiness while the other emphasizes missing the dance. Paragraphs can also be arranged in a cause and effect format. Since the format—before and after—is sequential, it is useful when authors wish to discuss the impact of choices. Researchers often apply this paragraph structure to the scientific method.

Transition Words

The writer should act as a guide, showing the reader how all the sentences fit together. Consider this example:

> Seat belts save more lives than any other automobile safety feature. Many studies show that airbags save lives as well. Not all cars have airbags. Many older cars don't. Air bags aren't entirely reliable. Studies show that in 15% of accidents, airbags don't deploy as designed. Seat belt malfunctions are extremely rare.

There's nothing wrong with any of these sentences individually, but together they're disjointed and difficult to follow. The best way for the writer to communicate information smoothly is with transition words. Here are examples of transition words and phrases that tie sentences together, enabling a more natural flow:

- To show causality: as a result, therefore, and consequently
- To compare and contrast: *however*, *but*, and *on the other hand*

- To introduce examples: *for instance*, *namely*, and *including*
- To show order of importance: *foremost*, *primarily*, *secondly*, and *lastly*

NOTE: This is not a complete list of transitions. There are many more that can be used; however, most fit into these or similar categories. The point is that the words should clearly show the relationship between sentences, supporting information, and the main idea.

Here is an update to the previous example using transition words. These changes make it easier to read and bring clarity to the writer's points:

> Seat belts save more lives than any other automobile safety feature. Many studies show that airbags save lives as well; however, not all cars have airbags. For instance, some older cars don't. Furthermore, air bags aren't entirely reliable. For example, studies show that in 15% of accidents, airbags don't deploy as designed, but, on the other hand, seat belt malfunctions are extremely rare.

Test takers should Also, be prepared to analyze whether the writer is using the best transition word or phrase for the situation. Take this sentence for example: "As a result, seat belt malfunctions are extremely rare." This sentence doesn't make sense in the context above because the writer is trying to show the contrast between seat belts and airbags, not the causality.

Logical Sequence

Even if the writer includes plenty of information to support their point, the writing is only coherent when the information is in a logical order. Logical sequencing is really just common sense, but it's also an important writing technique. First, the writer should introduce the main idea, whether for a paragraph, a section, or the entire piece. Then they should present evidence to support the main idea by using transitional language. This shows the reader how the information relates to the main idea and the sentences around it. The writer should then take time to interpret the information, making sure necessary connections are obvious to the reader. Finally, the writer can summarize the information in a closing section.

NOTE: Although most writing follows this pattern, it isn't a set rule. Sometimes writers change the order for effect. For example, the writer can begin with a surprising piece of supporting information to grab the reader's attention, and then transition to the main idea. Thus, if a passage doesn't follow the logical order, test takers should not immediately assume it's wrong. However, most writing usually settles into a logical sequence after a nontraditional beginning.

Introductions and Conclusions

Examining the writer's strategies for introductions and conclusions puts the reader in the right mindset to interpret the rest of the text. Test takers should look for methods the writer might use for introductions such as:

- Stating the main point immediately, followed by outlining how the rest of the piece supports this claim.
- Establishing important, smaller pieces of the main idea first, and then grouping these points into a case for the main idea.
- Opening with a quotation, anecdote, question, seeming paradox, or other piece of interesting information, and then using it to lead to the main point.
- Whatever method the writer chooses, the introduction should make their intention clear, establish their voice as a credible one, and encourage a person to continue reading.

Conclusions tend to follow a similar pattern. In them, the writer restates their main idea a final time, often after summarizing the smaller pieces of that idea. If the introduction uses a quote or anecdote to grab the reader's attention, the conclusion often makes reference to it again. Whatever way the writer chooses to arrange the conclusion, the final restatement of the main idea should be clear and simple for the reader to interpret. Finally, conclusions shouldn't introduce any new information.

Information or Ideas that can be Inferred

Inference questions require drawing a conclusion using reasoning and evidence. Making an **inference** requires careful reading of the passage to determine the author's intended meaning. The author's main idea or overall meaning may be directly stated in the passage, but in some cases, it is not. The **implied meaning** is, by definition, not explicitly stated in the passage, so it is necessary for readers to use details from the passage to decipher the author's implications. It is possible for readers to draw a logical conclusion about the author's intended meaning by using the facts and evidence presented in the passage.

The Premise

Inference questions are based on the premises provided in the passage. **Premises** are the facts or evidence presented by the author. These premises should be taken as fact, even if they are based on the author's opinion. In some cases, the reader may disagree with the premises presented, or even know them to be untrue, but it is important to view the premises as fact. This is what the author believes and wants the reader to believe, so the premises will help lead the reader to the most logical conclusion.

There are certain clue words that can indicate the premises in a passage. These clue words include:

- because
- for
- since
- as
- given that
- in that
- as indicated by
- owing to

While these words can help the reader discover the author's premises, making an inference requires reading between the lines to find the implied meaning of the passage. The implications of the facts are what lead the reader to a logical conclusion.

Question Types

An inference question may focus on a word's meaning or ask the reader to draw a conclusion based on the evidence presented. It is helpful for readers to know that a question calls for inference, so it is not confused with assumption.

Some clues to look for are questions that use statements like the following:

- If the previous statements are true, it logically follows that
- Must be true
- Author's conclusion
- Best supported by

It's important for test takers to remember that the facts presented should be taken as true, even if they aren't. When answering this type of question, answers that could be true, but not based on the facts presented in the passage, should be avoided. Instead, readers should look for the only answer that must be true based on the premises provided. Test takers should also avoid making assumptions, as this is a different type of question. Making an inference is about drawing a logical conclusion based on facts, not making assumptions.

Answer Types

Test takers should avoid answers that go too far in their value judgment. These answers are often distractors and can be identified by use of words like *always*, *never*, *only*, and *must*. These absolutes are tough to prove, and likely not to be inferred. The words to look for in the answers to inference questions are *some*, *most*, *can*, and *possibly*, because these are far more likely to indicate an inferred conclusion. Another distractor is an answer that is based on a different subject altogether. This is likely not the answer to an inference question and can typically be thrown out.

Sample Question

> Congress passed the Older Americans Act (OAA) in 1965 in response to concern by policymakers about a lack of community social services for older persons. The original legislation established authority for grants to States for community planning and social services, research and development projects, and personnel training in the field of aging. The law also established the Administration on Aging (AoA) to administer the newly created grant programs and to serve as the Federal focal point on matters concerning older persons.
>
> Although older individuals may receive services under many other Federal programs, today the OAA is considered to be the major vehicle for the organization and delivery of social and nutrition services to this group and their caregivers. It authorizes a wide array of service programs through a national network of 56 State agencies on aging, 629 area agencies on aging, nearly 20,000 service providers, 244 Tribal organizations, and 2 Native Hawaiian organizations representing 400 Tribes. The OAA also includes community service employment for low-income older Americans; training, research, and demonstration activities in the field of aging; and vulnerable elder rights protection activities. – Adapted from AOA.gov

Based on the above passage, which of the following must be true?

a. The OAA needs additional funding from the private sector.
b. Native Hawaiians are always underrepresented in the OAA.
c. The elderly are in need of protection of their rights.
d. Nutrition needs of the elderly are severely neglected in this country.

The best answer here is *C*. The author's main idea in this passage is that the OAA was created and exists to provide social services and protect the rights of the elderly. Based on this information, it can be logically inferred that the author believes the elderly need protection of their rights.

Choice *A* is incorrect because the passage mentions that the OAA is funded through grants, and there is no indication of a need for additional funding. It would be an assumption, not an inference, to conclude that more funding is needed from the private sector.

Choice *B* uses an absolute with the use of "never." Use of an absolute could be an indicator of an incorrect answer. While there are only two Native Hawaiian organizations identified as being represented by the OAA in the passage, it states that they represent 400 Tribes. This does not suggest an underrepresentation of this group in the OAA.

Choice *D* requires an assumption, not inference, based on the author's premises. The passage states that the OAA was created in response to a lack of services for the elderly. The OAA has become the biggest organization meeting the nutritional needs of the elderly, so it cannot be inferred that their nutritional needs are being neglected. This answer requires assumption, not inference, based on the author's premises.

The Application of Information in the Selection to a New Context

A natural extension of being able to make an inference from a given set of information is also being able to apply that information to a new context. This is especially useful in nonfiction or informative writing. Considering the facts and details presented in the text, readers should consider how the same information might be relevant in a different situation. The following is an example of applying an inferential conclusion to a different context:

> Often, individuals behave differently in large groups than they do as individuals. One example of this is the psychological phenomenon known as the bystander effect. According to the bystander effect, the more people who witness an accident or crime occur, the less likely each individual bystander is to respond or offer assistance to the victim. A classic example of this is the murder of Kitty Genovese in New York City in the 1960s. Although there were over thirty witnesses to her killing by a stabber, none of them intervened to help Kitty or contacted the police.

Considering the phenomenon of the bystander effect, what would probably happen if somebody tripped on the stairs in a crowded subway station?

a. Everybody would stop to help the person who tripped.
b. Bystanders would point and laugh at the person who tripped.
c. Someone would call the police after walking away from the station.
d. Few, if any, bystanders would aid the person who tripped.

This question asks readers to apply the information they learned from the passage, which is an informative paragraph about the bystander effect. According to the passage, this is a concept in psychology that describes the way people in groups respond to an accident—the more people that are present, the less likely any one person is to intervene. While the passage illustrates this effect with the example of a woman's murder, the question asks readers to apply it to a different context—in this case, someone falling down the stairs in front of many subway passengers. Although this specific situation is not discussed in the passage, readers should be able to apply the general concepts described in the paragraph. The definition of the bystander effect includes any instance of an accident or crime in front of a large group of people. The question asks about a situation that falls within the same definition, so the general concept should still hold true: amid a large crowd, few individuals are likely to actually respond to an accident. In this case, answer Choice *D* is the best response.

Principles that Function in the Selection

A **principle** can be defined as a fundamental truth that functions as the foundation of a system of belief, behavior, or reasoning. Expressed another way, a principle is a core truth that cannot be violated. The MCAT examiners write Critical Analysis and Reasoning Skills passages that rely on or express some principle, and the most common principle questions ask test takers to correctly identify the principle expressed in the passage. In addition, some question stems will provide a principle, state that it is true, and ask the test taker to select the answer choice that best describes how the stated principle impacts the passage. The Critical Analysis and Reasoning Skills section also might be composed of two passages, where one passage commonly states the principle, while the other applies it. Principle question stems are typically easy to identify since they will explicitly include the word *principle* or a synonym. Here is an example of a principle question stem:

> The reasoning in the passage most conforms to which of the following principles?

The overwhelming majority of principle questions will list the principles as answer choices, and the test taker should select the principle that best matches the passage.

The MCAT requires test takers to analyze and apply myriad concepts; however, determining a principle's validity will never be a question. If the author asserts the principle that all capitalist economic systems are doomed to fail and asks test takers to identify the principle, then they should select the answer stating that all capitalist systems are doomed to fail. No matter how sensational, the real-world validity of the principle is never in question. By their very definition, principles are outcome determinatives for any situation falling within its universe. Thus, the question that a test taker must always ask is: assuming this principle is true, how does it impact or match the given situation? If the principle is valid, which is assumed in the MCAT, and the specific circumstances fall within the principle's criteria, then the conclusion must adhere to the principle. As a result, answering principle questions is just a matter of matching the passage's specifics with the most appropriate principle.

The first step to interpreting principles is determining whether each principle is broad or narrow. Since everything covered by the principle is true, determining the confines will change how many situations the principle controls. Test takers should pay close attention to limiting language, or lack thereof, in the stated principle. Keywords to consider include: *all*, *every*, *any*, *some*, *never*, *none*, *no*, *anyone*, *everyone*, and any other similar words that describe an amount of something. Difference in language will decide whether some action or statement will, could, or could not happen, or be true. In addition, test takers should look for limitations on the group required for the principle to be activated. If the principle's stated limitation excludes some category or requires some characteristic, then it will not apply in situations not covered by the limitation. Consider the difference between the following principles:

- Every American will vote in the upcoming presidential election.
- All Americans interested in politics will vote in the upcoming presidential election.
- Some Americans will vote in the upcoming presidential election.
- No Americans will vote in the upcoming presidential election.

What do these principles say about an individual American? The first principle dictates that the simple fact that the individual is American necessitates that he or she will vote in the upcoming presidential election. As discussed at length above, the test taker must not consider external facts, such as the voting rate being substantially lower than one hundred percent in every American presidential election. This type of principle is outcome determinative for anyone who is an American. If you are an American, then you will vote in the upcoming presidential election. Although the second principle begins with *all*, it includes a limiting requirement, "interested in politics," that must be accounted for in the analysis.

It is unclear whether the individual American is interested in politics, and there is no way to find out that fact with the information provided; thus, this principle does not force any conclusion in this situation. The third principle only tells us that some Americans will vote; thus, it is both possible that the individual American will and will not vote, but no outcome is forced. The fourth principle is similar to the first principle since it is outcome determinative. The individual is American; no Americans will vote in the upcoming presidential election; thus, the individual will not be voting. This type of analysis should be used to determine what principle best matches the passage.

Principles can sometimes be converted into *if-then* statements, also known as **conditional statements**, which allow for inferences to be drawn. These inferences provide additional information that is useful for identifying the passage's principle. Before drawing an inference is possible, the principle must be converted into a conditional statement. For example:

> Original: Every American will vote in the upcoming presidential election.
>
> Conversion: If an individual is American, then that individual will vote in the upcoming presidential election.
>
> Representation: A → V (American → Vote)

In this scenario, the knowledge that an individual is American functions as a sufficient condition, since knowing that fact alone is sufficient to knowing something else—that individual will vote. Voting is referred to as the necessary condition since it necessarily must occur if the sufficient condition is triggered. Conditional statements can also be negated and flipped to reveal a second inference. This is known as the **contrapositive**. The example can be restated as the following:

> Contrapositive: If an individual will not vote in the upcoming presidential election, then that individual is not an American.
>
> Representation: ~~V~~ → ~~A~~ (~~Vote~~ → ~~American~~)

When writing the contrapositive, crossing out the symbol is shorthand for *not*. Depending on the complexity of the principle, as well as the test taker's familiarity with conditional statements, converting the principle might not be feasible in terms of time management. However, if possible, test takers should be cognizant of the effectiveness of conditional statements in evaluating principle questions.

Analogies to Claims or Arguments in the Selection

Analogous questions challenge test takers' understanding of the passage by asking questions involving the recognition of structurally similar arguments. Test takers often struggle with analogies to claims within a Critical Analysis and Reasoning Skills passage for two reasons. First, analogies inherently test abstract reasoning. The questions ask test takers to draw comparisons between situations that appear entirely unrelated on the surface. Emphasis is placed on logical structure rather than substantive content. For this reason, analogies to claims in the Critical Analysis and Reasoning Skills section are most similar to the parallel reasoning questions that appear in the logical reasoning section. Second, these questions take up a disproportionate amount of finite time relative to other question types.

Due to the abstract nature of these analogy questions, all of the answer choices must be given special scrutiny. It will likely be more difficult to immediately eliminate a choice, since every choice will form its own claim or element. Therefore, test takers must break down each answer choice into its corresponding elements and then compare those elements with the argument or claim from the passage. In addition, the smallest detail will often separate the correct answer from the next best option.

With that said, analogies to claims are not to be feared. Although admittedly cumbersome, they only require completing and repeating one of the most tested concepts on the MCAT—identifying conclusions and determining how premises operate to support those conclusions. The question stem will provide a quote or direct test takers to a set of lines from the passage. Sometimes the quote or line reference will isolate a single claim or argument from the passage, while other times the required interpretation will rely on the passage's broader context. This skill requires using abstract reasoning to draw analogies between situations, and the strongest analogy will typically prevail.

Analogies to claims questions will be easy to identify since *analogous* will almost always appear directly in the question stem. In less common instances, the question stem might include some derivation of application or ask what scenario is *most similar* to the logic deployed in the passage. Here is an example of an analogous question stem:

> Given Friedman's economic theory, as expressed between lines 32 and 45 in the passage, which one of the following is most analogous to the role monetary policy plays in his theory?

When initially reading through the passage, test takers need to pay close attention to differing theories, arguments, or claims, especially from competing sources. For example, a passage about economics might include arguments from two or more economists. In this scenario, the analogous question will always identify which of the competing arguments to analogize. Test takers should never stray from the constraints provided in the question stem. If the economics passage includes arguments from John Maynard Keynes, Milton Friedman, and Karl Marx, but the question only asks how Friedman's theory applies to different scenarios, only focus on the portion of the passage devoted to Friedman. For the purposes of this question, the theories of Keynes and Marx are irrelevant.

The abstract reasoning behind analogous questions forces test takers to compare the logical structure of claims and arguments. The MCAT often includes answer choices that closely mirror the substance of the passage, rather than its structure. Test takers must be careful not to fall for this trick—whether the passage and answer choice discuss the same substantive topic is irrelevant. As a result, test takers should be extremely cautious of answer choices that use similar language or cover identical topics as the claim in the passage. In fact, these type of similar substance answers are usually incorrect, functioning as a red herring to catch the less astute test takers who fail to analyze the structure.

The table below contains some general frameworks that MCAT examiners use to analogize between the passage and answer choices. These are not an exhaustive list of analogous situations included in the Critical Analysis and Reasoning Skills section; however, reviewing these examples provides a framework for thinking about patterns in analogous questions.

General Structure	Example of an Analogy
Cause and effect	A scientist meticulously attempts a variety of methods and ultimately cures a deadly disease. A student reads her textbook, watches class lectures, and listens to an audio recording from a panel of experts, and she achieves the highest grade in her class.
Part and whole (subset)	All whales are mammals but not all mammals are whales. All prosecutors are lawyers but not all lawyers are prosecutors.
Unintended consequence	A town passes legislation outlawing the hunting of deer to increase their population, but the exploding deer population eats all of the vegetation, and their population decreases. An airline invests in a new silent plane to attract more customers, but their business decreases as customers become irritated with the noise from the bathroom and side conversations that had previously been blocked out by the engine noise.
Confusing causation (especially with correlation)	Ice cream sales rise at the same time as the murder rate similarly increases, but the actual cause of both is more people outside during the summer. A textbook company doubles its sales at the same time the company moves its headquarters to a more prestigious location, but the actual cause of both is an increase in capital investment.
Performance relative to a defined standard	A teenager loses his driver's license after amassing too many points as a result of accidents and speeding tickets. A doctor loses his medical license after a series of patients win medical malpractice actions against him.

To answer analogous questions, the test taker should first reread the passage's discussion of the quote or lines referenced by the question stem. Next, the test taker should generally summarize the structure of the presented claim or argument. For example, many analogous questions ask what logical error the author committed, so the summary would be a short description of that error. This summary should be a slightly more detailed version of what appears in the chart's left column. Lastly, the test taker should make similar summaries for each answer choice, and then the closest match will be the correct answer.

The Impact of New Information on Claims or Arguments in the Selection

Critical Analysis and Reasoning Skills question stems will occasionally supplement the passage with new information in the answer choices. The new information will typically impact the conclusion of the entire passage or a supporting claim. The correct answer in a new information question will always do more than merely relate to the same substantive topic as the claim or argument in the passage; the new information will have a direct impact on the claim's plausibility or likelihood. Fortunately, new information questions are essentially strengthening or weakening questions, and the question stem will explicitly specify which of the two is being asked. Here is an example of a weakening question stem:

> Which of the following, if true, would most undermine the author's claim that *Infinite Jest* is the most rewarding book to read?

Here is an example of a strengthening question:

> Which of the following, if true, best supports the author's contention that capitalism is the most effective economic system?

Test takers should notice that the question stem includes the caveat "if true." All new information questions will include such a caveat, so the plausibility or validity of the new information should never be questioned based on real-world knowledge. The new information will likely involve an unaccounted-for fact, expert opinion, recent discovery, or some other substantive statement related to the passage. The next table includes the most common synonyms for *strengthen* or *weaken* to help identify new information questions.

Strengthen	**Weaken**
Support	Undermine
Fortify	Challenge
Buttress	Diminish
Reinforce	Impair
Fortify	Erode
Bolster	Call into question
Underpin	Lessen
Augment	Undercut
Supplement	Damage

The easiest type of new information question will simply ask which of the following statements weakens or strengthens the claim or argument. If the question stem does not include a modifier, such as *best* or *most*, then only one of the answer choices will weaken or strengthen the claim; it would be impossible for more than one answer choice to strengthen or weaken the claim in such a situation. This makes the question much more approachable, since only one answer choice will impact the argument in the right direction.

When the question does include the *best* or *most* modifier, then multiple answer choices will provide new information that impact the claim in the right direction. In this scenario, the test taker should immediately eliminate any answer choice that does the opposite. For example, if the question asks what best supports a claim, then test takers can eliminate any answer choice that weakens it. In addition, any answer choice that is neutral or irrelevant can be eliminated. Of the remaining answer choices, test takers should select the answer choice that is most relevant to the claim, which usually presents itself by directly addressing the conclusion or an important premise. Similarly, new information questions will occasionally come in the *except* variety. These questions are actually quite similar to the simple weaken or strengthen question, since there will only be one answer choice moving in the right direction. However, test takers should always make sure to read the question stem carefully, or else the question will be impossible to answer correctly.

Test takers often fret over new information questions, believing that the new information will completely fortify or totally deconstruct the argument. Although such extreme scenarios would actually be easier to answer, the correct answer will just make the argument more likely or less likely to be plausible. As with most of the other questions in the Critical Analysis and Reasoning Skills section, identifying conclusions and evaluating premises is by far the most important skill. The correct answers will almost always impact the conclusion by altering the premises.

For strengthen questions, test takers should review the claim or argument in the context of the passage and evaluate its logical strength. Where could the argument be improved? If the weakness is glaring, then the correct answer should be clear amongst the options. The test taker should look out for any new information that validates a prediction or proves a generalization mentioned in the passage. Another possible way to strengthen an argument occurs when the new information provides support for a previously unjustified assumption. In addition, answers to strengthen questions will sometimes come in the form of principles, as discussed above. In these instances, the principle will provide some generalization that impacts a specific statement from the passage. For example, the passage might rely on a supporting claim without any justification, and the principle will strengthen the argument by stating that the claim is always true under those circumstances.

One of the most common answers to strengthen questions is an answer choice that offers new information that will impact the claim by providing a missing link between premises. The original claim or argument might not have connected these two premises, or the new information might strengthen the bridge between premises and the conclusion. Strengthening connections between premises is common when the relevant argument or claim does not immediately appear to be weak or lacking in some way. In the case of already strong arguments, another common correct answer will rule out possible alternatives. For example, the premises might all be airtight, but they collectively lead to two equally plausible conclusions. In this case, the correct answer will rule out the alternative conclusion, and therefore strengthen the conclusion actually included in the claim or argument.

Similarly, in weaken questions, the correct answer will make the argument less plausible by showing that the premises do not necessarily lead to the stated conclusion. This occurs when an important premise is invalidated or eliminated in some way. Special attention should be paid to any premises, suppositions, or statements that rely on some fact being true. Test takers should also pay special attention to how the premises relate to each other in support of the conclusion. Does one premise connect multiple other premises to the argument? If so, then this is the type of premise that is often invalidated by the new information, and the argument will completely fall apart. The more premises that fall off from supporting the conclusion, the weaker the argument. In addition, any new information that invalidates an important prediction or disproves a relied upon generalization will often be the correct answer. Arguments or claims can also be weakened if the new information creates a scenario where an equally plausible alternative conclusion can be drawn. Furthermore, it is possible to weaken arguments by attacking a relied upon assumption.

MCAT Practice Test #1

Biological and Biochemical Foundations of Living Systems

1. Which statement about white blood cells is true?
    a. B cells are responsible for antibody production.
    b. White blood cells are made in the white/yellow cartilage before they enter the bloodstream.
    c. Platelets, a special class of white blood cell, function to clot blood and stop bleeding.
    d. Most white blood cells only activate during puberty, which explains why children and the elderly are particularly susceptible to disease.

2. Which location(s) in the digestive system is/are sites of chemical digestion?

    I. Mouth
    II. Stomach
    III. Small Intestine

    a. II only
    b. III only
    c. II and III only
    d. I, II, and III

3. What is the theory that certain physical and behavioral survival traits give a species an evolutionary advantage?
    a. Gradualism
    b. Evolutionary advantage
    c. Punctuated equilibrium
    d. Natural selection

4. Which event occurs first in receptor-mediated signal transduction involving receptors?
    a. Phosphorylation/dephosphorylation cascade
    b. Transcription factor activation by activated protein
    c. Ligand binding to a tyrosine kinase transmembrane protein
    d. Ion-gated channels open

5. Which cellular organelle is used for digestion to recycle materials?
    a. The Golgi apparatus
    b. The lysosome
    c. The centrioles
    d. The mitochondrion

6. Which of the following leads to diversity in meiotic division but not in mitotic division?
    a. Tetrad formation
    b. Disassembly of the mitotic spindle
    c. Extra/fewer chromosomes due to nondisjunction
    d. Fertilization by multiple sperm

7. Why do arteries have valves?
    a. They have valves to maintain high blood pressure so that capillaries diffuse nutrients properly.
    b. Their valves are designed to prevent backflow due to their low blood pressure.
    c. The valves have no known purpose and thus appear to be unnecessary.
    d. They do not have valves, but veins do.

8. If the pressure in the pulmonary artery is increased above normal, which chamber of the heart will be affected first?
   a. The right atrium
   b. The left atrium
   c. The right ventricle
   d. The left ventricle

9. What is the purpose of sodium bicarbonate when released into the lumen of the small intestine?
   a. It works to chemically digest fats in the chyme.
   b. It decreases the pH of the chyme to prevent harm to the small intestine.
   c. It works to chemically digest proteins in the chyme.
   d. It increases the pH of the chyme to prevent harm to the small intestine.

10. Which of the following describes a reflex arc?
   a. The storage and recall of memory
   b. The maintenance of visual and auditory acuity
   c. The autoregulation of heart rate and blood pressure
   d. A stimulus and response controlled by the spinal cord

11. Which of the following best describes the synthesis of the lagging strand of DNA?
   a. DNA polymerases synthesize DNA continuously after initially attaching to a primase.
   b. DNA polymerases synthesize DNA discontinuously in pieces called Okazaki fragments after initially attaching to primases.
   c. DNA polymerases synthesize DNA discontinuously in pieces called Okazaki fragments after initially attaching to RNA primers.
   d. DNA polymerases synthesize DNA discontinuously in pieces called Okazaki fragments, which are joined together in the end by a DNA helicase.

12. Which statement regarding the function of the different white blood cells is correct?
   a. B cells are responsible for antibody production.
   b. B cells inform T cells of the presence of foreign substances.
   c. Macrophages work directly on tumors and virus-infected cells.
   d. Both B cells and T cells differentiate into plasma cells.

13. Venous blood vessels carry blood from body tissues back to the heart and lungs. Venous blood is generally depleted of oxygen and nutrients. How is the blood in the hepatic portal vein able to support liver function?
   a. The liver makes its own energy, so additional nutrients are not necessary.
   b. The hepatic portal vein brings nutrients directly from the digestive tract to the liver.
   c. The hepatic artery brings metabolic nutrients to the liver.
   d. The gallbladder stores nutrients for the liver to use as needed.

14. Which of the following is NOT true regarding cell cycle checkpoints in mitosis?
   a. A cyclin/CDK pair is responsible for assembling mitotic machinery.
   b. Cyclin protein increases in interphase and is broken down during mitosis.
   c. CDK protein is equally expressed throughout the cell cycle.
   d. G_0 is a state that stimulates progression into S phase.

15. Which of the following is NOT a major function of the respiratory system in humans?
   a. To provide a large surface area for gas exchange of oxygen and carbon dioxide
   b. To help regulate the blood's pH
   c. To help cushion the heart against jarring motions
   d. To produce vocalization

16. Which of the following is NOT a function of the forebrain?
 a. To regulate blood pressure and heart rate
 b. To perceive and interpret emotional responses like fear and anger
 c. To perceive and interpret visual input from the eyes
 d. To integrate voluntary movement

17. What is the major difference between somatic and germline mutations?
 a. Somatic mutations usually benefit the individual, while germline mutations usually harm them.
 b. Since germline mutations only affect one cell, they are less noticeable than the rapidly-dividing somatic cells.
 c. Somatic mutations are not expressed for several generations, but germline mutations are expressed immediately.
 d. Germline mutations are usually inherited, while somatic mutations will affect only the individual.

18. What is the action of glucagon?
 a. It increases the cellular uptake of carbohydrates
 b. It stimulates insulin secretion by the beta cells in the pancreas
 c. It stimulates the liver to release stored glucose
 d. It increases the cellular absorption of insulin

19. The liver is responsible for many vital bodily functions. Which of the following functions is potentially harmful to the body?
 a. Conversion of ammonia to urea
 b. Breakdown of hemoglobin
 c. Cholesterol production
 d. Glycogen storage

20. What is the purpose of a catalyst?
 a. To increase a reaction's rate by increasing the activation energy
 b. To increase a reaction's rate by increasing the temperature
 c. To increase a reaction's rate by decreasing the activation energy
 d. To increase a reaction's rate by decreasing the temperature

21. Most catalysts found in biological systems are which of the following?
 a. Special lipids called cofactors
 b. Special proteins called enzymes
 c. Special lipids called enzymes
 d. Special proteins called cofactors

22. The cardiac cycle consists of diastole and systole. What are the specific events of the second diastole phase?
 a. The mitral valve closes, the aortic semilunar valve opens, and the ventricle contracts, sending blood into the aorta.
 b. Blood flows through the superior and inferior venae cavae into the right atrium. The right atrium contracts when stimulated by the impulse from the sinoatrial node, resulting in the movement of blood through the open tricuspid valve to the right ventricle.
 c. The impulse from atrioventricular node stimulates the right ventricle to contract. The tricuspid valve closes, and the pulmonary semilunar valve opens. Blood enters the pulmonary artery.
 d. Blood returns from the lungs to the left atrium through the pulmonary vein, the sinoatrial node triggers the mitral valve to open, the left atrium contracts, and the left ventricle fills with blood.

23. How do cellulose and starch differ?
   a. Cellulose and starch are proteins with different R groups.
   b. Cellulose is a polysaccharide made up of glucose molecules, and starch is a polysaccharide made up of galactose molecules.
   c. Cellulose and starch are both polysaccharides made up of glucose molecules, but they are connected with different types of bonds.
   d. Cellulose and starch are the same molecule, but cellulose is made by plants and starch is made by animals.

24. A mutation in the sequence of a protein causes the secondary structure to change. How did the mutation cause the change?
   a. The R group from the mutated amino acid interacts differently with other R groups.
   b. The R group from the mutated amino acid prevents the formation of hydrogen bonds between the atoms of the backbone of the protein.
   c. The mutation causes peptide bonds to change.
   d. All of the above

25. Which organelles have two layers of membranes?
   a. Nucleus, chloroplast, mitochondria
   b. Nucleus, Golgi apparatus, mitochondria
   c. ER, chloroplast, lysosome
   d. ER, nucleus, mitochondria

26. What organelle is the site of protein synthesis?
   a. Nucleus
   b. Smooth ER
   c. Rough ER
   d. Ribosome

27. Which of the following is an example of the "lock and key" model?
   a. Bacteria adhering to foreign cells
   b. Steroid hormones triggering protein synthesis
   c. Water and oxygen passing through the prokaryotic cell wall
   d. Enzymes breaking down nutrients into smaller units

28. Which of the following is an example of differentiation?
   a. A white blood cell ruptures after being infected by a virus
   b. A sperm fuses with an egg and forms a zygote
   c. A stem cell develops to become better suited to produce insulin
   d. A liver cell's DNA becomes damaged, so it enters the G0 stage

29. Which human cellular metabolic pathway is more energy-efficient and why?
   a. Anaerobic, because oxygen isn't depleted
   b. Aerobic, because all of the energy produced is used for ATP
   c. Anaerobic, because the process takes less time
   d. Aerobic, because more ATP is produced

30. Which of the following is directly transcribed from DNA and represents the first step in protein building?
   a. siRNA
   b. rRNA
   c. mRNA
   d. tRNA

31. What information does a genotype give that a phenotype does not?
    a. The genotype must include the proteins coded for by its alleles
    b. The genotype will always show an organism's recessive alleles
    c. The genotype must include the organism's physical characteristics
    d. The genotype shows what an organism's parents looked like

	T	*t*
T		
t		

32. Which statement is supported by the Punnett square above, if "T" = Tall and "t" = short?
    a. Both parents are homozygous tall.
    b. 100% of the offspring will be tall because both parents are tall.
    c. There is a 25% chance that an offspring will be short.
    d. The short allele will soon die out.

33. Two different bacterial cultures are grown from bacteria with the same genome sequence. Transcriptional analysis shows that Culture B is expressing genes that can metabolize lactose, but Culture A is not. How can this happen if they have the same genetic sequence?
    a. Someone mislabeled the tubes and the bacteria must have different genome sequences.
    b. Culture A is grown in the presence of lactose, which turns on a different set of genes.
    c. Culture B is grown in the presence of lactose, which turns on a different set of genes.
    d. B and C

34. Which of the following is NOT found in a human cell's genes?
    a. Sequences of amino acids to be transcribed into mRNA
    b. Lethal recessive traits like sickle cell anemia
    c. Mutated DNA
    d. DNA that codes for proteins that the cell doesn't use

35. What step happens first in protein synthesis?
    a. mRNA is pulled into the ribosome
    b. Exons are spliced out of mRNA in processing
    c. tRNA delivers amino acids
    d. mRNA makes a complementary DNA copy

36. Which of the following functions corresponds to the parasympathetic nervous system?
    a. It stimulates the fight-or-flight response.
    b. It increases heart rate.
    c. It stimulates digestion.
    d. It increases bronchiole dilation.

37. DNA must be created in a 5′ to 3′ direction. This causes which of the following?
   a. Shortening of telomeres
   b. Hydrogen bonds between nitrogen bases
   c. Primase binding
   d. Okazaki fragments to form on the leading strand

38. What term is used to describe a metabolic reaction that releases energy?
   a. Catabolic
   b. Carbolic
   c. Anabolic
   d. Endothermic

39. Which structure is found exclusively in eukaryotic cells?
   a. Cell wall
   b. Nucleus
   c. Cell membrane
   d. Vacuole

40. Which of these is NOT found in the cell nucleus?
   a. Golgi complex
   b. Chromosomes
   c. Nucleolus
   d. Chromatin

41. Which organelle digests and recycle cellular materials?
   a. Golgi apparatus
   b. Lysosome
   c. Centriole
   d. Mitochondria

42. The combination of alleles of an organism, when expressed, manifests as which of the following?
   a. An organism's genotype
   b. An organism's phenotype
   c. An organism's sex
   d. An organism's karyotype

43. Which of the following are the reproductive cells produced by meiosis?
   a. Genes
   b. Alleles
   c. Chromatids
   d. Gametes

44. What is the process of cell division in somatic cells called?
   a. Mitosis
   b. Meiosis
   c. Respiration
   d. Cytogenesis

45. When human cells divide by meiosis, how many chromosomes do the resulting cells contain?
   a. 96
   b. 54
   c. 46
   d. 23

46. Which of the following is a consequence of tetrad formation in meiosis?
   a. It causes diversity
   b. It determines the organism's sex
   c. It causes non-disjunction
   d. It causes transcription

47. What is an alteration in the normal gene sequence called?
   a. DNA mutation
   b. Gene migration
   c. Polygenetic inheritance
   d. Incomplete dominance

48. Blood type is a trait determined by multiple alleles, and two of them are co-dominant: I^A codes for A blood and I^B codes for B blood. The i allele codes for O blood and is recessive to both. If an A heterozygous individual and an O individual have a child, what is the probability that the child will have A blood?
   a. 25%
   b. 50%
   c. 75%
   d. 100%

49. What are the building blocks of DNA called?
   a. Helices
   b. Proteins
   c. Genes
   d. Nucleotides

50. Which statement is NOT true about RNA?
   a. It can be single-stranded.
   b. It has ribose sugar.
   c. It contains uracil.
   d. It only exists in three forms.

51. What is the term used for the set of metabolic reactions that converts the energy in chemical bonds to ATP?
   a. Photosynthesis
   b. Reproduction
   c. Active transport
   d. Cellular respiration

52. Which of the following regarding bacterial spores is NOT true?
   a. Spores allow survival during adverse conditions.
   b. Bacteria enter spore form during the lag phase.
   c. Not all bacteria are capable of producing spores.
   d. Spores can germinate into the vegetative form.

53. What is unique about retroviruses?
    a. They can create spores.
    b. They enter the host in RNA form then get converted to DNA form.
    c. They enter the host in DNA form then get converted to RNA form.
    d. They do not need a host to reproduce.

54. Which type of viruses undergo the lytic cycle once inside the host?
    a. Animal viruses
    b. Bacteriophages
    c. Retroviruses
    d. Lysogenic viruses

55. Which of the following correctly presents the order of steps in the lytic cycle?
    a. Attachment, penetration, biosynthesis, maturation, release
    b. Attachment, penetration, maturation, biosynthesis, release
    c. Penetration, attachment, biosynthesis, maturation, release
    d. Penetration, attachment, maturation, biosynthesis, release

56. Which of the following can move genetic material from the plasmid to the chromosome or from the chromosome to the plasmid?
    a. Reverse transcriptase
    b. Transposons
    c. Pili
    d. Sex pilus

57. Genetic variation can be introduced into bacteria through all EXCEPT which of the following ways?
    a. Mutation
    b. Binary fission
    c. Conjugation
    d. Transformation

58. Antibiotic resistance can spread rapidly through a bacterial population through which of the following processes?
    a. Conjugation
    b. Transformation
    c. Binary fission
    d. Transduction

59. By definition, competent bacteria can do which of the following?
    a. Transformation
    b. Transduction
    c. Conjugation
    d. Form a sex pilus

Chemical and Physical Foundations of Biological Systems

1. Water has many unique properties due to its unique structure. Which of the following does NOT play a role in water's unique properties?
   a. Hydrogen bonding between molecules
   b. Polarity within one molecule
   c. Molecules held apart in solid state
   d. Equal sharing of electrons

2. What's the current supplied from this 1.5V battery?

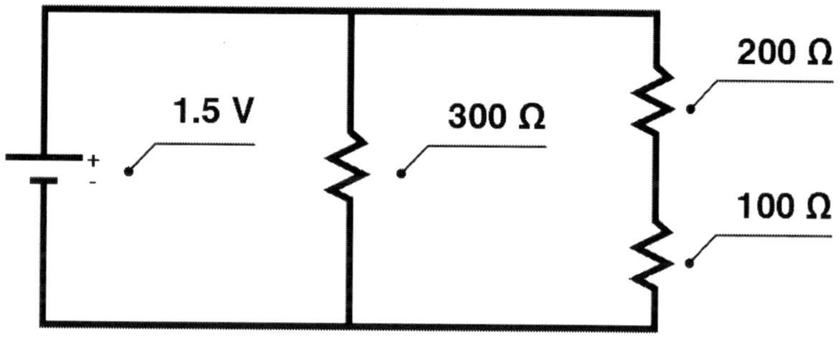

   a. 5 milliamps
   b. 10 milliamps
   c. 15 milliamps
   d. 20 milliamps

3. Which of the following must have an equal mass number?

   I. Isotopes
   II. Isotones
   III. Isobars

   a. I only
   b. I and II only
   c. II and III only
   d. III only

4. How are a sodium atom and a sodium isotope different?
   a. The isotope has a different number of protons.
   b. The isotope has a different number of neutrons.
   c. The isotope has a different number of electrons.
   d. The isotope has a different atomic number.

5. Which statement is true about nonmetals?
   a. They form cations.
   b. They form covalent bonds.
   c. They are mostly absent from organic compounds.
   d. They are all diatomic.

6. What is the basic unit of matter?
   a. Elementary particle
   b. Atom
   c. Molecule
   d. Photon

7. Which particle is responsible for all chemical reactions?
   a. Electrons
   b. Neutrons
   c. Protons
   d. Orbitals

8. Assuming a constant voltage source, what's the energy expended in this circuit in 30 minutes?

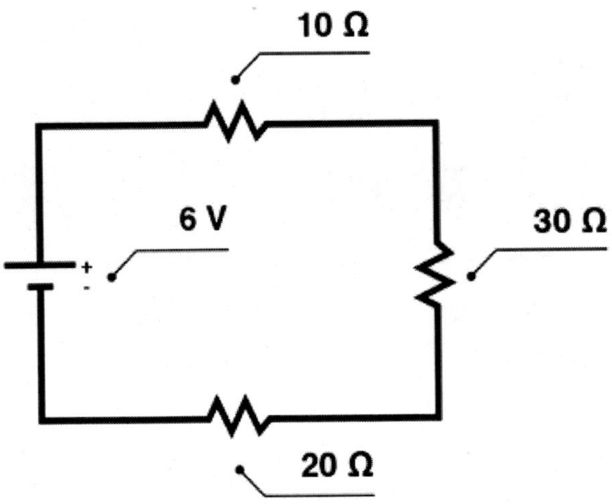

   a. 0.1 amp
   b. 1800 amp-seconds
   c. 0.3 watt-hours
   d. 100 J

9. How are similar chemical properties of elements grouped on the periodic table?
   a. In rows, according to their total configuration of electrons
   b. In columns, according to the electron configuration in their outer shells
   c. In rows, according to the electron configuration in their outer shells
   d. In columns, according to their total configurations of electrons

10. This circuit is built from single wires connected to five sockets, with four of five bulbs installed. Which bulbs in the circuit will light up?

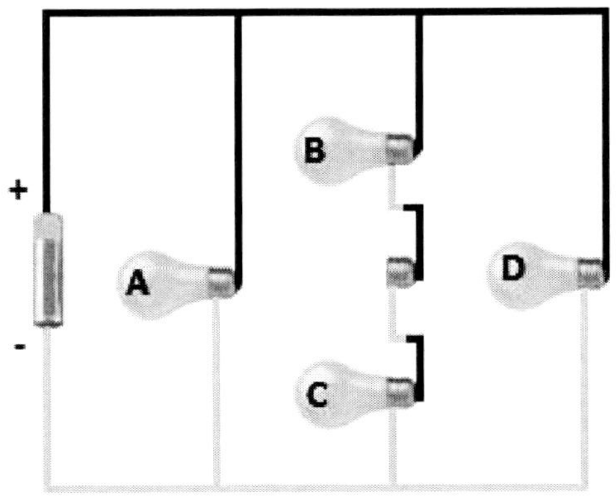

a. Only Bulb A
b. Only Bulb D
c. Bulbs A, B, C, and D
d. Bulbs A and D

11. The law of conservation of mass states which of the following?
a. All matter is equally created.
b. Matter changes, but is not created.
c. Matter can be changed, and new matter can be created.
d. Matter can be created, but not changed.

12. Which factor decreases the solubility of solids?
a. Heating
b. Agitation
c. Large Surface area
d. Decreasing solvent

13. What is the term for a homogeneous mixture that does not display the Tyndall effect?
a. Solvent
b. Suspension
c. Solution
d. Colloid

14. How does adding salt to water affect its boiling point?
a. It increases it.
b. It has no effect.
c. It decreases it.
d. It prevents it from boiling.

15. What is the effect of pressure on a liquid solution?
a. It decreases solubility.
b. It increases solubility.
c. It has little effect on solubility.
d. It has the same effect as with a gaseous solution.

16. Non-polar molecules must have which type of regions?
   a. Hydrophilic
   b. Hydrophobic
   c. Hydrolytic
   d. Hydrochloric

17. Which of these is a substance that increases the rate of a chemical reaction?
   a. Catalyst
   b. Brine
   c. Solvent
   d. Inhibitor

18. Based on collision theory, what is the effect of temperature on the rate of chemical reaction?
   a. Increasing the temperature slows the reaction.
   b. Decreasing the temperature speeds up the reaction.
   c. Increasing the temperature speeds up the reaction.
   d. Collision theory and temperature are unrelated.

19. What coefficients are needed to balance the following combustion equation?

$$\_\ C_2H_{10} + \_\ O_2 \rightarrow \_\ H_2O + \_\ CO_2$$

   a. 1:5:5:2
   b. 1:9:5:2
   c. 2:2:4:1
   d. 2:5:10:4

20. Which type of bonding results from transferring electrons between atoms?
   a. Ionic bonding
   b. Covalent bonding
   c. Hydrogen bonding
   d. Dipole interactions

21. Which substance is oxidized in the following reaction?

$$4\ Fe + 3\ O_2 \rightarrow 2\ Fe_2O_3$$

   a. Fe
   b. O
   c. O_2
   d. Fe_2O_3

22. Which statements are true regarding nuclear fission?

I. It is the splitting of heavy nuclei
II. It is utilized in power plants
III. It occurs on the sun

   a. I only
   b. II and III only
   c. I and II only
   d. III only

23. Which type of nuclear decay is occurring in the equation below?

$$U_{92}^{236} \rightarrow He_{2}^{4} + Th_{90}^{232}$$

a. Alpha
b. Beta
c. Gamma
d. Delta

24. Which statement is true about the pH of a solution?
a. A solution cannot have a pH less than 1.
b. The more hydroxide ions there are in the solution, the higher the pH will be.
c. If an acid has a pH of greater than -2, it is considered a weak acid.
d. A solution with a pH of 2 has ten times more hydrogen ions than a solution with a pH of 1.

25. Which radioactive particle is the most penetrating and damaging and is used to treat cancer in radiation therapy?
a. Alpha
b. Beta
c. Gamma
d. Delta

26. A car is traveling at a constant velocity of 25 m/s. How long does it take the car to travel 45 kilometers in a straight line?
a. 1 hour
b. 3,600 seconds
c. 1,800 seconds
d. 900 seconds

27. A ship is traveling due east at a speed of $1\ m/s$ against a current flowing due west at a speed of 0.5 m/s. How far has the ship travelled from its point of departure after two hours?
a. 1.8 kilometers west of its point of departure
b. 3.6 kilometers west of its point of departure
c. 1.8 kilometers east of its point of departure
d. 3.6 kilometers east of its point of departure

28. A car is driving along a straight stretch of highway at a constant speed of 60 km/hr when the driver slams the gas pedal to the floor, reaching a speed of 132 km/hr in 10 seconds. What's the average acceleration of the car after the pedal is floored?
a. 1 m/s^2
b. 2 m/s^2
c. 3 m/s^2
d. 4 m/s^2

29. A football is kicked so that it leaves the punter's toe at a horizontal angle of 45 degrees. Ignoring any spinning or tumbling, at what point is the upward vertical velocity of the football at a maximum?

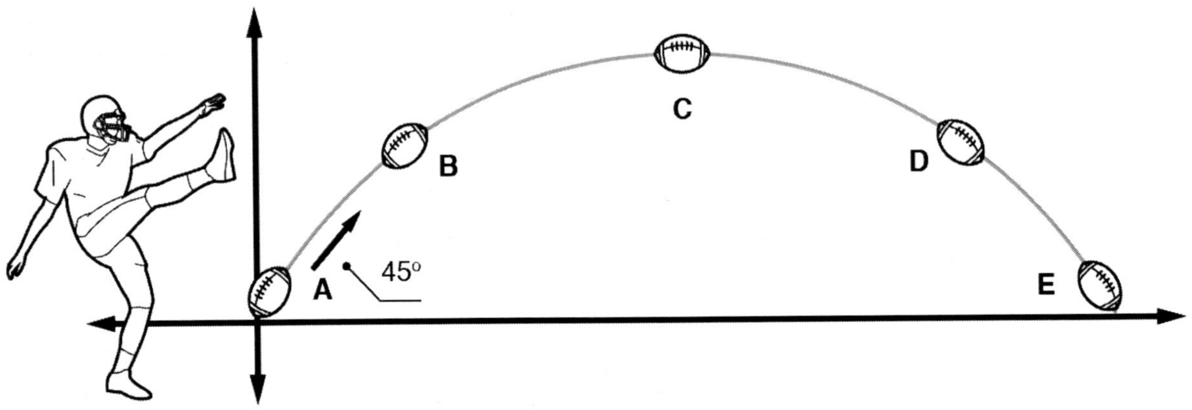

a. At Point A
b. At Point C
c. At Points B and D
d. At Points A and E

30. The skater is shown spinning in Figure (a), then bringing in her arms in Figure (b). Which sequence accurately describes what happens to her angular velocity?

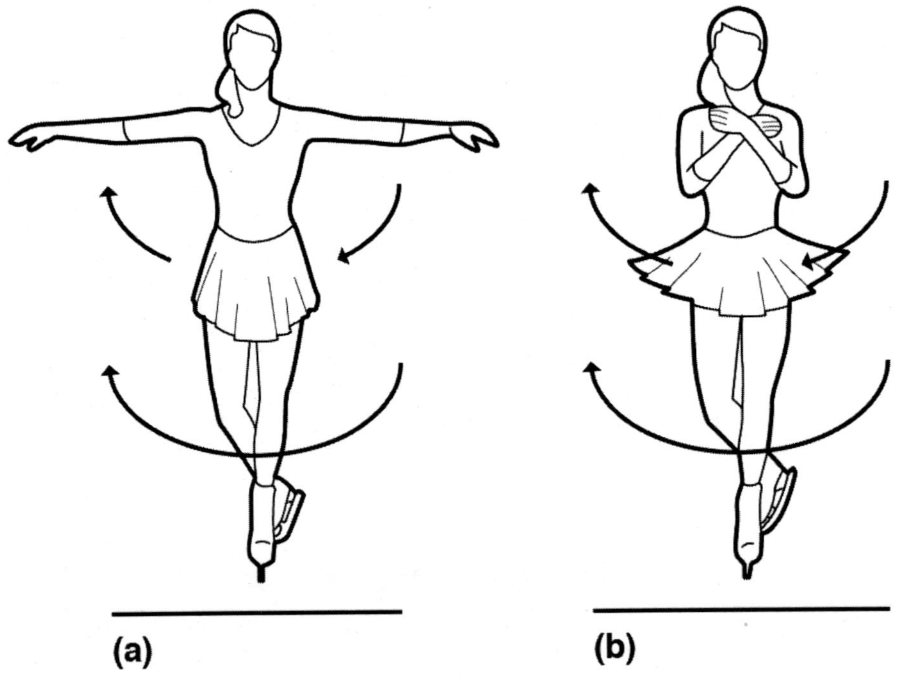

a. Her angular velocity decreases from (a) to (b).
b. Her angular velocity doesn't change from (a) to (b).
c. Her angular velocity increases from (a) to (b).
d. It's not possible to determine what happens to her angular velocity if her weight is unknown.

31. A cannonball is dropped from a height of 10 meters above sea level. What is its approximate velocity just before it hits the ground?

a. $9.81\ m/s$
b. $14\ m/s$
c. $32\ m/s$
d. It can't be determined without knowing the cannonball's mass

32.The pendulum is held at point A, and then released to swing to the right. At what point does the pendulum have the greatest kinetic energy?

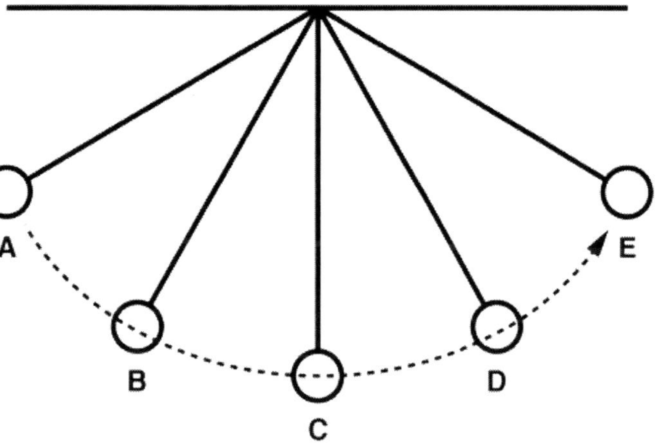

a. At Point B
b. At Point C
c. At Point D
d. At Point E

33. Which statement is true of the total energy of the pendulum?

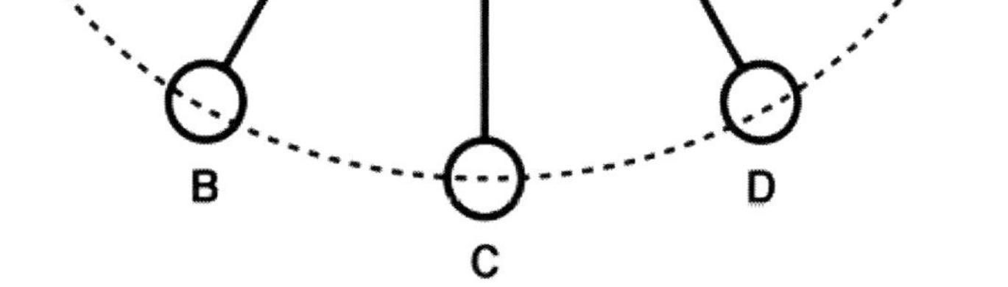

a. Its total energy is at a maximum and equal at Points A and E.
b. Its total energy is at a maximum at Point C.
c. Its total energy is the same at Points A, B, C, D, and E.
d. The total energy can't be compared without knowing the pendulum's mass.

34. How do you calculate the useful work performed in lifting a 10-kilogram weight from the ground to the top of a 2-meter ladder?

a. $10 \text{ kg} \times 2 \text{ m} \times 32 \text{ m/s}^2$
b. $10 \text{ kg} \times 2 \text{ m}^2 \times 9.81 \text{ m/s}$
c. $10 \text{ kg} \times 2 \text{ m} \times 9.81 \text{ m/s}^2$
d. It can't be determined without knowing the ground elevation

35. Closed Basins A and B each contain a 10,000-ton block of ice. The ice block in Basin A is floating in sea water. The ice block in Basin B is aground on a rock ledge (as shown). When all the ice melts, what happens to the water level in Basin A and Basin B?

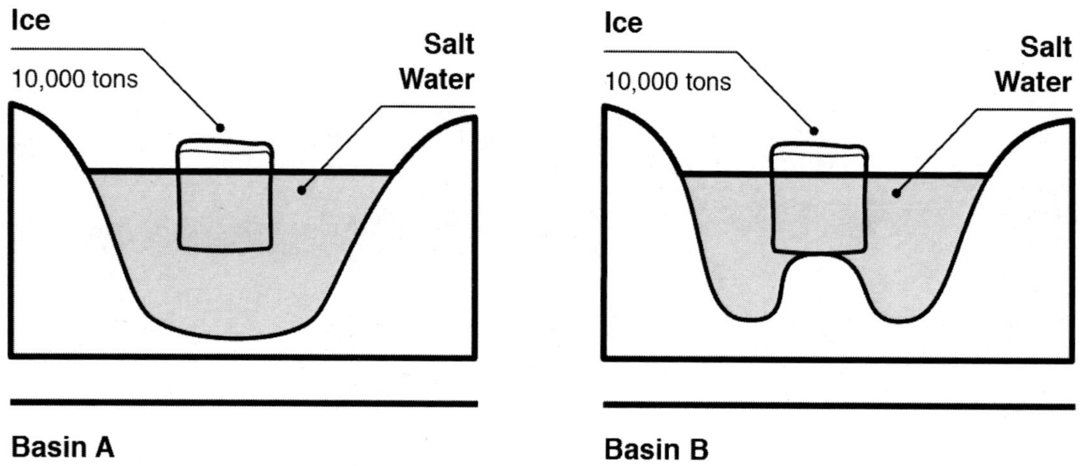

a. The water level rises in A but not in B.
b. The water level rises in B but not in A.
c. The water level rises in neither A nor B.
d. The water level rises in both A and B.

36. An official 10-lane Olympic pool is 50 meters wide by 25 meters long. How long does it take to fill the pool to the recommended depth of 3 meters using a pump with a 750 liter per second capacity?

a. 2,500 seconds
b. 5,000 seconds
c. 10,000 seconds
d. 100,000 seconds

37. Water is flowing in a rectangular canal 10 meters wide by 2 meters deep at a velocity of 3 m/s. The canal is half full. What is the flow rate?

a. $30 \text{ m}^3/\text{s}$
b. $60 \text{ m}^3/\text{s}$
c. $90 \text{ m}^3/\text{s}$
d. $120 \text{ m}^3/\text{s}$

38. When is a reaction spontaneous?
   a. If it is exothermic
   b. If ΔH and ΔS are positive
   c. If ΔG is less than zero
   d. If there is a low activation energy

Trial	[A]initial (M)	[B]initial (M)	R initial (M/sec)
1	2	2	3.2
2	6	6	9.1
3	2	6	2.9
4	4	8	5.9

39. For the equation $A + B \rightarrow C + D$, what is the rate constant considering the initial rates above?
   a. 0.5
   b. 1.5
   c. 3.0
   d. 6.0

40. Consider the reversible equation:

$$3\ A(g) + 4\ B(s) \rightarrow 3\ C(g) + 2\ D(g)$$

If pressure on the system were increased, what would happen to the reaction quotient Q?
   a. Q would increase
   b. Q would decrease
   c. Q would remain the same
   d. Q would immediately be equal to K

41. A solution has 4.3 grams/L of an organic substance, and the osmotic pressure of the is 12.2 atm at 23°C. What is the molar mass of the substance (in grams per mole)?
   a. 4.4
   b. 5.4
   c. 6.4
   d. 8.4

42. Under which extreme conditions do real gases behave like ideal gases?

I. High pressure
II. High temperature
III. Small volume

   a. I only
   b. II only
   c. III only
   d. I and II

43. If ΔH is negative, what process is occurring at point A?

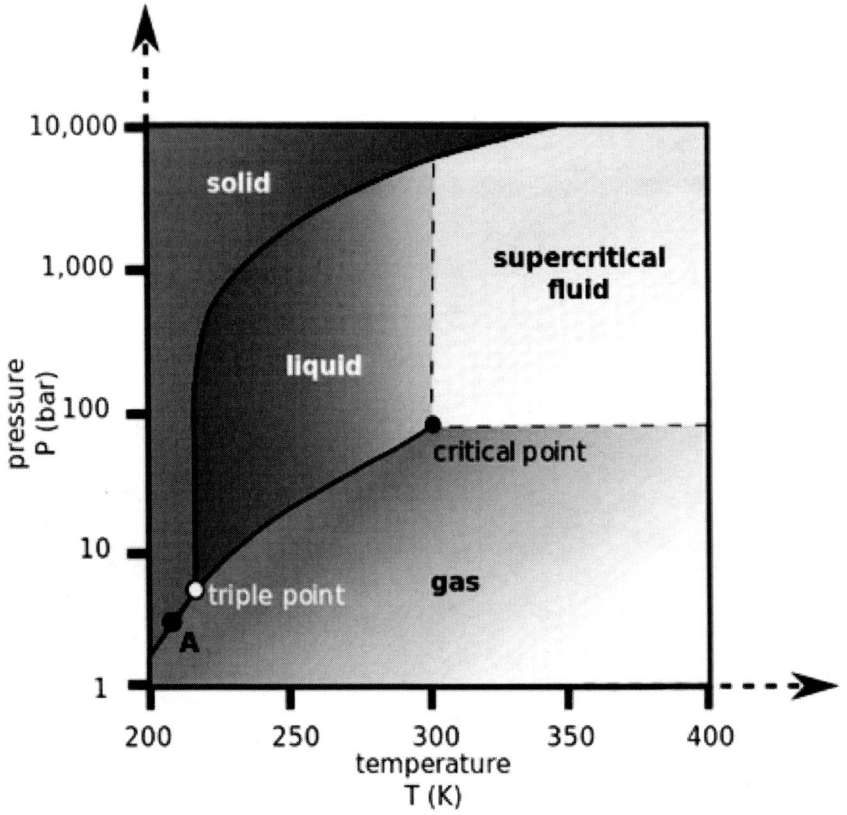

a. Melting
b. Condensation
c. Sublimation
d. Deposition

44. What is ΔH if 10.1g of water at -3˚C melts and stabilizes at 17˚C?

a. -3.3 kJ
b. 4.2 kJ
c. -12.5 kJ
d. 61.5 J

45. If 273g of oxygen are contained in a scuba tank, which on land has a pressure of 1.3 atm and a temperature of 28˚C, what is the volume of the tank?

a. 52,890L
b. 16,354L
c. 483L
d. 162L

46. The reaction below has the following observed mechanisms:

$$2A + B \leftrightarrow C$$

$$i. A + A \leftrightarrow C$$

$$ii. C + B \rightarrow 2D$$

Reversible reaction i is fast in both directions

Reaction ii is slow

What is the rate law for the reaction?

a. k[A]2[B][C]
b. k[B][C]
c. k[A]2[B]
d. k[A]2

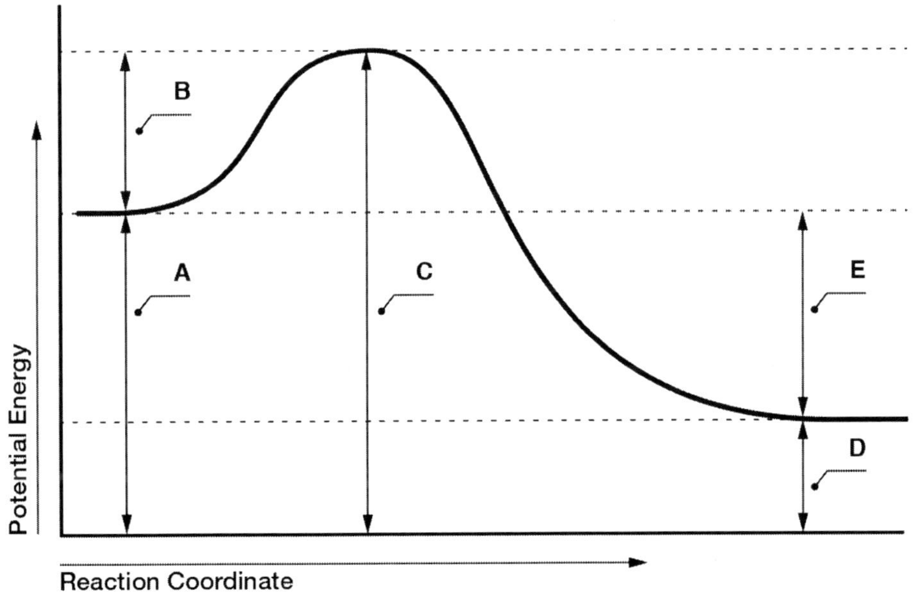

47. Which statements are true regarding the diagram above?

I. C represents ΔH
II. The reaction is exothermic
III. B would increase if an enzyme was added

a. I only
b. II only
c. I and II
d. II and III

48. A block of ice is contained inside a perfectly isolated system. Obeying the laws of thermodynamics, which of the following will happen to the that ice?
   a. It stays frozen.
   b. It completely melts.
   c. It partially melts.
   d. It melts and refreezes.

49. Which of the following is an exception to the second law of thermodynamics?
   a. A group of chickens roaming around a field
   b. Ice inside a perfectly closed system
   c. Water at zero Kelvin
   d. A perfect crystal at zero Kelvin

50. If substance A has a lower specific heat than substance B, which of the following is true of substance A?
   a. Substance A is harder to heat up.
   b. Substance A is easier to heat up.
   c. Substance A is easier to melt.
   d. Substance B is easier to melt.

51. If energy is applied in the form of heat to a set quantity of gas and pressure is held constant, according to the ideal gas law, which of these will most likely happen?
   a. The temperature returns to the original temperature.
   b. The gas escapes.
   c. The volume of the gas increases.
   d. The internal energy of the gas increases.

52. For a certain given reaction, if the reactants have low entropy compared to their products, which of the following situations would most likely yield a spontaneous reaction?
   a. At very low temperature
   b. It will always be spontaneous, regardless of temperature.
   c. At very high temperature
   d. The reaction is endothermic.

53. When Gibbs free energy is very negative for a chemical reaction, which of the following is the best description of that reaction?
   a. It is exothermic.
   b. It will favor the reactants.
   c. K will be large.
   d. It is spontaneous.

54. At the critical point of a phase change diagram, the element exists in what phases?
   a. Gas only
   b. Gas and solid
   c. Liquid only
   d. Liquid and gas

55. Which of the following would be considered isotopes?

I. 2H
II. H+
III. H

a. I only
b. I and II only
c. I and III only
d. None of the above

56. Which of the following releases the most energy?

a. Nuclear fusion
b. Splitting of an unstable nucleus
c. Nuclear fission
d. Radioactive decay

57. Given the rate of a reaction, rate = k(X)2(Y)3, which increase will decrease the rate?

a. Adding a catalyst to the reaction
b. Doubling the concentration of both reactions
c. Doubling X and halving Y
d. Doubling Y and halving X

58. When is it possible to increase the boiling point temperature of a substance?

a. Decrease pressure
b. Increase pressure
c. It is impossible
d. Increase the rate of temperature change

59. Which of the following elements has the largest atomic radius?

a. Lithium
b. Helium
c. Potassium
d. Boron

Psychological, Social, and Biological Foundations of Behavior

1. What is the last stage in Freud's model of the five stages of human development?

a. Latent stage
b. Adult stage
c. Genital stage
d. Self-actualization stage

2. In Erikson's eight stages of development, Identity versus Role Confusion begins at age 12 and contains all EXCEPT which of the following challenges?

a. Working through and understanding multiple changes and demands placed upon the child as he or she moves toward adulthood
b. Increasing understanding of sexual, hormonal, and other physical changes that are occurring
c. Finding a long-term partner and starting a family
d. Assessing one's talents, sexual preferences, and vocational interests

3. According to Piaget, the process by which old ideas or beliefs must be replaced with new ones due to obtaining new and more factual information is called which of the following?
   a. Schemas
   b. Assimilation
   c. Object permanence
   d. Accommodation

4. Ivan Pavlov is best known in the field of psychology for his concepts regarding which of the following?
   a. Classical conditioning
   b. Training dogs to behave obediently
   c. Development of sexual identity and orientation
   d. How positive reinforcement helps children develop

5. According to B.F. Skinner, providing positive reinforcement increases the likelihood that a desired behavior will be repeated. Which of the following is NOT a form of positive reinforcement when working with children?
   a. A trip to the park with Mom following a week of good behavior
   b. Praise in response to a task well done
   c. Taking away TV and computer privileges for a week
   d. Putting a colorful sticker on a poster each time the child goes to bed on time

6. In Skinner's theory of operant conditioning, the term *shaping* refers to which of the following?
   a. Attempts to change behavior through a series of small shocks
   b. Changing behavior through rewarding the person each time an approximation of the desired behavior occurs
   c. Exploring superstitions that might impact one's willingness to make behavioral changes
   d. Giving a person a reward only when the desired behavior is perfected

7. In the field of personality theories, which researcher proposed that personality develops from striving to become the best one can be, combined with the importance of self-perception?
   a. Erik Erikson
   b. Sigmund Freud
   c. Carl Rogers
   d. Gordon Allport

8. The process of social development as defined by Lev Vygotsky suggests that one's development in life is deeply impacted by:
   a. Income status
   b. Birth order and gender
   c. The variety of social institutions, such as family, school, or church, to which someone is exposed throughout life
   d. Physical stamina and overall health

9. Those who research self-image throughout the life cycle report which of the following?
   a. Most people's self-image tends to peak around the age of 60.
   b. Adolescents, compared to other age groups, have the highest likelihood of a positive self-image.
   c. There is very little change in one's self-image once middle school is completed.
   d. Young adults who are completing high school and entering the workforce or college show an increase in self-image.

10. One's cultural background is based primarily upon which of the following?
    a. The color of one's skin
    b. Whether one lives in an urban or rural society
    c. The prevalence of racism in one's current environment
    d. A combination of factors, including where one was born, at what point in time one was born, and the sociological practices and standards in which one was raised

11. One's culture, race, and ethnicity can significantly influence self-image because of which of the following?
    a. Sometimes, entire groups of people are negatively judged solely on skin color or religious affiliation.
    b. Some people find racially-biased jokes humorous.
    c. Racial profiling by law enforcement and the courts can lead to higher conviction rates and longer prison sentence for minority groups.
    d. All of the above

12. Which of the following is an example of indirect discrimination?
    a. An employer tosses a resume in the trash because the name on it is commonly held by persons of the Muslim religion.
    b. A school requires all students to come to school on Saturday for a makeup day despite having Jewish students who observe Saturday as a day of rest.
    c. A restaurant owner refuses to serve a customer because the customer is black.
    d. A landlord tells an interracial couple seeking an apartment that there are no vacancies, even though there are several empty units ready to be rented.

13. Which of these statements regarding the impact of being a woman is NOT true?
    a. Women earn $0.90 on the dollar compared to men.
    b. Women are not proportionally represented in management positions.
    c. Women who are pregnant may be passed over when interviewing for a new job or applying for a promotion.
    d. Women are more likely than men to be the victims of sexual assault.

14. An indication that self-image is affected by growing old in our society is evidenced by which of the following?
    a. Only 15% of US families reporting living in multigenerational households
    b. People experiencing a decrease in self-esteem and self-image as they enter their retirement years
    c. Most people showing great respect and appreciating the wisdom of elders in their lives
    d. Many of today's most successful entertainers being over the age of 65

15. Why is the impact of sexual orientation on self-image sometimes felt more intensely in small towns or rural areas?
    a. People living in small or isolated communities do not have as much opportunity to interact with persons with diverse sexual orientations; therefore, LGBT persons may be seen as different or unacceptable.
    b. People living in small or rural communities tend to be more conservative in their political views than those residing in larger urban areas where gay bars, restaurants, or shopping areas are not uncommon and even provide a good source of revenue to the community.
    c. LGBT persons living in small communities do not have strong ties with a support group of persons with a similar orientation, whereas this is more easily accessible in larger cities.
    d. All of the above

16. All EXCEPT which of the following are true of an area with an extremely high population density?
    a. Competition for resources is intense.
    b. Greater strain on public services exists.
    c. More people live in rural areas.
    d. More people live in urban areas.

17. All EXCEPT which of the following are negative demographic indicators?
    a. High infant mortality rates
    b. Low literacy rates
    c. High population density
    d. Low life expectancy

18. Which of the following best describes ethnic groups?
    a. Subgroups within a population who share a common history, language, or religion
    b. Divisive groups within a nation's boundaries seeking independence
    c. People who choose to leave a location
    d. Any minority group within a nation's boundaries

19. Which of the following could be considered a pull factor for a particular area?
    a. High rates of unemployment
    b. Low GDP
    c. Educational opportunity
    d. High population density

20. Which of the following best describes the process of globalization?
    a. The integration of the world's economic systems into a singular entity
    b. The emergence of powerful nations seeking world dominance
    c. The absence of nation-states who seek to control certain areas
    d. Efforts to establish a singular world government for the world's citizens

21. Which nerve pathway is the simplest, and bypasses the brain?
    a. Autonomic
    b. Reflex arc
    c. Somatic
    d. Sympathetic

22. Which of the following is a function of the parasympathetic nervous system?
    a. Stimulating the fight-or-flight response
    b. Increasing heart rate
    c. Stimulating digestion
    d. Increasing bronchiole dilation

23. Which of the following is the type of neuron that transmits signals from the CNS to effector tissues and organs?
    a. Motor
    b. Sensory
    c. Interneuron
    d. Reflex

24. Which statement regarding brain structure is NOT true?
    a. The corpus callosum connects the hemispheres.
    b. Broca's and Wernicke's areas are associated with speech and language.
    c. The cerebellum is important for long-term memory storage.
    d. The brainstem is responsible for involuntary movement.

25. What are the functions of the hypothalamus?

    I. Regulate body temperature.
    II. Send stimulatory and inhibitory instructions to the pituitary gland.
    III. Receive sensory information from the brain.

    a. I and II
    b. I and III
    c. II and III
    d. I, II, and III

26. What is the major difference between absolute and relative poverty?
    a. Absolute poverty presents humans with a higher risk of death than relative poverty.
    b. Absolute poverty affects only developed countries.
    c. Relative poverty presents humans with more severe circumstances.
    d. Relative poverty affects only underdeveloped countries.

27. Why do some scholars believe meritocracy is a myth?
    a. Meritocracy is an outdated philosophy.
    b. The traditional definition of meritocracy is "a society built on fiction."
    c. Meritocracy cannot always exist thanks to social reproduction and inheritance.
    d. Hard work is a myth.

28. Which of the following is the best definition for racialization?
    a. Prejudice or oppression based on racial standards, beliefs, and practices
    b. Racial genocide carried out on minority group by a majority group
    c. The process by which society becomes more racist in its beliefs and practices
    d. The process of categorizing and separating people in society based on race or distinguishing physical characteristics

29. Why do some scholars consider the term *cult* to be a pejorative term?
    a. The term conjures up notions of brainwashing, ritual suicide, and illicit practices
    b. The term explains that it is a religious group that is less organized than sects or churches
    c. The term refers to highly-organized and bureaucratized institutions filled with corruption
    d. The term reminds people of institutions like the Roman Catholic Church

30. Which of the following is the best example of environmental injustice?
    a. The designation of a National Park for conservation purposes
    b. High lead levels in the water system of a low-income community
    c. Social activists picket to include a threatened animal on the endangered species list
    d. The discovery of bacteria that feed on sulfur emissions from oceanic vents

31. Which of the following can be considered factors contributing to globalization?

I. Travel advances
II. Technological advances
III. Communication advances
IV. Social media and the Internet

a. I & II
b. IV
c. I, II, & III
d. All of the above

32. What of the following are examples of vertical mobility?

I. Taking a job that is more satisfying, but pays the same salary
II. Getting promoted
III. Filing for bankruptcy
IV. Taking a job that is more satisfying, but pays less

a. I & II
b. II, III, & IV
c. I, III, & IV
d. All of the above

33. What are some ways in which people can be segregated?

I. Gender
II. Race
III. Socioeconomic status
IV. Age

a. I
b. I & II
c. I, II, & III
d. All of the above

34. Which of the following can be best defined as "social and/or economic changes that affect a person during their lifetime?"

a. Intragenerational mobility
b. Intergenerational mobility
c. Social reproduction
d. Vertical mobility

35. Which of the following can be considered a type of immigration status?

I. Undocumented resident
II. Deferred action
III. Asylum
IV. Temporary visitors

a. I only
b. I & II
c. I, II, & III
d. All of the above

36. Neuronal communication is which type of process?
a. Chemical process
b. Electrical process
c. Electrochemical process
d. Psychological process

37. Which of the following tends to be highly genetic with individual differences showing as early as infancy?
a. Temperament
b. Cleanliness
c. Food preferences
d. Language

38. Which of the following refers to the changes that may occur in which the expression or activation of genes is altered?
a. Adigenetics
b. Epigenetics
c. Supergenetics
d. Eugenics

39. Approximately what percentage of people in the United States struggle with mental illness in a given year?
a. 20-25%
b. 4-8%
c. 10-15%
d. 75-80%

40. What category of psychological disorders is characterized by a mood that fluctuates between mania and depression?
a. Manic-depressive disorder
b. Anxiety disorders
c. Trauma-related disorders
d. Bipolar disorders

41. High levels of dopamine are associated with which of the following?
a. Parkinson's disease
b. Alzheimer's disease
c. Schizophrenia
d. Personality disorders

42. What is one social factor that influences hunger motivation?
    a. Lateral area of the hypothalamus
    b. Body perception
    c. Coercion
    d. Metabolism

43. Which term refers to when someone influences another person to do a greater behavior or action, by first getting them to agree to a small step?
    a. Door-in-face phenomenon
    b. Central route to persuasion
    c. Foot-in-door phenomenon
    d. Role-playing

44. What is it called when a group of people gather with others who hold similar beliefs and they become stronger in those shared beliefs?
    a. Group polarization
    b. Group dynamics
    c. Groupthink
    d. Group deindividuation

45. Which type of social norm is characterized by a moral or ethical component?
    a. Taboos
    b. Group norms
    c. Folkways
    d. Mores

46. Which deviance theory explains deviance as a learned behavior?
    a. Labeling theory
    b. Differential association
    c. Strain theory
    d. Observational learning

47. What is habituation?
    a. When a person or animal adapts to the new habitat in which they live
    b. When a person or animal shows a decreased response to a stimulus after a period of time
    c. When a person or animal develops new personal habits
    d. When a person or animal shows an increased response to a stimulus

48. Which experiment illustrated modeling?
    a. The Bobo Doll experiment
    b. The Stanford Prison Experiment
    c. The Asch Conformity Study
    d. The Milgram Obedience Study

49. What term best describes a feeling of personal worth or value?
    a. Self-identity
    b. Self-concept
    c. Self-efficacy
    d. Self-esteem

50. What term best describes someone mistakenly attributing a person's observed behaviors to disposition rather than situation?
   a. Disposition attribution error
   b. Situation attribution error
   c. Behavior attribution error
   d. Fundamental attribution error

51. Which of the following is a usually negative belief about others based on prejudging with limited information and faulty assumptions?
   a. Stereotype
   b. Prejudice
   c. Discrimination
   d. Ethnocentrism

52. A woman who struggles with balancing the needs of her sick mother and fulfilling the expectations of her office is probably dealing with which of the following?
   a. Role confusion
   b. Role strain
   c. Role conflict
   d. Role transformation

53. What is the dramaturgical approach?
   a. A view that compares human behavior and social interaction to actors on a stage
   b. The dramatic expression of emotions
   c. A theatrical style that integrates aspects of psychology and sociology
   d. Persuading someone to comply with a request using expressive actions

54. Which of the following is NOT a principle contributor to attraction?
   a. Familiarity
   b. Similarity
   c. Conformity
   d. Physical attractiveness

55. What is a biological contributor to aggressive behaviors?
   a. An increased level of serotonin
   b. Higher levels of testosterone
   c. Modeling
   d. Observational learning

56. What is the sensory threshold?
   a. The smallest amount of stimulus required for an individual to feel a sensation
   b. The amount of stimulus required for an individual to feel pain
   c. The amount of stimulus required to cause an individual to move away from the stimulus
   d. The place where the stimulus is coming from

57. How many neurons generally make up a sensory pathway?
   a. 1
   b. 2
   c. 3
   d. 4

58. In which part of the eye does visual processing begin?
    a. Cornea
    b. Optic nerve
    c. Retina
    d. Eyelid

59. Sour foods release which type of ion that then cause a person to sense sourness on the tongue?
    a. Potassium
    b. Sodium
    c. Calcium
    d. Hydrogen

Critical Analysis and Reasoning Skills

Questions 1–6 are based on the following passage:

Dana Gioia argues in his article that poetry is dying, now little more than a limited art form confined to academic and college settings. Of course, poetry remains healthy in the academic setting, but the idea of poetry being limited to this academic subculture is a stretch. New technology and social networking alone have contributed to poets and other writers' work being shared across the world. YouTube has emerged to be a major asset to poets, allowing live performances to be streamed to billions of users. Even now, poetry continues to grow and voice topics that are relevant to the culture of our time. Poetry is not in the spotlight as it may have been in earlier times, but it's still a relevant art form that continues to expand in scope and appeal.

Furthermore, Gioia's argument does not account for live performances of poetry. Not everyone has taken a poetry class or enrolled in university—but most everyone is online. The Internet is a perfect launching point to get all creative work out there. An example of this was the performance of Buddy Wakefield's "Hurling Crowbirds at Mockingbars." Wakefield is a well-known poet who has published several collections of contemporary poetry. One of my favorite works by Wakefield is "Crowbirds," specifically his performance at New York University in 2009. Although his reading was a campus event, views of his performance online number in the thousands. His poetry attracted people outside of the university setting.

Naturally, the poem's popularity can be attributed both to Wakefield's performance and the quality of his writing. "Crowbirds" touches on themes of core human concepts such as faith, personal loss, and growth. These are not ideas that only poets or students of literature understand, but all human beings: "You acted like I was hurling crowbirds at mockingbars / and abandoned me for not making sense. / Evidently, I don't experience things as rationally as you do" (Wakefield 15-17). Wakefield weaves together a complex description of the perplexed and hurt emotions of the speaker who is undergoing a separation from a romantic interest. The line "You acted like I was hurling crowbirds at mockingbars" conjures up an image of someone confused, seemingly out of their mind ... or in the case of the speaker, passionately trying to grasp at a relationship that is fading. The speaker is looking back and finding the words that described how he wasn't making sense. This poem is particularly human and gripping in its message, but the entire effect of the poem is enhanced through the physical performance.

At its core, poetry is about addressing issues and ideas in the world. Part of this is also addressing the perspectives that are exiguously considered. Although the platform may look different, poetry continues to have a steady audience due to the emotional connection the poet shares with the audience.

1. Which of the following best explains how the passage is organized?
   a. The author begins with a long definition of the main topic and then proceeds to prove how that definition has changed over the course of modernity.
   b. The author presents a puzzling phenomenon and uses the rest of the passage to showcase personal experiences in order to explain it.
   c. The author contrasts two different viewpoints and then builds a case showing preference for one over the other.
   d. The passage is an analysis of another theory that the author has no stake in.

2. The author of the passage would likely agree most with which of the following?
   a. Buddy Wakefield is a genius and is considered at the forefront of modern poetry.
   b. Poetry is not irrelevant; it is an art form that adapts to the changing times while containing its core elements.
   c. Spoken word is the zenith of poetic forms and the premier style of poetry in this decade.
   d. Poetry is on the verge of vanishing from our cultural consciousness.

3. Which of the following words, if substituted for the word exiguously in the last paragraph, would LEAST change the meaning of the sentence?
   a. Indolently
   b. Inaudibly
   c. Interminably
   d. Infrequently

4. Which of the following is most closely analogous to the author's opinion of Buddy Wakefield's performance in relation to modern poetry?
   a. Someone's refusal to accept that the Higgs Boson will validate the Standard Model
   b. An individual's belief that soccer will lose popularity within the next 50 years
   c. A professor's opinion that poetry contains the language of the heart, while fiction contains the language of the mind
   d. A student's insistence that psychoanalysis is a subset of modern psychology

5. What is the primary purpose of the passage?
   a. To educate readers on the development of poetry and describe the historical implications of poetry in media
   b. To disprove Dana Gioia's stance that poetry is becoming irrelevant and is only appreciated in academia
   c. To inform readers of the brilliance of Buddy Wakefield and to introduce them to other poets that have influenced contemporary poetry
   d. To prove that Gioia's article does have some truth to it and to shed light on its relevance to modern poetry

6. What is the author's main reason for including the following quote in the passage:

> "You acted like I was hurling crowbirds at mockingbars / and abandoned me for not making sense. / Evidently, I don't experience things as rationally as you do."

a. The quote opens up an opportunity to disprove Gioia's views.
b. The quote demonstrates that people are still writing poetry even if the medium has changed in current times.
c. The quote proves that poets still have an audience to write for even if the audience looks different than it did centuries ago.
d. The quote illustrates the complex themes poets continue to address, which still draw listeners and appreciation.

Questions 7–14 are based on the following passage:

In the quest to understand existence, modern philosophers must question if humans can fully comprehend the world. Classical western approaches to philosophy tend to hold that one can understand something, be it an event or object, by standing outside of the phenomena and observing it. It is then by unbiased observation that one can grasp the details of the world. This seems to hold true for many things. Scientists conduct experiments and record their findings, and thus many natural phenomena become comprehensible. However, several of these observations were possible because humans used tools in order to make these discoveries.

This may seem like an extraneous matter. After all, people invented things like microscopes and telescopes in order to enhance their capacity to view cells or the movement of stars. While humans are still capable of seeing things, the question remains if human beings have the capacity to fully observe and see the world in order to understand it. It would not be an impossible stretch to argue that what humans see through a microscope is not the exact thing itself but rather a human interpretation of it.

This would seem to be the case in the "business of the holes" experiment conducted by Richard Feynman. To study the way electrons behave, Feynman set up a barrier with two holes and a plate. The plate was there to indicate how many times the electrons would pass through the hole(s). Rather than casually observing the electrons acting under normal circumstances, Feynman discovered that electrons behave in two totally different ways depending on whether or not they are observed. The electrons that were observed had passed through either one of the holes or were caught on the plate as particles. However, electrons that weren't observed acted as waves instead of particles and passed through both holes. This indicated that electrons have a dual nature. Electrons seen by the human eye act like particles, while unseen electrons act like waves of energy.

This dual nature of the electrons presents a conundrum. While humans now have a better understanding of electrons, the fact remains that people cannot entirely perceive how electrons behave without the use of instruments. We can only observe one of the mentioned behaviors, which only provides a partial understanding of the entire function of electrons. Therefore, we're forced to ask ourselves whether the world we observe is objective or if it is subjectively perceived by humans. Or, an alternative question: can man understand the world only through machines that will allow them to observe natural phenomena?

Both questions humble man's capacity to grasp the world. However, those ideas don't consider that many phenomena have been proven by human beings without the use of machines, such as the existence of gravity. Like all philosophical questions, whether man's reason and observation alone can understand the universe can be approached from many angles.

7. The word *extraneous* in paragraph two can be best interpreted as meaning which one of the following?
   a. Indispensable
   b. Bewildering
   c. Superfluous
   d. Exuberant

8. What is the author's motivation for writing the passage?
   a. To bring to light an alternative view on human perception by examining the role of technology in human understanding
   b. To educate the reader on the latest astroparticle physics discovery and offer terms that may be unfamiliar to the reader
   c. To argue that humans are totally blind to the realities of the world by presenting an experiment that proves that electrons are not what they seem on the surface
   d. To reflect on opposing views of human understanding

9. Which of the following most closely resembles the way in which paragraph four is structured?
   a. It offers one solution, questions the solution, and then ends with an alternative solution.
   b. It presents an inquiry, explains the details of that inquiry, and then offers a solution.
   c. It presents a problem, explains the details of that problem, and then ends with more inquiries.
   d. It gives a definition, offers an explanation, and then ends with an inquiry.

10. For the classical approach of understanding to hold true, which of the following is required?

a. A telescope
   b. A recording device
   c. Multiple witnesses must be present
   d. The person observing must be unbiased

11. Which best describes how the electrons in the experiment behaved like waves?
   a. The electrons moved up and down like actual waves.
   b. The electrons passed through both holes and then onto the plate.
   c. The electrons converted to photons upon touching the plate.
   d. Electrons were seen passing through one hole or the other.

12. The author mentions gravity in the last paragraph in order to do what?
   a. To show that different natural phenomena test man's ability to grasp the world
   b. To prove that since man has not measured it with the use of tools or machines, humans cannot know the Applied nature of gravity
   c. To demonstrate an example of natural phenomena humans discovered and understood without the use of tools or machines
   d. To show an alternative solution to the nature of electrons that humans have not thought of yet

13. Which situation best parallels the revelation of the dual nature of electrons discovered in Feynman's experiment?
   a. A man is born color-blind and grows up observing everything in lighter or darker shades. With the invention of special goggles he puts on, he discovers that there are other colors in addition to different shades.
   b. The coelacanth was thought to be extinct, but a live specimen was just recently discovered. There are now two living species of coelacanth known to man, and both are believed to be endangered.
   c. In the Middle Ages, blacksmiths added carbon to iron, thus inventing steel. The consequences of this important discovery would have its biggest effects during the Industrial Revolution.
   d. In order to better examine and treat broken bones, the x-ray machine was invented and put to use in hospitals and medical centers.

14. Which statement about technology would the author likely disagree with?
   a. Technology can help expand the field of human vision.
   b. Technology renders human observation irrelevant.
   c. Developing tools used in observation and research indicates growing understanding of our world itself.
   d. Studying certain phenomena necessitates the use of tools and machines.

Questions 15–19 are based on the following passage:

The Middle Ages were a time of great superstition and theological debate. Many beliefs were developed and practiced, while some died out or were listed as heresy. Boethianism is a Medieval theological philosophy that attributes sin to gratification and righteousness with virtue and God's providence. Boethianism holds that sin, greed, and corruption are means to attain temporary pleasure, but they inherently harm the person's soul as well as other human beings.

In *The Canterbury Tales,* we observe more instances of bad actions punished than goodness being rewarded. This would appear to be some reflection of Boethianism. In the "Pardoner's Tale," all three thieves wind up dead, which is a result of their desire for wealth. Each wrongdoer pays with their life, and they are unable to enjoy the wealth they worked to steal. Within his tales, Chaucer gives reprieve to people undergoing struggle, but he also interweaves stories of contemptible individuals being cosmically punished for their wickedness. The thieves idolize physical wealth, which leads to their downfall. This same theme and ideological principle of Boethianism is repeated in the "Friar's Tale," in which the summoner character attempts to gain further wealth by partnering with a demon. The summoner's refusal to repent for his avarice and corruption leads to the demon dragging his soul to Hell. Again, we see the theme of the individual who puts faith and morality aside in favor for a physical prize. The result, of course, is that the summoner loses everything.

The examples of the righteous being rewarded tend to appear in a spiritual context within the *Canterbury Tales*. However, there are a few instances where we see goodness resulting in physical reward. In the "*Prioress's Tale*," we see corporal punishment for barbarism and a reward for goodness. The Jews are punished for their murder of the child, giving a sense of law and order (though racist) to the plot. While the boy does die, he is granted a lasting reward by being able to sing even after his death, a miracle that marks that the murdered youth led a pure life. Here, the miracle represents eternal favor with God.

Again, we see the theological philosophy of Boethianism in Chaucer's *The Canterbury Tales* through acts of sin and righteousness and the consequences that follow. When pleasures of the world are sought instead of God's favor, we see characters being punished in tragic ways. However, the absence of worldly lust has its own set of consequences for the characters seeking to obtain God's favor.

15. What would be a potential reward for living a good life, as described in Boethianism?
   a. A long life sustained by the good deeds one has done over a lifetime
   b. Wealth and fertility for oneself and the extension of one's family line
   c. Vengeance for those who have been persecuted by others who have a capacity for committing wrongdoing
   d. God's divine favor for one's righteousness

16. What might be the main reason why the author chose to discuss Boethianism through examining *The Canterbury Tales*?
   a. *The Canterbury Tales* is a well-known text.
   b. *The Canterbury Tales* is the only known fictional text that contains use of Boethianism.
   c. *The Canterbury Tales* presents a manuscript written in the medieval period that can help illustrate Boethianism through stories and show how people of the time might have responded to the idea.
   d. Within each individual tale in *The Canterbury Tales*, the reader can read about different levels of Boethianism and how each level leads to greater enlightenment.

17. What "ideological principle" is the author referring to in the middle of the second paragraph when talking about the "Friar's Tale"?
   a. The principle that the act of ravaging another's possessions is the same as ravaging one's soul
   b. The principle that thieves who idolize physical wealth will be punished in an earthly sense as well as eternally
   c. The principle that fraternization with a demon will result in one losing everything, including their life
   d. The principle that a desire for material goods leads to moral malfeasance punishable by a higher being

18. Which of the following words, if substituted for the word *avarice* in paragraph two, would LEAST change the meaning of the sentence?
   a. Perniciousness
   b. Pithiness
   c. Parsimoniousness
   d. Precariousness

19. Based on the passage, what view does Boethianism take on desire?
   a. Desire does not exist in the context of Boethianism.
   b. Desire is a virtue and should be welcomed.
   c. Having desire is evidence of demonic possession.
   d. Desire for pleasure can lead toward sin.

Questions 20–27 are based on the following passages:

Passage I

Lethal force, or deadly force, is defined as any action that is intended or likely to cause death or serious harm to another individual. The law holds that lethal force is only accepted when you or another person are in immediate and unavoidable danger of death or severe bodily harm. For example, a person could be beating someone in such a way that the victim is suffering severe trauma that could result in death or serious harm. This would be an instance where lethal force would be acceptable and possibly the only way to save the victim from irrevocable damage.

Another example of when to use lethal force would be when someone enters your home with a deadly weapon. The intruder's presence and possession of the weapon indicate mal-intent and the ability to inflict death or severe injury upon you and your loved ones. Again, lethal force can be used in this situation. Lethal force can also be applied to prevent the harm of another individual. If a woman is being brutally assaulted and is unable to fend off an attacker, lethal force can be used to defend her as a last-ditch effort. If she is in immediate jeopardy of rape, harm, and/or death, lethal force could be the only response that could effectively deter the assailant.

The key to understanding the concept of lethal force is the term *last resort*. Deadly force cannot be taken back; it should be used only to prevent severe harm or death. The law does distinguish whether the means of one's self-defense is fully warranted or if the individual goes out of control in the process. If you continually attack the assailant after they are rendered incapacitated, this would be causing unnecessary harm, and the law can bring charges against you. Likewise, if you kill an attacker unnecessarily after defending yourself, you can be charged with murder. This would move lethal force beyond necessary defense, making it no longer a last resort but rather a use of excessive force.

Passage II

Assault is an unlawful and intentional threat or attempt that causes reasonable apprehension in another individual, either by an imminent threat or by initiating offensive contact. Assaults can vary, encompassing threatening body language and even provocative language.

Let's look at an example. A homeowner is angered because his neighbor blows fallen leaves onto his freshly mowed lawn. Irate, the homeowner gestures a fist to his neighbor and threatens to bash his head in for littering on his lawn. The homeowner's physical motions and verbal threats herald a physical threat against the other neighbor. These factors classify the homeowner's reaction as an assault. If the angry neighbor hits the threatening homeowner in retaliation, that would constitute an assault and battery as well because he physically hit the homeowner.

Assault also centers on the involvement of weapons in a conflict. If someone fires a gun at another person, this could be interpreted as an assault unless the shooter acted in self-defense. If an individual drew a gun or a knife on someone with the intent to harm them, that would be considered assault. However, it's also considered an assault if someone simply aims a weapon, loaded or not, at another person in a threatening manner.

20. What is the purpose of the second passage?
    a. To inform the reader about what assault is and how it is committed
    b. To inform the reader about how assault is a minor example of lethal force
    c. To disprove the previous passage concerning lethal force
    d. The author is recounting an incident in which they were assaulted

21. Using lethal force would be legal in which of the following situations, according to the passages?
    a. A disgruntled cashier yells obscenities at a customer.
    b. A thief is seen running away with stolen cash.
    c. A man is attacked in an alley by another man with a knife.
    d. A woman punches another woman in a bar.

22. Given the information in the passages, which of the following must be true about assault?
    a. Assault charges are more severe than unnecessary use of force charges.
    b. There are various forms of assault.
    c. Smaller, weaker people cannot commit assaults.
    d. Assault is justified only as a last resort.

23. Which of the following, if true, would most seriously undermine the explanation proposed by the author of Passage I in the third paragraph?
   a. An instance of lethal force in self-defense is not absolutely absolved from blame. The law considers the necessary use of force at the time it is committed.
   b. An individual who uses lethal force under necessary defense is in direct compliance of the law under most circumstances.
   c. Lethal force in self-defense should be forgiven in all cases for the peace of mind of the primary victim.
   d. The use of lethal force is not evaluated on the intent of the user, but rather the severity of the primary attack that warranted self-defense.

24. Based on the passages, what can be inferred about the relationship between assault and lethal force?
   a. An act of lethal force always leads to a type of assault.
   b. An assault will result in someone using lethal force.
   c. An assault with deadly intent can lead to an individual using lethal force to preserve their well-being.
   d. If someone uses self-defense in a conflict, it is called deadly force; if actions or threats are intended, it is called assault.

25. Which of the following best describes the way the passages are structured?
   a. Both passages open by defining a legal concept and then continue to describe situations that further explain the concept.
   b. Both passages begin with situations, introduce accepted definitions, and then cite legal ramifications.
   c. Passage I presents a long definition, while Passage II begins by showing an example of assault.
   d. Both cite specific legal doctrines and proceed to explain the rulings.

26. What can be inferred about the role of intent in lethal force and assault?
   a. Intent is irrelevant. The law does not take intent into account.
   b. Intent is vital for determining the lawfulness of using lethal force.
   c. Intent is very important for determining both lethal force and assault; intent is examined in both parties and helps determine the severity of the issue.
   d. The intent of the assailant is the main focus for determining legal ramifications; it is used to determine if the defender was justified in using force to respond.

27. The author uses the example in the second paragraph of Passage II in order to do what?
   a. To demonstrate two different types of assault by showing how each specifically relates to the other
   b. To demonstrate a single example of two different types of assault, then adding in the third type of assault in the example's conclusion
   c. To prove that the definition of lethal force is altered when the victim in question is a homeowner and his property is threatened
   d. To suggest that verbal assault can be an exaggerated crime by the law and does not necessarily lead to physical violence

Questions 28–33 are based upon the following passage:

> Fellow-citizens, pardon me, allow me to ask, why am I called upon to speak here to-day? What have I, or those I represent, to do with your national independence? Are the great principles of political freedom and of natural justice, embodied in that Declaration of Independence, extended to us? And am I, therefore, called upon to bring our humble offering to the national altar, and to confess the benefits and express devout gratitude for the blessings resulting from your independence to us?
>
> Would to God, both for your sakes and ours, that an affirmative answer could be truthfully returned to these questions! Then would my task be light, and my burden easy and delightful. For

who is there so cold, that a nation's sympathy could not warm him? Who so obdurate and dead to the claims of gratitude, that would not thankfully acknowledge such priceless benefits? Who so stolid and selfish, that would not give his voice to swell the hallelujahs of a nation's jubilee, when the chains of servitude had been torn from his limbs? I am not that man. In a case like that, the dumb my eloquently speak, and the lame man leap as an hart.

But, such is not the state of the case. I say it with a sad sense of the disparity between us. I am not included within the pale of this glorious and anniversary! Your high independence only reveals the immeasurable distance between us. The blessings in which you, this day, rejoice, are not enjoyed in common. The rich inheritance of justice, liberty, prosperity, and independence, bequeathed by your fathers, is shared by you, not by me. The sunlight that brought life and healing to you, has brought stripes and death to me. This Fourth [of] July is yours, not mine. You may rejoice, I must mourn. To drag a man in fetters into the grand illuminated temple of liberty, and call upon him to join you in joyous anthems, were inhuman mockery and sacrilegious irony. Do you mean, citizens, to mock me, by asking me to speak to-day? If so, there is a parallel to your conduct. And let me warn you that it is dangerous to copy the example of a nation whose crimes, towering up to heaven, were thrown down by the breath of the Almighty, burying that nation in irrecoverable ruin! I can to-day take up the plaintive lament of a peeled and woe-smitten people!

"By the rivers of Babylon, there we sat down. Yea! We wept when we remembered Zion. We hanged our harps upon the willows in the midst thereof. For there, they that carried us away captive, required of us a song; and they who wasted us required of us mirth, saying, Sing us one of the songs of Zion. How can we sing the Lord's song in a strange land? If I forget thee, O Jerusalem, let my right hand forget her cunning. If I do not remember thee, let my tongue cleave to the roof of my mouth."

Excerpt from "What to the Slave is the Fourth of July?" by Frederick Douglass, Rochester, New York July 5, 1852.

28. What is the tone of the first paragraph of this passage?
    a. Incredulous
    b. Inclusive
    c. Contemplative
    d. Nonchalant

29. Which word is NOT a synonym for "obdurate" as it is used in the sentence below?

    Who so obdurate and dead to the claims of gratitude, that would not thankfully acknowledge such priceless benefits?

    a. Callous
    b. Stubborn
    c. Contented
    d. Hardened

30. What is the central purpose of this text?
    a. To demonstrate the author's extensive knowledge of the Bible
    b. To address the hypocrisy of the Fourth of July holiday
    c. To convince wealthy landowners to adopt new holiday rituals
    d. To explain why minorities often relished the notion of segregation in government institutions

31. Which statement serves as evidence for the answer to question 30 above?
    a. By the rivers of Babylon, there we sat down.
    b. Fellow-citizens, pardon me, allow me to ask, why am I called upon to speak here to-day?
    c. I can to-day take up the plaintive lament of a peeled and woe-smitten people!
    d. The rich inheritance of justice, liberty, prosperity, and independence, bequeathed by your fathers, is shared by you, not by me.

32. The statement below features an example of which of the following literary devices:

    Oh pity! Your high independence only reveals the immeasurable distance between us.

    a. Assonance
    b. Parallelism
    c. Amplification
    d. Hyperbole

33. Why does the speaker include the following quote from the Bible?

    "By the rivers of Babylon, there we sat down. Yea! we wept when we remembered Zion. We hanged our harps upon the willows in the midst thereof. For there, they that carried us away captive, required of us a song; and they who wasted us required of us mirth, saying, 'Sing us one of the songs of Zion.' How can we sing the Lord's song in a strange land? If I forget thee, O Jerusalem, let my right hand forget her cunning. If I do not remember thee, let my tongue cleave to the roof of my mouth."

    a. To connect with the audience on a religious level
    b. To prove to the audience that injustices have been committed
    c. To support his claim of paralleled conduct
    d. To call on the citizens to join him in joyous anthems

Questions 34–39 are based upon the following passage:

Four score and seven years ago our fathers brought forth on this continent, a new nation, conceived in Liberty, and dedicated to the proposition that all men are created equal.

Now we are engaged in a great civil war, testing whether that nation, or any nation so conceived and so dedicated, can long endure. We are met on a great battle-field of that war. We have come to dedicate a portion of that field, as a final resting place for those who here gave their lives that that nation might live. It is altogether fitting and proper that we should do this.

But, in a larger sense, we can not dedicate—we can not consecrate—we can not hallow—this ground. The brave men, living and dead, who struggled here, have consecrated it, far above our poor power to add or detract. The world will little note, nor long remember what we say here, but it can never forget what they did here. It is for us the living, rather, to be dedicated here to the unfinished work which they who fought here have thus far so nobly advanced. It is rather for us to be here dedicated to the great task remaining before us—that from these honored dead we take increased devotion to that cause for which they gave the last full measure of devotion—that we here highly resolve that these dead shall not have died in vain—that this nation, under God, shall have a new birth of freedom—and that government of the people, by the people, for the people, shall not perish from the earth.

Excerpt from Abraham Lincoln's Address Delivered at the Dedication of the Cemetery at Gettysburg, November 19, 1863.

34. The best description for the phrase *four score and seven years ago* is which of the following?
    a. A unit of measurement
    b. A period of time
    c. A literary movement
    d. A statement of political reform

35. What is the setting of this text?
    a. A battleship off of the coast of France
    b. A desert plain on the Sahara Desert
    c. A battlefield in North America
    d. The residence of Abraham Lincoln

36. Which war is Abraham Lincoln referring to in the following sentence?

    Now we are engaged in a great civil war, testing whether that nation, or any nation so conceived and so dedicated, can long endure.

    a. World War I
    b. The War of the Spanish Succession
    c. World War II
    d. The American Civil War

37. What message is the speaker trying to convey through this address?
    a. The audience should perpetuate the ideals of freedom that the soldiers died fighting for.
    b. The audience should honor the dead by establishing an annual memorial service.
    c. The audience should form a militia that would overturn the current political structure.
    d. The audience should forget the lives that were lost and discredit the soldiers.

38. Which rhetorical device is being used in the following passage?

    ...we here highly resolve that these dead shall not have died in vain—that this nation, under God, shall have a new birth of freedom—and that government of the people, by the people, for the people, shall not perish from the earth.

    a. Antimetabole
    b. Antiphrasis
    c. Anaphora
    d. Epiphora

39. What is the effect of Lincoln's statement in the following passage?

    But, in a larger sense, we can not dedicate—we can not consecrate—we can not hallow—this ground. The brave men, living and dead, who struggled here, have consecrated it, far above our poor power to add or detract.

    a. His comparison emphasizes the great sacrifice of the soldiers who fought in the war.
    b. His comparison serves as a reminder of the inadequacies of his audience.
    c. His comparison serves as a catalyst for guilt and shame among audience members.
    d. His comparison suggests that the dedication ceremony was inappropriate.

Questions 40–45 are based upon the following passage:

My Good Friends,—When I first imparted to the committee of the projected Institute my particular wish that on one of the evenings of my readings here the main body of my audience should be composed of working men and their families, I was animated by two desires; first, by the wish to have the great pleasure of meeting you face to face at this Christmas time, and accompany you myself through one of my little Christmas books; and second, by the wish to have an opportunity of stating publicly in your presence, and in the presence of the committee, my earnest hope that the Institute will, from the beginning, recognize one great principle—strong in reason and justice—which I believe to be essential to the very life of such an Institution. It is, that the working man shall, from the first unto the last, have a share in the management of an Institution which is designed for his benefit, and which calls itself by his name.

I have no fear here of being misunderstood—of being supposed to mean too much in this. If there ever was a time when any one class could of itself do much for its own good, and for the welfare of society—which I greatly doubt—that time is unquestionably past. It is in the fusion of different classes, without confusion; in the bringing together of employers and employed; in the creating of a better common understanding among those whose interests are identical, who depend upon each other, who are vitally essential to each other, and who never can be in unnatural antagonism without deplorable results, that one of the chief principles of a Mechanics' Institution should consist. In this world, a great deal of the bitterness among us arises from an imperfect understanding of one another. Erect in Birmingham a great Educational Institution, properly educational; educational of the feelings as well as of the reason; to which all orders of Birmingham men contribute; in which all orders of Birmingham men meet; wherein all orders of Birmingham men are faithfully represented—and you will erect a Temple of Concord here which will be a model edifice to the whole of England.

Contemplating as I do the existence of the Artisans' Committee, which not long ago considered the establishment of the Institute so sensibly, and supported it so heartily, I earnestly entreat the gentlemen—earnest I know in the good work, and who are now among us—by all means to avoid the great shortcoming of similar institutions; and in asking the working man for his confidence, to set him the great example and give him theirs in return. You will judge for yourselves if I promise too much for the working man, when I say that he will stand by such an enterprise with the utmost of his patience, his perseverance, sense, and support; that I am sure he will need no charitable aid or condescending patronage; but will readily and cheerfully pay for the advantages which it confers; that he will prepare himself in individual cases where he feels that the adverse circumstances around him have rendered it necessary; in a word, that he will feel his responsibility like an honest man, and will most honestly and manfully discharge it. I now proceed to the pleasant task to which I assure you I have looked forward for a long time.

Excerpt from Charles Dickens' speech in Birmingham in England on December 30, 1853 on behalf of the Birmingham and Midland Institute.

40. Which word is most closely synonymous with the word patronage as it appears in the following statement:

...that I am sure he will need no charitable aid or condescending patronage;

a. Auspices
b. Aberration
c. Acerbic
d. Adulation

41. Which term is most closely aligned with the definition of the term working man as it is used in the following quotation?

> You will judge for yourselves if I promise too much for the working man, when I say that he will stand by such an enterprise with the utmost of his patience, his perseverance, sense, and support...

a. Plebian
b. Viscount
c. Entrepreneur
d. Proletariat

42. Which of the following statements most closely correlates with the definition of the term *working man* as it is defined in Question 41?

a. A working man is not someone who works for institutions or corporations, but someone who is well-versed in the workings of the soul.
b. A working man is someone who is probably not involved in social activities because the physical demand for work is too high.
c. A working man is someone who works for wages among the middle class.
d. The working man has historically taken to the field, to the factory, and now to the screen.

43. Based upon the contextual evidence provided in the passage above, what is the meaning of the term *enterprise* in the third paragraph?

a. Company
b. Courage
c. Game
d. Cause

44. The speaker addresses his audience as *My Good Friends.* What kind of credibility does this salutation give to the speaker?

a. The speaker is an employer addressing his employees, so the salutation is a way for the boss to bridge the gap between himself and his employees.
b. The speaker's salutation is one from an entertainer to his audience, and he uses this friendly language to connect to his audience before a serious speech.
c. The salutation is used ironically to give a somber tone to the serious speech that follows.
d. The speech is one from a politician to the public, so the salutation is used to grab the audience's attention.

45. According to the passage, what is the speaker's second desire for his time in front of the audience?

a. To read a Christmas story
b. For the working man to have a say in his institution, which is designed for his benefit
c. To have an opportunity to stand in their presence
d. For the life of the institution to be essential to the audience as a whole

Questions 46–51 are based upon the following passage:

> MANKIND being originally equals in the order of creation, the equality could only be destroyed by some subsequent circumstance; the distinctions of rich, and poor, may in a great measure be accounted for, and that without having recourse to the harsh, ill-sounding names of oppression and avarice. Oppression is often the CONSEQUENCE, but seldom or never the MEANS of riches; and though avarice will preserve a man from being necessitously poor, it generally makes him too timorous to be wealthy.

But there is another and greater distinction, for which no truly natural or religious reason can be assigned, and that is, the distinction of men into KINGS and SUBJECTS. Male and female are the distinctions of nature, good and bad the distinctions of heaven; but how a race of men came into the world so exalted above the rest, and distinguished like some new species, is worth enquiring into, and whether they are the means of happiness or of misery to mankind.

In the early ages of the world, according to the scripture chronology, there were no kings; the consequence of which was, there were no wars; it is the pride of kings which throw mankind into confusion. Holland without a king hath enjoyed more peace for this last century than any of the monarchical governments in Europe. Antiquity favors the same remark; for the quiet and rural lives of the first patriarchs hath a happy something in them, which vanishes away when we come to the history of Jewish royalty.

Government by kings was first introduced into the world by the Heathens, from whom the children of Israel copied the custom. It was the most prosperous invention the Devil ever set on foot for the promotion of idolatry. The Heathens paid divine honors to their deceased kings, and the Christian world hath improved on the plan, by doing the same to their living ones. How impious is the title of sacred majesty applied to a worm, who in the midst of his splendor is crumbling into dust!

As the exalting one man so greatly above the rest cannot be justified on the equal rights of nature, so neither can it be defended on the authority of scripture; for the will of the Almighty, as declared by Gideon and the prophet Samuel, expressly disapproves of government by kings. All anti-monarchical parts of scripture have been very smoothly glossed over in monarchical governments, but they undoubtedly merit the attention of countries which have their governments yet to form. "Render unto Caesar the things which are Caesar's" is the scripture doctrine of courts, yet it is no support of monarchical government, for the Jews at that time were without a king, and in a state of vassalage to the Romans.

Now three thousand years passed away from the Mosaic account of the creation, till the Jews under a national delusion requested a king. Till then their form of government (except in extraordinary cases, where the Almighty interposed) was a kind of republic administered by a judge and the elders of the tribes. Kings they had none, and it was held sinful to acknowledge any being under that title but the Lord of Hosts And when a man seriously reflects on the idolatrous homage which is paid to the persons of kings, he need not wonder that the Almighty, ever jealous of his honor, should disapprove of a form of government which so impiously invades the prerogative of heaven.

The following is an excerpt from Common Sense by Thomas Payne. iBooks.

46. According to the passage, what role does avarice, or greed, play in wealth and poverty?
    a. Avarice makes a man poor.
    b. Avarice is the consequence of wealth.
    c. Avarice prevents a man from being poor, but makes him too fearful to be wealthy.
    d. Avarice is what drives a person to be wealthy.

47. Of these distinctions, which does the author believe to be beyond natural or religious reason?
    a. Good and bad
    b. Male and female
    c. Human and animal
    d. Kings and subjects

48. According to the passage, what are the Heathens responsible for?
    a. Government by kings
    b. Quiet and rural lives of patriarchs
    c. Paying divine honors to their living kings
    d. Equal rights of nature

49. Which of the following best states Paine's rationale for the denouncement of monarchy?
    a. It is against the laws of nature.
    b. It is against the equal rights of nature and is denounced in scripture.
    c. Despite scripture, a monarchical government is unlawful.
    d. Neither the law nor scripture denounce monarchy.

50. Based on the passage, what is the best definition of the word *idolatrous*?
    a. Worshipping kings
    b. Being deceitful
    c. Sinfulness
    d. Engaging in illegal activities

51. What is the essential meaning of the following passage:

    > And when a man seriously reflects on the idolatrous homage which is paid to the persons of kings, he need not wonder that the Almighty, ever jealous of his honor, should disapprove of a form of government which so impiously invades the prerogative of heaven.

    a. God disapproves of the irreverence of a monarchical government.
    b. With careful reflection, men should realize that heaven is not promised.
    c. God will punish those that follow a monarchical government.
    d. Belief in a monarchical government cannot coexist with belief in God.

Answer Explanations

Biological and Biochemical Foundations of Living Systems

1. A: When activated, B cells create antibodies against specific antigens. White blood cells are generated in the red bone marrow, not in cartilage. Platelets are not a type of white blood cell and are typically cell fragments produced by megakaryocytes. White blood cells are active throughout nearly all of one's life and have not been shown to specially activate or deactivate because of life events like puberty or menopause.

2. D: Mechanical digestion is physical digestion of food and breaking or tearing it into smaller pieces using force. Mechanical digestion occurs in the stomach and mouth. Chemical digestion involves chemically changing the food and breaking it down into small organic compounds that can be utilized by the cell to perform functions or build other molecules. The salivary glands in the mouth secrete amylase, which breaks down starch and begins chemical digestion. The stomach contains enzymes, such as pepsinogen/pepsin and gastric lipase, which chemically digest protein and fats, respectively. The small intestine continues to digest protein using the enzymes trypsin and chymotrypsin. It also digests fats, with the help of bile from the liver and lipase from the pancreas. These organs act as exocrine glands because they secrete substances through ducts. Carbohydrates are digested in the small intestine with the help of pancreatic amylase, gut bacterial flora and fauna, and brush border enzymes like lactose. Brush border enzymes are contained in the towel-like microvilli in the small intestine, which soak up nutrients.

3. D: Charles Darwin developed the theory of natural selection, which explains the evolutionary process. He postulated that heritable genetic differences could aid an organism's chance of survival in its environment. The organisms with favorable traits pass genes to their offspring, and because they have more reproductive success than those that do not contain the adaptation, the favorable gene spreads throughout the population. Those that do not contain the adaptation often extinguish, so their genes are not passed on. In this way, nature "selects" for the organisms that have more fitness in their environment. Birds with bright-colored feathers and cacti with spines are examples of "fit" organisms.

4. C: Ligand binding to a tyrosine kinase transmembrane protein. Tyrosine kinase transmembrane proteins are just one example of a receptor protein. There are also G protein-coupled receptors and ion channel receptors. Regardless of the type of receptor, ligand binding is the first step. Choice *D* is incorrect because, prior to ion-gated channels opening, a ligand would need to bind to the receptor to induce the conformational change. Choice *A* occurs after ligand binding and Choice *B* is a response that is much farther downstream (it's an effect of signal transduction).

5. B: The cell structure responsible for cellular digestion and waste removal is the lysosome. Lysosomes are like recycle bins. They are filled with digestive enzymes that facilitate catabolic reactions to regenerate monomers. The Golgi apparatus is designed to tag, package, and ship out proteins destined for other cells or locations. The centrioles typically play a large role only in cell division when they ratchet the chromosomes from the mitotic plate to the poles of the cell. The mitochondria are involved in energy production and are the powerhouses of the cell.

6. A: Crossing over, or genetic recombination, is the rearrangement of chromosomal sections in tetrads during meiosis. A result of this process is that each gamete has a different combination of alleles than the other gametes. The disassembly of the mitotic spindle happens only after telophase and is not related to diversity. While nondisjunction does cause diversity in division and is highly noticeable in gametes formed through meiosis, it can also happen through mitotic division in somatic cells. Although an egg fertilized by multiple sperm would lead to interesting diversity in the offspring (and possibly fraternal twins), this is not strictly a byproduct of meiotic division.

7. D: Veins have valves, but arteries do not. Valves in veins are designed to prevent backflow since they are the furthest blood vessels from the pumping action of the heart and steadily increase in volume (which decreases the available pressure). Capillaries diffuse nutrients properly because of their thin walls and high surface area and are not particularly dependent on positive pressure.

8. C: The blood leaves the right ventricle through a semilunar valve and goes through the pulmonary artery to the lungs. Any increase in pressure in the artery will eventually affect the contractibility of the right ventricle. Blood enters the right atrium from the superior and inferior venae cavae veins, and blood leaves the right atrium through the tricuspid valve to the right ventricle. Blood enters the left atrium from the pulmonary veins carrying oxygenated blood from the lungs. Blood flows from the left atrium to the left ventricle through the mitral valve and leaves the left ventricle through a semilunar valve to enter the aorta.

9. D: Sodium bicarbonate, a very effective base, functions chiefly to increase the pH of the chyme. Chyme leaving the stomach has a very low pH due to the high amounts of acid that are used to digest and break down food. If this is not neutralized, the walls of the small intestine will be damaged and may form ulcers. Sodium bicarbonate is produced by the pancreas and released in response to pyloric stimulation so that it can neutralize the acid. It has little to no digestive effect.

10. D: A reflex arc is a simple nerve pathway involving a stimulus, a synapse, and a response that is controlled by the spinal cord—not the brain. The knee-jerk reflex is an example of a reflex arc. The stimulus is the hammer touching the tendon, which reaches the synapse in the spinal cord by an afferent pathway. The response is the resulting muscle contraction, which reaches the muscle by an efferent pathway. None of the remaining processes are simple reflexes. Memories are processed and stored in the hippocampus in the limbic system. The visual center is located in the occipital lobe, while auditory processing occurs in the temporal lobe. The sympathetic and parasympathetic divisions of the autonomic nervous system control heart rate and blood pressure.

11. C: The lagging strand of DNA falls behind the leading strand because of its discontinuous synthesis. DNA helicase unzips the DNA helices so that synthesis can take place, and RNA primers are created by the RNA primase for the polymerases to attach to and build from. The lagging strand is synthesizing DNA in a direction that is hard for the polymerase to build, so multiple primers are laid down so that the entire length of DNA can be synthesized simultaneously, piecemeal. These short pieces of DNA being synthesized are known as Okazaki fragments and are joined together by DNA ligase.

12. A: When activated, B cells create antibodies against specific bacteria. T cells directly attack cells that are infected with bacteria or viruses. Macrophages alert the B cells to the presence of foreign cells. In addition, by the process of phagocytosis, macrophages surround and ingest the invading cells, rendering them harmless.

13. B: The hepatic portal vein brings newly absorbed nutrients to the liver from the digestive system. The hepatic artery brings oxygen to the liver. The liver cannot make its own energy without the "raw ingredients" supplied by the digestive system. The gallbladder stores bile that is made by the liver. When food is consumed, the gallbladder secretes the bile through the common bile duct to add in digestion.

14. D: G0 is a state that stimulates progression into S phase. G0 is actually a checkpoint that involves cells exiting the cell cycle, such as mature neurons and damaged cells that may undergo apoptosis. Therefore, Choice *D* is the untrue statement. Choices A, B, and C refer to the Maturation Promoting Factor (MPF), which is a cyclin/CDK pair that forms in G2 when rising levels of cyclin bind to and activate an ever-present cyclin dependent kinase.

15. C: Although the lungs may provide some cushioning for the heart when the body is violently struck, this is not a major function of the respiratory system. Its most notable function is that of gas exchange for oxygen and carbon dioxide, but it also plays a vital role in the regulation of blood pH. The aqueous form of carbon dioxide, carbonic acid, is a major pH buffer of the blood, and the respiratory system directly controls how much carbon dioxide stays and is released from the blood through respiration. The respiratory system also enables vocalization and forms the basis for the mode of speech and language used by most humans.

16. A: The forebrain contains the cerebrum, the thalamus, the hypothalamus, and the limbic system. The limbic system is chiefly responsible for the perception of emotions through the amygdala, while the cerebrum interprets sensory input and generates movement. The occipital lobe receives visual input, while the primary motor cortex in the frontal lobe is the controller of voluntary movement. The hindbrain, specifically the medulla oblongata and brain stem, control and regulate blood pressure and heart rate.

17. D: Germline mutations in eggs and sperm are permanent, they can be on the chromosomal level, and they will be inherited by offspring. Somatic mutations cannot affect eggs and sperm, and therefore are not inherited by offspring. Mutations of either kind are rarely beneficial to the individual, but do not necessarily harm them. Germline cells divide much more rapidly than do somatic cells, and a mutation in a sex cell would promulgate and affect many thousands of its daughter cells.

18. C: Glucagon is released by the alpha cells of the pancreas when blood glucose levels fall below normal. Glucagon then stimulates the liver to convert stored glycogen to glucose. The glucose is then released to the circulating blood, increasing the serum glucose level. This is the process of glycogenolysis. Insulin secretion will further decrease the blood glucose level. Insulin is not absorbed by the cells. It remains in the circulating blood volume, stimulating the cellular absorption of glucose.

19. C: Cholesterol is necessary for the formation of cellular membranes, vitamin D, and some hormones. However, overproduction of cholesterol may contribute to cardiovascular disease. Hemoglobin is processed in order to store iron for use as needed. Ammonia, which is toxic, is converted to urea, which is then excreted by the kidneys. Glycogen is stored until the body requires additional glucose to maintain blood sugar levels.

20. C: A catalyst functions to increase reaction rates by decreasing the activation energy required for a reaction to take place. Inhibitors would increase the activation energy or otherwise stop the reactants from reacting. Although increasing the temperature usually increases a reaction's rate, this is not true in all cases, and most catalysts do not function in this manner.

21. B: Biological catalysts are termed enzymes; enzymes are proteins with conformations that specifically manipulate reactants into positions that decrease the reaction's activation energy. Lipids do not usually affect reactions, and while cofactors can aid or be required for the proper functioning of enzymes, they do not make up the majority of biological catalysts.

22. D: In the second diastolic phase, the blood returns to the left atrium and then is pumped into the left ventricle. Choice *A* is the definition of the second systolic phase. Choice *B* is the definition of the first diastolic phase, and Choice *C* is the definition of the first systolic phase.

23. C: Cellulose and starch are both polysaccharides, which are long chains of glucose molecules. However, they are connected by different types of bonds, which gives them different structures and different functions.

24. B: The secondary structure is formed from hydrogen bonds between the backbone atoms in the protein chain. Some R groups allow these interactions to form, and others prevent them. A mutation can cause the secondary structure to change when it changes an R group from one that allows these interactions to one that prevents these interactions.

25. A: The nucleus, chloroplast, and mitochondria are all bound by two layers of membranes. The Golgi apparatus, lysosome, and ER only have one membrane layer.

26. D: Proteins are synthesized on ribosomes. The ribosome uses messenger RNA as a template, and transfer RNA brings amino acids to the ribosome, where they are synthesized into peptide strands using the genetic code provided by the mRNA.

27. B: The "lock and key" model of hormone secretion states that only cells with specific receptors can benefit from hormonal influence. Steroid hormones are capable of triggering protein synthesis by binding to receptor proteins in the cell's nucleus, resulting in the formation of other hormones or enzymes. Bacteria adhere to foreign cells by phagocytosis.

28. C: When cells differentiate, they specialize from a general cell into one with more specific functions. The best example of this is when pluripotent cells like stem cells differentiate during development to become a certain kind of cell that makes a certain kind of protein. Choice *A* references cell lysis, Choice *B* references fertilization, and Choice *D* references cell senescence.

29. D: Aerobic respiration produces 36 molecules of ATP, and anaerobic respiration, through fermentation, produces only 4 molecules of ATP per molecule of glucose. Oxygen is not present in the anaerobic pathway, so it can't be depleted. The anaerobic pathway has far fewer steps than the anaerobic pathway, so it takes less time. Only about half of the energy produced by the aerobic pathway is used to form ATP. The remaining energy is dissipated as heat.

30. C: mRNA is directly transcribed from DNA before being taken to the cytoplasm and translated by rRNA into a protein. tRNA transfers amino acids from the cytoplasm to the rRNA for use in building these proteins. siRNA is a special type of RNA which interferes with other strands of mRNA, typically by causing them to get degraded by the cell rather than translated into protein.

31. B: Since the genotype is a depiction of the specific alleles that an organism's genes code for, it includes recessive genes that may or may not be physically expressed. The genotype does not have to name the proteins that its alleles code for; indeed, some of them may be unknown. The phenotype is the physical, visual manifestations of a gene, not the genotype. The genotype does not necessarily include any information about the organism's physical characteristics. Although some information about an organism's parents can be obtained from its genotype, its genotype does not actually show the parents' phenotypes.

32. C: One in four offspring (or 25%) will be short, so all four offspring cannot be tall. Although both of the parents are tall, they are hybrid or heterozygous tall, not homozygous. Although it may seem intuitive that the short allele will be expressed by lower numbers of the population than the tall allele, it still appears in 75% of the offspring (although its effects are masked in 2/3 of those). Besides, conditions could favor the recessive allele and kill off the tall offspring.

	T	*t*
T	*TT*	*Tt*
t	*Tt*	*tt*

Both parents are mixed hybrids
so offspring are a 3:1 ratio

33. C: Gene expression can be influenced by the environment. Lactose metabolism is regulated by the presence of lactose. Bacteria that have the genes to metabolize lactose will turn them off if lactose is not present but will turn them on if lactose is present.

34. A: Human genes are strictly DNA and do not include proteins or amino acids. A human's genome and collection of genes will include even their recessive traits, mutations, and unused DNA.

35. D: All statements are true, but nothing can happen without the message being available; thus, Choice *D* must occur first. After the copy is made in transcription (D), Choice *B* occurs because mRNA has to be processed before it is exported into the cytoplasm. Once it has reached the cytoplasm, Choice *A* occurs as mRNA is pulled into the ribosome. Finally, Choice *C* occurs, and tRNA delivers amino acids one at a time until the full polypeptide has been created. At that point, the baby protein (polypeptide) will be processed and folded in the ER and Golgi.

36. C: The parasympathetic nervous system is related to calm, peaceful times without stress that require no immediate decisions. It relaxes the fight-or-flight response, slows heart rate to a comfortable pace, and decreases bronchiole dilation to a normal size. On the other hand, the sympathetic nervous system is in charge of the fight-or-flight response and works to increase blood pressure and oxygen absorption.

37. A: Shortening of telomeres. Choices B and C both occur, but they have nothing to do with the direction of DNA synthesis. Choice *D* is untrue because Okazaki fragments are due to the directional synthesis of DNA, but they form on the lagging strand.

38. A: Catabolic reactions release energy and are exothermic. Catabolism breaks down complex molecules into simpler molecules. Anabolic reactions are just the opposite—they absorb energy in order to form complex molecules from simpler ones. Proteins, carbohydrates (polysaccharides), lipids, and nucleic acids are complex organic molecules synthesized by anabolic metabolism. The monomers of these organic compounds are amino acids, monosaccharides, triglycerides, and nucleotides.

39. B: The structure exclusively found in eukaryotic cells is the nucleus. Animal, plant, fungi, and protist cells are all eukaryotic. DNA is contained within the nucleus of eukaryotic cells, and they also have membrane-bound organelles that perform complex intracellular metabolic activities. Prokaryotic cells (archaea and bacteria) do not have a nucleus or other membrane-bound organelles and are less complex than eukaryotic cells.

40. A: The Golgi complex, also known as the Golgi apparatus, is not found in the nucleus. Chromosomes, the nucleolus, and chromatin are all found within the nucleus of the cell. The Golgi apparatus is found in the cytoplasm and is responsible for protein maturation, which is the process of proteins folding into their secondary, tertiary, and quaternary configurations. The structure appears folded in membranous layers and is easily visible with microscopy. The Golgi apparatus packages proteins in vesicles for export out of the cell or to their cellular destination.

41. B: The cell structure responsible for cellular storage, digestion, and waste removal is the lysosome. Lysosomes are like recycle bins. They are filled with digestive enzymes that facilitate catabolic reactions to regenerate monomers.

42. B: Phenotypes are observable traits, such as eye color, hair color, blood type, etc. They can also be biochemical or have physiological or behavioral traits. A genotype is the collective gene representation of an individual, whether the genes are expressed or not. Alleles are different forms of the same gene that code for specific traits, like blue eyes or brown eyes. In simple genetics, there are two forms of a gene: dominant and recessive. More complex genetics involves co-dominance, multiple alleles, and sex-linked genes. The other answer choices are incorrect because sex is determined by the presence of an entire chromosome (the Y chromosome), and a karyotype is an image of all of an individual's chromosomes.

43. D: Reproductive cells are referred to as gametes: egg (female) and sperm (male). These cells have only 1 set of 23 chromosomes and are haploid so that when they combine during fertilization, the zygote has the correct diploid number (46). Reproductive cell division is called meiosis, which is different from mitosis, the type of division process for body (somatic) cells.

44. A: The process of cell division in somatic cells is called mitosis. In interphase, which precedes mitosis, cells prepare for division by copying their DNA. Once mitotic machinery has been assembled in interphase, mitosis occurs, which has four distinct phases: prophase, metaphase, anaphase, and telophase, followed by cytokinesis, which is the final splitting of the cytoplasm. The two diploid daughter cells are genetically identical to the parent cell.

45. D: Human gametes each contain 23 chromosomes. This is referred to as a haploid, which is a cell that has half the number of chromosomes as the original germ cell (46). Germ cells are diploid precursors of the haploid egg and sperm. Meiosis has two major phases, each of which is characterized by sub-phases similar to mitosis. In meiosis I, the DNA of the parent cell is duplicated in interphase, just like in mitosis. Starting with prophase I, things become a little different. Two homologous chromosomes form a tetrad, cross over, and exchange genetic content. Each shuffled chromosome of the tetrad migrates to the cell's poles, and two haploid daughter cells are formed. In meiosis II, each daughter undergoes another division more similar to mitosis (except for the fact that there is no interphase), resulting in four genetically-different cells, each with only half of the chromosomal material of the original germ cell.

46. A: The crossing over, or rearrangement of chromosomal sections in tetrads during meiosis, results in each gamete having a different combination of alleles than other gametes. Choice *B* is incorrect because the presence of a Y chromosome determines an organism's sex. Choice *C* is incorrect because it is improper separation in anaphase, not recombination, that causes non-disjunction. Choice *D* is incorrect because transcription is an entirely different process involved in protein expression.

47. A: An alteration in the normal gene sequence is called a DNA point mutation. Mutations can be harmful, neutral, or even beneficial. Sometimes, as seen in natural selection, a genetic mutation can improve fitness, providing an adaptation that will aid in survival. DNA mutations can happen as a result of environmental damage, for example, from radiation or chemicals. Mutations can also happen during cell replication as a result of incorrect pairing of complementary nucleotides by DNA polymerase. There are also chromosomal mutations as well, where entire segments of chromosomes can be deleted, inverted, duplicated, or sent or received from a different chromosome.

48. B: The child has a two out of four chance (50%) of having type A blood since the dominant allele IA is present in two of the four possible offspring. The type O blood allele is masked by the type A blood allele since it is recessive. Test takers can sketch out a Punnett square to better visualize.

49. D: A nucleotide is a five-carbon sugar with a phosphate group and a nitrogenous base (adenine, guanine, cytosine, and thymine). DNA is a double helix and looks like a spiral ladder. Each side has a sugar/phosphate backbone, and the rungs of the ladder that connect the sides are the nitrogenous bases. Adenine always pairs with thymine via two hydrogen bonds, and cytosine always pairs with guanine via three hydrogen bonds. The weak hydrogen bonds are important because they allow DNA to easily be opened for replication and transcription.

50. D: There are actually many different types of RNA. The three involved in protein synthesis are messenger RNA (mRNA), ribosomal RNA (rRNA), and transfer RNA (tRNA). Others, including small interfering RNA, microRNA, and Piwi-interacting RNA, are being investigated. Their known functions include gene regulation and facilitating chromosome wrapping and unwrapping. RNA, unlike DNA, can be single stranded (mRNA, specifically), has a ribose sugar (rather than deoxyribose, like in DNA), and contains uracil (in place of thymine in DNA).

51. D: Cellular respiration is the term used for the set of metabolic reactions that converts the energy in chemical bonds to ATP. All cellular respiration starts with glycolysis in the cytoplasm, and in the presence of oxygen, the process will continue to the mitochondria. In a series of oxidation/reduction reactions, primarily glucose will be broken down so that the energy contained within its bonds can be transferred to the smaller ATP molecules. It's like having a $100 bill (glucose) as opposed to having 100 $1 bills. This is beneficial to the organism because it allows energy to be distributed throughout the cell very easily in smaller allotments as needed, so that less is wasted.

When glucose is broken down, its electrons and hydrogen atoms are involved in oxidative phosphorylation in order to make ATP, while its carbon and oxygen atoms are released as carbon dioxide. Anaerobic respiration does not occur frequently in humans, but during rigorous exercise, lack of available oxygen in the muscles can lead to anaerobic ATP production in a process called lactic acid fermentation. Alcohol fermentation, which occurs in yeast, is another type of anaerobic respiration. Anaerobic respiration is much less efficient than aerobic respiration, as it has a net yield of two ATP, while aerobic respiration's net yield exceeds 30 ATP.

52. B: Not all bacteria are capable of producing spores, but those that can have a developed an advantage to survive during unfavorable environmental conditions. This most frequently occurs during the final stage of the bacterial growth cycle—decline or death. During this stage, the death rate of the population exceeds the new cell production rate because the environment and resources cannot support the population. By surviving as a spore, the bacteria can flourish back to vegetative form when the adverse conditions subside.

53. B: Opposite to the normal flow of information in a cell, retroviruses enter the host cell in RNA form and then must get converted to DNA form via an enzyme called reverse transcriptase. Like all viruses, they need a host cell to reproduce. Viruses do not produce spores.

54. B: Bacteriophages are DNA viruses that inject into the host bacterial cell, where they can undergo the lytic cycle and sometimes the lysogenic cycle, depending on the specific type of bacteriophage. Bacteriophages only infect bacteria. Animal viruses affect animal cells, retroviruses are a type of RNA virus, and lysogenic viruses are not an accepted term. Certain bacteriophages can enter the lysogenic cycle.

55. A: The order of steps in the lytic cycle is attachment, penetration, biosynthesis, maturation, and release. In attachment, the bacteriophage comes in contact with the host cell as the capsid binds with the receptor. During penetration, the viral DNA enters the host cell. If a bacteriophage is capable of undergoing the lysogenic cycle, that cycle takes place after penetration. If not, biosynthesis occurs, and the components of the virus are synthesized to be assembled during the fourth stage, maturation. In the final stage, called the release, the virus leaves the host via lysis, immediately killing the host.

56. B: Transposons can move genetic material from the plasmid to the chromosome or vice versa. Reverse transcriptase is the enzyme that retroviruses produce to facilitate the conversion of RNA to DNA once inside the host cell. Pili are tiny protein projections on the surface of some bacterial cells, which aid in the cell's ability to form attachments to other cells. The sex pilus is the connection that forms during conjugation.

57. B: Genetic variation can be introduced into bacteria through mutation, conjugation, or transformation, but not binary fission. In the process of binary fission, each daughter cell is genetically identical to the parent cell. For this reason, binary fission is a type of asexual reproduction. The single chromosome of the parent cell is replicated and then passed on to each of the two daughter cells. Variation can be introduced with conjugation and transformation because both processes involve the bacteria "mating" with another bacteria cell or picking up genetic material from their environment.

58. A: Antibiotic resistance can spread rapidly through conjugation. Conjugation is the process by which some bacterial cells can replicate their plasmid and pass it to another cell through a direct physical connection. Plasmids typically encode for antibiotic resistance. When the cell that contains the plasmid bridges to the other cell in a connection called a sex pilus, the copy of the plasmid is transferred so that both cells then contain the plasmid. Therefore, an additional cell over baseline conditions has gained the ability to be resistant to an antibiotic. The process of conjugation is very rapid, so resistance can spread quickly throughout a bacterial population.

59. A: Competent bacteria can perform the process of transformation, wherein they can absorb and incorporate foreign DNA from their environment into their own chromosomal DNA. Some bacteria are naturally competent, while others, under certain laboratory conditions, can become competent. Transduction is a term used with viral replication and is the process by which some portion of the host cell's chromosome gets packaged and transferred out of the cell in the new copy of the virus, and then gets incorporated into the next host cell when the virus delivers its viral DNA.

Chemical and Physical Foundations of Biological Systems

1. D: In water, the electronegative oxygen pulls in the electrons of the two hydrogen atoms, making the oxygen slightly negatively-charged and the hydrogen atoms slightly positively-charged. This unequal sharing is called "polarity." This polarity is responsible for the slightly-positive hydrogen atoms from one molecule being attracted to a slightly-negative oxygen in a different molecule, creating a weak intermolecular force called a hydrogen bond, so Choices A and B are true. Choice *C* is also true, because this unique hydrogen bonding creates intermolecular forces that allow molecules with low enough kinetic energy (at low temperatures) to be held apart at "arm's length" (really, the length of the hydrogen bonds). This makes ice less dense than liquid, which explains why ice floats. Choice *D* is the only statement that is false, so it is the correct answer.

2. B: The answer is 10 milliamps. First work on the right-hand leg of the circuit with the two resistors in series. The equivalent resistance is the sum of the series components, or 300 ohms. Now work on the two remaining resistors in parallel:

$$\frac{1}{R_{eq}} = \frac{1}{\frac{1}{R_1} + \frac{1}{R_2}} = \frac{1}{\frac{1}{300\Omega} + \frac{1}{300\Omega}}$$

So,

$$R_{eq} = 150\Omega \text{ and i} = \frac{1.5\ V}{150\Omega} = .01 \text{ amps} = 10 \text{ milliamps}$$

3. D: Isotones are atoms of different elements that have the same number of neutrons. Isotones will have different mass numbers, as will isotopes, which are atoms of the same element that have a different number of neutrons. Isobars are atoms that have the same number of nucleons (protons and neutrons), and therefore, they must have the same mass number.

4. B: Choices A and D both suggest a different number of protons, which would make a different element. It would no longer be a sodium atom if the proton number or atomic number were different, so those are both incorrect. An atom that has a different number of electrons is called an ion, so Choice *C* is incorrect as well.

5. B: If nonmetals form ionic bonds, they will fill their electron orbital (and become an anion) rather than lose electrons (and become a cation), due to their smaller atomic radius and higher electronegativity than metals. Choice *A* is, therefore, incorrect. There are some nonmetals that are diatomic (hydrogen, oxygen, nitrogen, and halogens), but that is not Applied for all of them; thus, Choice *D* is incorrect. Organic compounds are carbon-based due to carbon's ability to form four covalent bonds. In addition to carbon, organic compounds are also rich in hydrogen, phosphorus, nitrogen, oxygen, and sulfur, so Choice *C* is incorrect as well.

6. B: The basic unit of matter is the atom. Each element is identified by a letter symbol for that element and an atomic number, which indicates the number of protons in that element. Atoms are the building block of each element and are comprised of a nucleus that contains protons and neutrons. Orbiting around the nucleus at varying distances are negatively charged electrons. An electrically neutral atom contains equal numbers of protons and electrons. Atomic mass is the combined mass of protons and neutrons in the nucleus. Electrons have such negligible mass that they are not considered in the atomic mass. Although the nucleus is compact, the electrons orbit in energy levels at great relative distances to it, making an atom mostly empty space.

7. A: Nuclear reactions involve the nucleus, and chemical reactions involve electron behavior alone. If electrons are transferred between atoms, they form ionic bonds. If they are shared between atoms, they form covalent bonds. Unequal sharing within a covalent bond results in intermolecular attractions, including hydrogen bonding. Metallic bonding involves a "sea of electrons," where they float around non-specifically, resulting in metal ductility and malleability, due to their glue-like effect of sticking neighboring atoms together. Their metallic bonding also contributes to electrical conductivity and low specific heats, due to electrons' quick response to charge and heat, given to their mobility. Their floating also results in metals' property of luster as light reflects off the mobile electrons. Electron movement in any type of bond is enhanced by photon and heat energy investments, increasing their likelihood to jump energy levels. Valence electron status is the ultimate contributor to electron behavior as it determines their likelihood to be transferred or shared.

8. C: The answer is 0.3 watt-hours. The equivalent resistance is the sum of the three resistors in series, or 60 ohms. The Voltage is 6 Volts. The instantaneous power,

$$P = \frac{I^2}{R} = 0.6 \text{ W}$$

Multiplying 0.6 Watts times 0.5 hours gives 0.3 Watt-hours.

9. B: On the periodic table, the elements are grouped in columns according to the configuration of electrons in their outer orbitals. The groupings on the periodic table give a broad view of trends in chemical properties for the elements. The outer electron shell (or orbital) is most important in determining the chemical properties of the element. The electrons in this orbital determine charge and bonding compatibility. The number of electron shells increases by row from top to bottom. The periodic table is organized with elements that have similar chemical behavior in the columns (groups or families).

10. D: The answer is Bulbs A and D. The empty socket in the center leg of the circuit provides an infinite resistance, so no current flows in that leg. Bulbs A and D receive current, so they light up.

11. B: The law of conservation of mass states that matter cannot be created or destroyed, but that it can change forms. This is important in balancing chemical equations on both sides of the arrow. Unbalanced equations will have an unequal number of atoms of each element on either side of the equation and violate the law.

12. D: Solids all increase solubility with Choices A-C. Powdered hot chocolate is an example to consider. Heating (A) and stirring (B) make it dissolve faster. Regarding Choice *C*, powder is in chunks that collectively result in a very large surface area, as opposed to a chocolate bar that has a very small relative surface area. The small, surface area form dramatically increases solubility. Decreasing the solvent (most of the time, water) will decrease solubility.

13. C: A solution is the term for a homogeneous mixture. A solution contains a solute (particle) dissolved in solvent (water). Solutions have the smallest solutes of the mixtures, dissolving very easily, and the solute is spread out evenly, or homogeneous. A colloid has medium-sized particles that are somewhat evenly spread out, but their major difference from solutions is that they have the Tyndall effect. Because their particles are larger, they will reflect light that will appear as a beam (Tyndall). The sun's rays are an example of Tyndall; the light is reflecting off of the large gas particles in the atmosphere. A suspension has very large particles that actually settle, creating a heterogeneous mixture.

14. A: When salt is added to water, it increases its boiling point. This is an example of a colligative property, which is any property that changes the physical property of a substance. This particular colligative property of boiling point elevation occurs because the extra solute dissolved in water reduces the surface area of the water, impeding it from vaporizing. If heat is applied, though, it gives water particles enough kinetic energy to vaporize. This additional heat results in an increased boiling point. Other colligative properties of solutions include the following: their melting points decrease with the addition of solute, and their osmotic pressure increases (because it creates a concentration gradient that was otherwise not there).

15. C: Pressure has little effect on the solubility of a liquid solution because liquid is not easily compressible; therefore, increased pressure won't result in increased kinetic energy. Pressure increases solubility in gaseous solutions, since it causes them to move faster.

16. B: Non-polar molecules have hydrophobic regions that do not dissolve in water. Oil is a non-polar molecule that repels water. Polar molecules combine readily with water, which is, itself, a polar solvent. Polar molecules are hydrophilic or "water-loving" because their polar regions have intermolecular bonding with water via hydrogen bonds. Some structures and molecules are both polar and non-polar, like the phospholipid bilayer. The phospholipid bilayer has polar heads that are the external "water-loving portions" and hydrophobic tails that are immiscible in water. Polar solvents dissolve polar solutes, and non-polar solvents dissolve non-polar solutes. One way to remember these is "Like dissolves like."

17. A: A catalyst increases the rate of a chemical reaction by lowering the activation energy. Enzymes are biological protein catalysts that are utilized by organisms to facilitate anabolic and catabolic reactions. They speed up the rate of reaction by making the reaction easier (perhaps by orienting a molecule more favorably upon induced fit, for example). Catalysts are not used up by the reaction and can be used repeatedly.

18. C: Increasing temperature increases the rate of reactions due to increases in the kinetic energy of atoms and molecules. This increased movement results in increased collisions between reactants (with each other as well as with enzymes), which is the cause of the rate increase.

19. C: 2:2:4:1 are the coefficients that follow the law of conservation of matter. The coefficient times the subscript of each element should be the same on both sides of the equation.

20. A: Ionic bonding is the result of electrons transferred between atoms. When an atom loses one or more electrons, a cation, or positively-charged ion, is formed. An anion, or negatively-charged ion, is formed when an atom gains one or more electrons. Ionic bonds are formed from the attraction between a positively-charged cation and a negatively-charged anion. The bond between sodium and chlorine in table salt, or sodium chloride (NaCl), is an example of an ionic bond.

21. A: Oxidation is when a substance loses electrons in a chemical reaction, and reduction is when a substance gains electrons. Any element by itself has a charge of 0, as iron and oxygen do on the reactant side. In the ionic compound formed, iron has a +3 charge, and oxygen has a -2 charge. Because iron had a zero charge that then changed to +3, it means that it lost three electrons and was oxidized. Oxygen, which gained two electrons, was reduced.

22. C: Fission occurs when heavy nuclei are split, and it is currently an energy source that fuels power plants. Fusion, on the other hand, is the combining of small nuclei and produces far more energy, and it is the nuclear reaction that powers stars like the sun. Harnessing the extreme energy released by fusion has proven impossible so far, which is unfortunate since its waste products are not radioactive, while waste produced by fission typically is.

23. A: Alpha decay involves a helium particle emission (with two neutrons). Beta decay involves emission of an electron or positron, and gamma is just high-energy light emissions.

24. B: Choice *A* is false because it is possible to have a very strong acid with a pH between 0 and 1. Choice *C* is false because the pH scale is from 0 to 14, and -2 is outside the boundaries. Choice *D* is false because a solution with a pH of 2 has ten times fewer hydronium ions than a pH of 1 solution.

25. C: Gamma is the lightest radioactive decay with the most energy, and this high energy is toxic to cells. Due to its weightlessness, gamma rays are extremely penetrating. Alpha particles are heavy and can be easily shielded by skin.

Beta particles are electrons and can penetrate more than alpha particles because they are lighter. Beta particles can be shielded by plastic.

26. C: The answer is 1,800 seconds:

$$45\text{km} \times \frac{1{,}000 \text{ m}}{1 \text{ km}} \times \frac{1\ s}{25 \text{ m}} = 1{,}800 \text{ seconds}$$

27. D: The ship is traveling faster than the current, so it will be east of the starting location. Its net forward velocity is 0.5 m/s which is 1.8 km/hr, or 3.6 kilometers in two hours.

28. B: First, find the change in speed.

$$132 \text{ km/hr} - 60 \text{ km/hr} = 72 \text{ km/hr}$$

Then, convert this value to meters per second.

$$\frac{72 \text{ km}}{1 \text{ hr}} \times \frac{1000 \text{ m}}{1 \text{ km}} \times \frac{1 \text{ hr}}{3{,}600 \text{ s}} = 20 \text{ m/s}$$

Average acceleration is found by dividing the change in velocity (or speed with a given direction) by the change in time.

$$a = \frac{\Delta v}{\Delta t} = \frac{20 \text{ m/s}}{10 \text{ s}} = 2 \text{ m/s}^2$$

Therefore, the average acceleration after the engine is floored is 2 m/s^2.

29. A: The answer is that the upward velocity is at a maximum when it leaves the punter's toe. The acceleration due to gravity reduces the upward velocity every moment thereafter. The speed is the same at points A and E, but the velocity is different. At point E, the velocity has a maximum negative value.

30. C: Her angular velocity increases from (a) to (b) as she pulls her arms in close to her body and reduces her moment of inertia.

31. B: The answer is 14 m/s. Remember that the cannonball at rest, y meters off the ground, has a potential energy of $PE = mgy$. As it falls, the potential energy is converted to kinetic energy until (at ground level) the kinetic energy is equal to the total original potential energy:

$$\frac{1}{2}mv^2 = mgy$$

Rearranged to solve for velocity, the equation is:

$$v = \sqrt{2gy}$$

This makes sense because all objects fall at the same rate, so the velocity *must* be independent of the mass; thus, Choice *D* is incorrect. Plugging the values into the equation gives a result of about 14.142 m/s, which is rounded to 14 m/s. Remember, the way to figure this quickly is to approximate g as 10 m/s^2 rather than 9.81 m/s^2.

32. B: The answer is at Point C, the bottom of the arc. The bottom of the arc must have the greatest kinetic energy because it is the point with the least potential energy, since the total energy is equivalent to the sum of both potential and kinetic energy.

33. C: This question isn't difficult, but it must be read carefully. Choice *A* is wrong. Even though the potential energy is at a maximum at Points A and E, the total energy is not. The total energy is the same at all points. Choice *B* is wrong. The kinetic energy is at a maximum at point C, but not the total energy. The correct answer is Choice *C*. The total energy is conserved, so it's the same at all points on the arc. Choice *D* is wrong. The motion of a pendulum is independent of the mass. Just like how all objects fall at the same rate, all pendulum bobs swing at the same rate, dependent on the length of the cord.

34. C: The answer is $10 \text{ kg} \times 2 \text{ m} \times 9.81 \text{ m/s}^2$. This question requires careful reading. Choice *D* is incorrect because it isn't necessary to know the ground elevation. The potential energy is measured with respect to the ground, and the ground (or datum elevation) can be set to any arbitrary value.

35. B: The answer is that the water level rises in B but not in A. Why? Because ice is not as dense as water, so a given mass of water has less volume in a solid state than in a liquid state. Thus, it floats. As the mass of ice in Basin A melts, its volume (as a liquid) is reduced. In the end, the water level doesn't change. The ice in Basin B isn't floating. It's perched on high ground in the center of the basin. When it melts, water is added to the basin and the water level rises.

36. B: The volume is:

$$3 \times 25 \times 50 = 3{,}750 \text{ m}^3$$

The volume divided by the flow rate gives the time. Since the pump capacity is given in liters per second, it's easier to convert the volume to liters. 1,000 liters equals 1 cubic meter:

$$t = \frac{3{,}750{,}000 \text{ L}}{750 \text{ L/s}} = 5{,}000 \text{ s}$$

37. A: The answer is $30 \frac{m^3}{s}$. One of the few equations that must be memorized is the flow rate formula, $Q = v \times A$, to find volumetric flow rates. This represents the volume of fluid passing through a channel in a given timeframe, which is equivalent to the velocity of a fluid passing through a fixed area, as shown below:

$$Q = v \times A$$

$$Q = \frac{s}{t} \times s^2$$

$$Q = \frac{s^3}{t}$$

$$Q = \frac{V}{t}$$

The length of the canal is unnecessary because the flow rate can be found from the velocity at a two-dimensional slice of the canal. The area of flow is $1\, m \times 10\, m$ because the canal is only half full of water, therefore:

$$Q = 3\, \frac{m}{s} \times 10\, m^2 = 30\, \frac{m^3}{s}.$$

38. C: The definition of a spontaneous reaction is that Gibbs free energy (ΔG) is less than zero. The equation for ΔG is: $\Delta G = \Delta H - T\Delta S$. Choice *A* can be spontaneous, but is not always, so this is not the correct choice. Exothermic reactions have a negative enthalpy and provide high energy, which suggests spontaneity, but spontaneity is determined by entropy as well. Entropy is not specified here. If entropy is negative and low enough, there will not be enough kinetic energy to do work, even if enthalpy provides some energy. This scenario would be non-spontaneous. If entropy is positive, particles are moving quickly. With the energy given off in the chemical reaction and the high kinetic energy of the particles, this reaction is spontaneous. Choice *B* is false because even though a positive value for entropy is favorable, a positive value for enthalpy is endothermic and unfavorable. If the energy absorbed by the reaction exceeds the kinetic energy available, the reaction is not spontaneous. Only in higher temperatures where there is a large amount of entropy and kinetic energy could this reaction be spontaneous. Choice *D* is false because enthalpy and entropy are not related to activation energy.

39. B: Finding rate constant requires the following calculations:

Rate of trial #1 $= k[A] \times [B]y = k[2] \times [2]y$

Rate of trial #2 $= k[A] \times [B]y = k[6] \times [6]y$

Rate of trial #3 $= k[A] \times [B]y = k[2] \times [6]y$

Rate of trial #4 $= k[A] \times [B]y = k[4] \times [8]y$

To solve for x:

#2 divided by #3 $= k[6] \times \frac{[6]y}{k[2]} \times [6]y$

The rate of #2 divided by #3 $= \frac{9.1}{2.9} =$ about 3

The two are equal, so 3 is equal to $3x$ (since k and $6y$ cancel); $x = 1$

To solve for y:

#3 divided by #1 $= k[2] \times \frac{[6]y}{k[2]} \times [2]y$

The rate of #3 divided by #1 $= \frac{2.9}{3.2} =$ about 1

The two are equal, so 1 is equal to $3x$ (since k and $2x$ cancel)

$y = 0$ (zero rates do not go in rate laws)

$\text{Rate} = k[A]\ 1\ [2B]\ 0 = k[A]$

Solve for k:

Trial #2: Rate is 9.1 and [A] is 6

$9.1 = k[6]$

$k = 1.5$

40. B: Q would decrease. Pressure will affect the collision of gas particles, so it is important to look at the coefficients on the reactant and product side. Because there are 5 moles of gas on the product side and 3 moles of gas on the reactant side, increasing pressure will have a greater increase in product collisions, altering the reaction so that the reactants are favored. Because the quotient represents the products over the reactants, because the products are decreasing, the quotient will decrease as well, making Choices *A*, *C*, and *E* incorrect. Over time, once the reaction reaches equilibrium, Q will be equal to K, but this will not happen immediately, so Choice *D* is incorrect.

41. D: See calculations below.

Givens:

- $i = 1$, van't Hoff factor accounts for disassociation. This is an organic molecule, so the value is 1
- $\pi = 12.2 \text{ atm}$
- $R = \text{constant } (0.0821 \text{ L atm})/(\text{mol K})$
- $T = 296K\ (23°C + 273)$

Unknown:

M = Molarity is measured in moles per liter, and the amount given is in grams. This poses a problem. Because it is an unknown, there is no way to convert the amount to moles because the formula (and therefore molar mass) is unknown.

What we do know is that for any substance, grams can be converted to moles by dividing by the molar mass. For example, 365 grams of hydrochloric acid can be converted to moles by utilizing the molar mass of HCl (36.5 grams), as demonstrated below.

Amount in moles: $365 \text{ g HCl} \times 1 \text{ mole HCl}/36.5 \text{ g HCl} = 10 \text{ g HCl}$

Knowing this, we can make M, our unknown, equal to $4.3 \text{ g/L} \times 1/y$ and solve for y (molar mass)

$$\pi = iMRT$$

Using the equation above, solve for y:

$$12.2 \text{ atm} = \frac{4.3 \text{ g}}{\text{L} \times \text{y}} \times \frac{0.0821\text{L atm}}{\text{mol K}} \times 293\text{K}$$

$$12.2 \text{ atm} = \frac{103 \text{ g} \times \text{atm}}{y \times \text{mol}}$$

$$y = \frac{103 \text{ atm}}{12.2 \text{ atm}} \times \text{g/mol}$$

$$y = 8.44 \times \text{g/mol}$$

$$Molar\ mass = 8.44 \text{ g/mol}$$

42. B: At high temperatures, gas particles have high kinetic energy and behave like ideal gases due to low intermolecular forces, so II is correct. However, increased pressure and smaller volume bring the particles closer together, and the proximity results in significant intermolecular forces. The small volume also makes the actual mass of the gas particles proportionally larger, and therefore significant. Options I and III are incorrect due to the significant volume and intermolecular forces that come with high pressure and small volume.

43. D: If ΔH is negative, energy is being released in an exothermic reaction. Because the boundary is between gas and solid, gas must be releasing kinetic energy to become a solid in the process of deposition. The line between the solid and gas shows sublimation and deposition. The line between solid and liquid shows freezing and melting. The line between liquid and gas shows condensation and vaporization. The critical point represents the point where gas particles have too much energy to ever condense into a liquid, and the triple point is when the solid, liquid, and gas phases are in equilibrium.

44. B: The answer has to be a positive number because the reaction is endothermic. Calculations to find the value are shown below:

ICE	MELTING	WATER
$Q = mc\Delta T$	$Q = m\Delta Hfus$	$Q = mc\Delta T$
$10.1 \text{ g} \times 2.09 \text{ J/g}^\circ\text{C} \times 3^\circ\text{C} = 63.3 \text{ J}$	$10.1 \text{ g} \times 1 \text{ mol}/18 \text{ g} \times 6{,}010 \text{ J}/(\text{g} \times {}^\circ\text{C}) = 3372 \text{ J}$	$10.1 \text{ g} \times 4.18 \text{ J/g}^\circ\text{C} \times 17^\circ\text{C} = 723 \text{ J}$

$$63.3 \text{ J} + 3372 \text{ J} + 723 \text{ J} = 4200 \text{ J or } 4.2 \text{ kJ}$$

45. D: The wide range of answers options accounts for common mistakes (forgetting to convert to Kelvin, using the wrong gas constant, and forgetting to convert grams to moles). See calculations below for the correct answer.

Givens:

- $T = 28^\circ\text{C} + 273 = 301\text{K}$
- $P = 1.3 \text{ atm}$
- $R = .0821 \text{ L} \times \text{atm}/(\text{mol} \times \text{K})$
- $n = 273 \text{ g}$ (molar mass of diatomic oxygen is 32 g/mol, so grams must be converted to moles: $273 \text{ g} \times 1 \text{ mol}/32 \text{ g} = 8.5 \text{ moles}$)

$$PV = nRT$$

Using the equation above, solve for V: $V = 8.5 \text{ mol} \times .0821 \text{ L} \times \text{atm}/(\text{mol} \times \text{K}) \times 301 \text{ K}/1.3 \text{ atm} = 162 \text{ L}$

46. C: See calculations below.

The rate-limiting step is step 2, and its rate law is: k2[C] [B]

[C] is not part of the original equation, so it cannot be included in the rate law

According to first reaction: $\text{k1[A]2} = \text{k} - \text{1[C]}$

By substitution: $\text{k1/ k} - \text{1[A] 2} = \text{[C]}$

Substitute [C] in rate-limiting step 2 formula: $\text{k2} \times \text{k1 /k} - \text{1 [A]2 [B]} = \text{k[A]2[B]}$

47. B: Of the choices, *II* is true and the reaction is exothermic since the products have lower potential energy than the reactants, indicating that energy was released. *I* is not true because E is the energy given off (ΔH) because some of the energy from the potential energy of the reactants are conserved in the formation of product. *III* is untrue because adding an enzyme would decrease the activation energy.

48. A: Remember that a perfectly isolated system, which is theoretical, stops any energy transfer between the inside and outside environment. And if no energy can ever be created, that perfectly isolated system will not receive any heat/energy from the outside and thus, the ice will stay frozen.

49. D: Zero Kelvin is a theoretical temperature, where it is cold enough to stop molecules from moving. If the crystal is imperfect and has any asymmetry or non-conformity, it inherently has disorder. Therefore, water, which forms an imperfect ice crystal, still obeys the second law.

50. B: The specific heat is the energy required to raise 1 gram of a substance by 1 degree C. It does not specify the melting point of that substance, making Choices C and D incorrect.

51. C: The ideal gas law states: $\mathrm{PV} = \mathrm{nRT}$, therefore, with constant pressure (P) and amount of gas (n), increasing V is the only way to balance the increased temperature. Choice *B* is wrong because we are assuming that the quantity of gas also stays the same, so this is not the best answer.

52. C: When a reaction has reactants with lower entropy than its products, it means some form of energy must be applied to it (either from external heat [endothermic] or from an exothermic reaction), thus, eliminating Choices A and D. Choice *B* is incorrect because temperature does affect the spontaneity of the reaction described.

53. D: When Gibbs free energy is very negative, the reaction favors the products and may go to completion. Gibbs free energy does not define if a reaction is endothermic or exothermic. And Choice *C* is incorrect because a reaction that favors the products will produce a very large Kc.

54. D: The critical point represents when there is such high pressure and temperature that the gas particles have too much kinetic energy that it is impossible for them to condense. The high temperature wants to vaporize the liquid, but the high pressure condenses the gas into a liquid.

55. C: An isotope is an atom of the same element with the same electron charge. Therefore, H+ is not an isotope of 2H nor H, because it has a positive charge while the other two choices are neutral.

56. A: Nuclear fusion is the reaction that releases the most energy (modern day nuclear power plants can split atoms, but not fuse because it takes such high pressure). Choices B and C are the same, thus eliminating them. Choice *D* does release energy but not nearly as much as the other choices.

57. C: Adding a catalyst or doubling the concentration of both reactants will increase the rate. Now, the question is a mathematic problem – decreasing Y (because it has a much higher exponential effect) will counteract any change in the concentration of X.

58. B: Increasing pressure is the best way to increase the temperature at which a liquid goes from liquid phase to gas phase. Choice *C* is incorrect (pressure cookers work by increasing the pressure and allowing its contents to reach a higher temperature and cook faster).

59. C: Of the choices, potassium has the largest atomic radius. Remember that the atomic radius generally increases when moving down the periodic table and from the right to the left.

Psychological, Social, and Biological Foundations of Behavior

1. C: The Genital stage starts in adolescence and lays the groundwork for future life relationships. As one enters adolescence, sexual identity and orientation begin to develop. Values regarding sexuality, views about the opposite sex, and the process of interacting with others on a more intimate level occur. These more mature elements of relationship-building lay the foundation for future relationships, but not only from a sexual standpoint. Choice *A*, the Latent stage, occurs from age 6 to puberty, and it is a time when the child's sexual energy becomes somewhat dormant. Choices B and D are not included in Freud's model of human development.

2. C: Developing a long-term relationship and starting a family are concepts more closely associated with stage six of Erikson's model, Intimacy versus Isolation, which occurs from age 18 through age 40. During this period, one is faced with the challenge of coming to terms with sexual preference, choosing a career path, and determining where, with whom, and how one plans to live. Long-term, future-oriented thinking is required. This phase is important, in that if not successfully mastered, the following phases—Generativity versus Stagnation and Ego Integrity versus Despair—may lead to emotional pain and anxiety in later life.

3. D: Accommodation occurs when one recognizes that previous beliefs were incorrect or no longer beneficial, based upon learning and integrating new information. Accommodation should occur throughout one's life as new information enters the consciousness and the process of assimilation occurs. If one is unable to accommodate new ideas, then it is difficult to grow emotionally and intellectually. If an individual continues to insist that using a yellow legal pad and an encyclopedia is just as efficient as using a computer to complete a complex research project, accommodation has failed to occur. This forces the person to work at a "snail's pace" in comparison to using technology to more quickly and accurately complete the task. Choice *A* is incorrect in that schemas are a set of thoughts and ideas that fit together and present the person with a belief, or even a script, for life. Choice *B* is incorrect because assimilation refers to the process of integrating the new information gained through accommodation. Choice *C* refers to object permanence, a process in which an infant learns that even though a person or object leaves the room, that person still exists, and this understanding reduces anxiety and fear of abandonment.

4. A: Pavlov developed the theory of classical conditioning in which it has been demonstrated that pairing one stimulus with another produces specific responses in animals and humans. In his famous experiment, he noted that when feeding a dog and simultaneously pairing that feeding with the sound of a bell, the ringing of the bell eventually became associated with feeding time. Soon, a behavioral change was noted. The dog salivated with the sound of the bell, even when no food was provided. This demonstrated that people and animals can learn things through pairing one stimulus with another. Although dog training was part of his research, Choice *B* is wrong as it was not the focus of his research. Choice *C* reflects one of Erikson's stages of development, and Choice *D* relates more to the function of behavioral theory devised by B.F. Skinner.

5. C: Taking away privileges for a week is a form of punishment for negative behavior, not a reward for positive behavior. While punishment can be an effective means for changing behavior, research indicates it is less desirable than positive reinforcement. Choices A, B, and D are all forms of positive reinforcement in which a person is rewarded for performing a specific behavior correctly.

6. B: Changing behavior through rewards for approximation of desired behavior is the correct answer. Skinner demonstrated that behavior can be learned by rewarding actions that are similar to the desired behavior. If one wants to teach a dog to chase and catch a Frisbee thrown to the end of a field, the dog must first be rewarded for sniffing the Frisbee, then grasping the Frisbee, and then catching it when thrown four feet, then six, then ten. This process is called successive approximation. Choice *A* refers to a form of behavioral change through punishment. Choice *C* refers to superstitions, meaning that one can sometimes be confused as to which behavior is soliciting the reward. Some athletes wear the same pair of "lucky" socks each game, thinking this behavior leads to the reward of winning. In reality, the behavior that leads to the win can be anything from practicing harder to playing a team that is not highly skilled; therefore, the behavior is superstitious. Choice *D* is a poor form of teaching a person to learn a new behavior because it may take much trial and error before perfection is achieved.

7. C: Carl Rogers emphasized reaching one's greatest potential and the interplay between this potential and one's perception of self. Erikson and Freud theorized that one must achieve certain developmental challenges before moving to the next level of human growth. Allport, on the other hand, believed one's destiny depended on the possession of certain clusters of personality traits. Therefore, Choices A, B, and D are wrong. Rogers focused on the concept that humans are driven by their own need to develop into the best person they can become.

8. C: Vygotsky believed individuals are shaped by the formal and informal social groups in which they interact. These institutions teach values, how to behave in relationships, how closely one must follow rules and laws, and, in general, what is important in life. A child growing up hungry and neglected will have a very different view of life than one who is cherished and provided with love, support, and material needs. Choices A, B, and D all impact the quality of one's life, but Vygotsky leaned toward a more global explanation of social development that encompasses multiple social factors.

9. A: Self-image does change throughout the life cycle, and while this varies from individual to individual, age 60 often represents a change in roles from being an actively engaged parent and successful member of the workforce to an empty nester who will soon face retirement. In our society where youth, beauty, and wealth are revered, there is often a shortage of several of these attributes when one enters their 60s. Even those who are physically fit will begin to experience physical changes, such as less energy, more body fat, and the onset of a variety of medical conditions that prevent one from doing some of the things that were once simple, such as lifting a three-year-old grandchild. Gracefully accepting these changes is difficult and painful. Choices B, C, and D all represent stages that consist of great change and challenging transitions and often fail to correlate with a positive self-image.

10. D: Culture is a complex and multi-faceted concept and is related to when, where, and with whom one was raised. Those in the mental health field should be constantly vigilant about a client's cultural practices because these strongly impact beliefs, ethics, and behavior. Choice *D* is the best answer because it does not constitute an aspect of cultural identity as easily as when, where, and how one was raised.

11. D: All of the statements are true. Research demonstrates that members of minority groups are more likely to be pulled over for minor violations; receive longer sentences; be under-represented in important professions, such as medicine, politics, and entertainment; and are more likely to live at or under the poverty level than those in the majority group. Most people have heard derogatory jokes or slurs about various minority groups.

12. B: Indirect discrimination relates to laws and policies that are applied equally but have negative consequences for certain groups. The other three answers are examples of direct discrimination since the actions are based on individual biases rather than organizational decisions. In those three scenarios, people are purposefully discriminating against others. In Choice *B*, the school administrators may not have even considered the negative consequence for Jewish students.

13. A: Choice *A* is an untrue statement. Women earn approximately $0.77 on the dollar when compared to male counterparts. Choices, B, C, and D are true statements regarding the status of women in American society. Women are more likely to be discriminated against in the workplace when pregnant, are more likely than male gender to be sexually assaulted, and are not well-represented in management positions.

14. B: American culture places great value on social status, earning capacity, and productivity, all of which tend to diminish in later life. When one enters retirement, there is a sense of feeling less valued by the rest of society. Only 3% of families are multigenerational, not 15%. Choices C and D are both incorrect. There are not a lot of older entertainers in our culture compared to the number of younger ones. In American culture, the respect of elders is not emphasized in the same way it is in some other cultures, such as Asian or Native American ones.

15. D: Studies show that larger urban areas provide more resources and tend to be more accepting of various populations than those communities with less exposure to people or groups who are culturally, racially, or sexually diverse. Smaller communities do not have many places for LGBT persons to comfortably congregate, such as a gay coffee shop or club. Smaller communities tend to be more politically conservative than larger cities, especially those like San Francisco or New York, where there are many gay establishments and community organizations. Larger urban areas tend to be more accepting of diversity in general.

16. C: Population density, which is the total number of people divided by the total land area, generally tends to be much higher in urban areas than rural ones. This is true due to high-rise apartment complexes, sewage and freshwater infrastructure, and complex transportation systems, allowing for easy movement of food from nearby farms. Consequently, competition among citizens for resources is certainly higher in high-density areas, as are greater strains on infrastructure within urban centers.

17. C: Although it can place a strain on some resources, population density is not a negative demographic indicator. For example, New York City, one of the most densely populated places on Earth, enjoys one of the highest standards of living in the world. Other world cities such as Tokyo, Los Angeles, and Sydney also have tremendously high population densities and high standards of living. High infant mortality rates, low literacy rates, and low life expectancies are all poor demographic indicators that suggest a low quality of life for the citizens living in those areas.

18. A: Although some ethnic groups throughout the world do engage in armed conflicts, the vast majority do not. Most ethnic groups tend to live in relative harmony with others from whom they are different. Ethnic groups are simply a group of people with a religious, cultural, economic, or linguistic commonality. Additionally, ethnic groups don't always choose to leave places. Many have called certain locations home for centuries. Also, some ethnic groups actually comprise the majority in some countries and are not always minority groups.

19. C: Pull factors are reasons people immigrate to a particular area. Obviously, educational opportunities attract thousands of people on a global level and on a local level. For example, generally, areas with strong schools have higher property values, due to the relative demand for housing in those districts. The same is true for nations with better educational opportunities. Unemployment, low GDP, and incredibly high population densities may serve to deter people from moving to a certain place and can be considered push factors.

20. A: Globalization refers to the cooperation and integration of economies, cultures, and societies through trade, communication, and movement of people and ideas. As a result, it has put students and workers in direct conflict with one another despite their relative level of physical separation. For example, students who excel in mathematics and engineering may be recruited by multinational firms who want the best talent for their business despite where they are educated. Furthermore, products produced in other nations are also in competition with global manufacturers to ensure quality craftsmanship at an affordable price. Globalization does not refer to world domination, an absence of nation-states, or a singular world government.

21. B: The reflex arc is the simplest nerve pathway. The stimulus bypasses the brain, going from sensory receptors through an afferent (incoming) neuron to the spinal cord. It synapses with an efferent (outgoing) neuron in the spinal cord and is transmitted directly to muscle. The classic example of a reflex arc is the knee-jerk response. Tapping on the patellar tendon of the knee stimulates the quadriceps muscle of the thigh, resulting in contraction of the muscle and extension of the knee.

22. C: The sympathetic nervous system initiates the "fight-or-flight" response and is responsible for body changes that direct all available energy towards survival. Digestion is completely sacrificed so that energy can be diverted to increase heart rate and breathing (thus, bronchiole dilation). The liver is stimulated to release glycogen to provide available energy. The parasympathetic system is responsible for stimulating everyday activities like digestion.

23. A: Motor neurons transmit signals from the central nervous system (CNS) to effector tissues and organs, such as skeletal muscle and glands. Sensory neurons carry impulses from receptors in the extremities to the CNS. Interneurons relay impulses from neuron to neuron.

24. C: The cerebellum is important for balance and motor coordination. Aside from the brainstem and cerebellum, the outside portion of the brain is the cerebrum, which is the advanced operating system of the brain that is responsible for learning, emotion, memory, perception, and voluntary movement. The amygdala (involved in emotions), language areas, and corpus callosum all exist within the cerebrum.

25. D: The hypothalamus is the link between the nervous and endocrine systems. It receives information from the brain and sends signals to the pituitary gland, instructing it to release or inhibit the release of hormones. Aside from its endocrine function, it controls body temperature, hunger, sleep, and circadian rhythms, and it is part of the limbic system.

26. A: Absolute poverty affects human beings in a way that poses a higher risk of disease or death. Absolute poverty can affect people living in both developed and underdeveloped countries, although it is more prevalent amongst residents of underdeveloped countries. Thus, Choice *B* is not wholly true. Relative poverty is less severe than absolute poverty and occurs most often in countries that have solid infrastructures. Choices C and D can be eliminated because they do not convey the greater risk of death that accompanies absolute poverty and they make inaccurate statements about relative poverty.

27. C: Meritocracy can be destroyed or undermined by the inheritance of wealth and privilege within families. Social reproduction—the privileges and inequalities that are passed on from one generation to the next—limits the capacity of societies striving to be meritocratic. The answer is not Choice *A* because meritocracy is a philosophy that still drives modern values such as the "American Dream." It is not an outdated philosophy. The definition of meritocracy is "any form of social stratification or social mobility that appears to be dependent upon personal merit." It is not traditionally defined as a "society built on fiction," though, as mentioned, many scholars see it as a myth. Since Choice *B* is false according to traditional definitions, it must be eliminated. Choice *D* is not correct because, logically speaking, hard work is a reality that continues to exist in a meritocratic society even when the social stratification is reinforced by the myth of "pulling yourself up by your bootstraps."

28. D: Racialization is best defined as "process of categorizing and separating people in society based on race, or physical characteristics that distinguish them from other groups." Although racialization can lead to prejudice (A), genocide (B), or increased racism (C), it is not best defined by these phenomena.

29. A: Cults have traditionally been associated with brainwashing, ritual suicide, and illicit practices. Cults are loosely-organized, and not as bureaucratized as sects or churches, but Choice *B* does not necessarily explain the pejorative association. Choice *C* is inaccurate. Cults are typically not highly-organized. They are experimental small groups with loose organization. Choice *D* is also inaccurate because the Roman Catholic Church is typically categorized as an ecclesia rather than a cult.

30. B: Environmental injustice refers to the ways in which minority statuses, human segregation, and location can directly affect the health of certain marginalized communities. Choice *B*—high lead levels in the water system of a low-income community—is the best example of the ways in which a minority status may affect the infrastructure of a poorer, black community like the one living in Flint, Michigan. The rest of the answers refer to forms of environmental justice (C), environmental conservation (A), or environmental discovery (D).

31. D: Globalization has traditionally been linked to advances in travel, technology, and communication, and advanced computer technologies such as social media and the Internet. These interrelated advances have brought the world and its varying economies "closer together," so to speak. Choices A, B, and C do not suffice because they do not consider all variables or factors.

32. B: Vertical mobility refers to any kind of social or economic mobility that may increase or decrease the general standing of living for a person or family. Upward vertical mobility may occur when a person or family's social and/or economic standing increases as a result of personal entrepreneurship, marriage, college graduation, or a job promotion. Downward vertical mobility may occur with dropping out of school, loss of a job, inability to earn a college degree, taking a lower paying job, health issues, or even divorce. Choice *B* is correct because II (getting promoted), III (filing for bankruptcy), and IV (taking a lower-paying job for personal reasons) can all lead to vertical movements. A promotion is an example of upward vertical mobility. Filing for bankruptcy and taking a lower-paying job, on the other hand, can lead to downward vertical mobility. Choice *I*—taking a job that is more satisfying, but pays the same salary—is an example of horizontal mobility rather than vertical mobility.

33. D: People can be segregated by gender (I), race (II), socioeconomic status (III), and age (IV). Thus, Choice *D*—all of the above—is the best answer. Patriarchal households and societies tend to segregate based on gender. Likewise, even the most developed nations, such as the United States, play host to some of the most racially and socioeconomically segregated neighborhoods in the world. The high concentration of elderly people in nursing homes and retirement communities represents an extreme example of age segregation, while separating Thanksgiving dinner into parent tables and kid tables would be a mild example of age segregation.

34. A: Intragenerational mobility refers to "social and/or economic changes that affect a person during their lifetime." Thus, Choice *A* is the best answer. Intergenerational mobility (B) is a term used to describe the vertical mobility of children in relationship to their parents or an entire younger generation in relationship to an older generation; it reveals long-term changes in history, highlighting broad-sweeping superstructural shifts such as industrialization, urbanization, gentrification, and/or suburbanization. Social reproduction (C) refers to the privileges and inequalities that are passed on from one generation to the next. Vertical mobility refers to any kind of social or economic mobility that may increase or decrease the general standing of living for a person or family.

35. C: Immigration status describes the citizenship and/or resident status of an immigrant or immigrant family. Types of immigrant statuses differ according to the laws of the state. In some countries, immigrants may obtain work visas, asylum (III), or deferred action (II) with regards to their resident/citizenship status. Conversely, some immigrants maintain an "undocumented status" (I), meaning they unlawfully immigrated to a nation without going through the legal channels to obtain work visas, asylum, deferred action, or citizenship. Currently, in the United States of America, there is an ongoing debate regarding the status of millions of undocumented residents residing on U.S. soil. Choice *C*—Choices I, II, & III—is best because temporary visitors (IV) are not technically considered immigrants. For instance, if a U.S. citizen crosses the southern international border between the U.S. and Mexico to visit a small Mexican town, then that person is not usually considered an immigrant but merely a traveler or temporary visitor. There is no permanence associated with their migration.

36. C: Neuronal communication happens via an electrochemical process. When a neuron is depolarized, an electrical impulse is sent through the neuron and neurotransmitters are released into the synapse between neurons. Neurotransmitters are chemical messengers that bind onto the receptor sites of the post-synaptic neuron, causing the next cell to fire.

37. A: Temperament, which consists of the basic and innate components of personality, has been shown to be highly genetic and individual variations can be viewed as early as infancy. Although personality is more influenced by environmental factors as it develops, temperament is highly genetic. Differences in cleanliness, food preferences, and language cannot be identified from infancy, nor are they genetically influenced in the way that temperament is.

38. B: Epigenetics is when the expression of genes is changed but the overall genetic sequence remains the same. These genetic adaptations can be passed on to the next generations. The other terms are not related to this topic.

39. A: Approximately 20-25 percent of the population in the United States struggles with a mental disorder in any given year. That is 1 out of every 4 or 5 people. It is estimated that a smaller percentage, 4-8, struggle with a severe or serious mental illness. The United States has a high level of mental disorders as compared to other countries.

40. D: Bipolar disorder was formerly called manic-depressive disorder and is characterized by fluctuations in mood, from bouts of depression to periods of mania or euphoria. There are different types of bipolar disorder, some types having milder forms of mania or depression than others. Anxiety disorders are characterized by persistent worry, anxiety, or fear. Trauma-related disorders develop in reaction to stressful and traumatic experiences that a person has endured.

41. C: Schizophrenia is highly genetic and is associated with high levels of dopamine in the brain. Parkinson's disease is correlated to low levels of dopamine, so treatments for schizophrenia can sometimes cause Parkinson's disease. Alzheimer's disease is associated with a deficit in the neurotransmitter acetylcholine rather than dopamine. There has been no strong link connecting dopamine to personality disorders.

42. B: Body perception, a social construct that dictates norms around what is attractive or unattractive, socially influences a person's hunger motivation. Coercion is not a factor in hunger motivation. Both the lateral hypothalamus and the metabolism are examples of biological motivations rather than social factors.

43. C: The foot-in-door phenomenon is when a person persuades someone to do a greater act after having agreed to something small. Once they have agreed to the more minor action or favor, they are more likely to agree to something bigger. The central route to persuasion is a means of persuasion based on the actual arguments, message, or characteristics. The door-in-face phenomenon is the opposite of foot-in-door in that a person first asks for a big request and when that is denied, he or she requests something smaller. Role-playing is a way in which behavior influences attitude because the mere act of playing a role can powerfully influence a person to take on the feelings and attitudes of the role.

44. A: Group polarization refers to the phenomenon that when people gather with others who hold similar beliefs, they will become stronger in their shared beliefs. They also tend to make more extreme decisions than they would as individuals. Groupthink occurs when members of a group are unwilling to share ideas in opposition to the group and thus, a decision is made without having adequately considered all possibilities and options. Group dynamics covers a whole range of topics related to how groups influence and interact with one another. Deindividuation is when an individual loses sense of self and responsibility when caught up in the anonymity and emotion of a crowd.

45. D: Mores are social norms that are particularly characterized by a moral component. They are often established through religious systems, and violations of mores are likely to lead to formal or informal sanction. Folkways are the daily customs and traditions of a society. Taboos are the behaviors that are so strictly forbidden by a society that ostracism may occur if a person violates them.

46. B: Differential association asserts that deviant behavior has been learned through observation of others. Labeling theory looks at the power of labels in marking certain behavior as deviant. Strain theory assigns blame to the society structure for the deviant behavior. Observational learning does not apply in this context, as it covers a much broader range of behaviors than just deviance.

47. B: When a person or animal shows a decreased response to a stimulus after a period of time, it is considered habituation. Something that may at first provoke a response will, after time and repeated exposure to the stimulus, cease to yield the same response. None of the other answers are in any way related to habituation.

48. A: In the Bobo Doll experiment children were asked to observe adults who were acting violently toward a blow-up doll. The children who observed the violent behavior later acted more violently toward the doll. This illustrated the idea of modeling. The Stanford Prison experiment looked at the power of role-playing on attitudes and behaviors. Asch's conformity study explored the idea of how people conform to the behaviors of others. Milgram's obedience study examined the extent to which people would obey those in authority.

49. D: Self-esteem is the term that best describes a feeling of personal worth or value. Self-efficacy refers to a person's feelings of competency to perform or achieve a particular task. Self-identity and self-concept have to do with one's overall view of self.

50. D: The fundamental attribution error occurs when someone mistakenly attributes observed behavior to someone's disposition rather than their situation. For example, if someone is observed to become very angry in public, the fundamental attribution error would attribute being in public to them having an angry disposition rather than the fact that a close family member just died.

51. B: Prejudice is most often a negative belief about others and is based on prejudging without all the facts. Unfortunately, prejudice can, and is, shown toward people due to their race, gender, sexual orientation, religion, and many other factors. The other terms are similar and connected but distinct from prejudice. Stereotyping is the labeling and categorizing of people based on their group membership. Discrimination is negative action taken against people based on prejudice. Ethnocentrism is the tendency to view everything from one's culture as superior to other cultures.

52. C: Role conflict occurs when there is a conflict between the different responsibilities of roles played by the same person. This woman is dealing with a conflict between her work responsibilities and her responsibilities in the role of daughter. Role strain would be if someone has difficulty dealing with the different responsibilities within one role, such as managing several different assignments at work. The other terms are unrelated.

53. A: The dramaturgical approach is a view of presentation of self that compares human behavior and social interactions to that of actors on a stage. It proposes that humans act as a front stage self, presenting themselves for an audience, or as a backstage self, engaging in actions that are not intended for an audience.

54. C: Conformity is not associated with attraction. Similarity, familiarity, and physical attractiveness all contribute to someone liking or being drawn to another person.

55. B: Higher levels of testosterone have been connected to higher levels of aggression and men tend to show more aggression than women. An increased level of serotonin is not associated with aggression. Modeling and observational learning are both considered environmental factors that lead to aggressive behaviors.

56. A: The sensory threshold is the smallest amount of stimulus that is required for an individual to experience one of the senses. For example, during a hearing test, the sensory threshold would be the quietest sound that a person could detect. This threshold is an important indicator of whether a person's senses are working within a normal range.

57. C: Generally, all sensory pathways that extend from the sensory receptor to the brain are composed of three long neurons called the primary, secondary, and tertiary neurons. The primary one stretches from the sensory receptor to the dorsal root ganglion of the spinal nerve, and the secondary one stretches from the cell body of the primary neuron to the spinal cord or the brain stem. The tertiary one stretches from the cell body of the secondary one into the thalamus. Each type of sense, such as touch, hearing, and vision, has a different pathway designed specifically for that sensation.

58. C: Visual processing begins in the retina. When an individual sees an image, it is taken in through the cornea and lens and then transmitted upside down onto the retina. The cells in the retina process what is being seen and then send signals to the ganglion cells, whose axons make up the optic nerve. The optic nerve cells connect the retina to the brain, which is where the processing of the visual information is completed and the images are returned to their proper orientation.

59. D: Sourness is sensed on the tongue when sour foods or drinks release a hydrogen ion. Saltiness is sensed when sodium ions are transported across the membrane of the taste bud through sodium ion channels. The sensory pathways of the sweet and bitter taste sensations are the result of a more complicated ion flow along the sensory pathways.

Critical Analysis and Reasoning Skills

1. C: Choice *A* is incorrect because the introduction does not contain an impartial definition, but rather, an opinion. Choice *B* is incorrect. There is no puzzling phenomenon given, as the author doesn't mention any peculiar cause or effect that is in question regarding poetry. Choice *D* does contain another's viewpoint at the beginning of the passage; however, to say that the author has no stake in this argument is incorrect because the author uses personal experiences to build their case.

2. B: Choice *B* accurately describes the author's argument in the text: that poetry is not irrelevant. While the author does praise, and even value, Buddy Wakefield as a poet, the author never heralds him as a genius. Eliminate Choice *A*, as it is an exaggeration. Not only is Choice *C* an exaggerated statement, but the author never mentions spoken word poetry in the text. Choice *D* is incorrect because this statement contradicts the writer's argument.

3. D: Exiguously means not occurring often, or occurring rarely, so Choice *D* would least change the meaning of the sentence. Choice *A*, indolently, means unhurriedly, or slow, and does not fit the context of the sentence. Choice *B*, inaudibly, means quietly or silently. Choice *C*, interminably, means endlessly, or all the time, and is the opposite of the word exiguously.

4. D: A student's insistence that psychoanalysis is a subset of modern psychology is the most analogous option. The author of the passage tries to insist that performance poetry is a subset of modern poetry, and therefore, tries to prove that modern poetry is not "dying," but thriving on social media for the masses. Choice *A* is incorrect, as the author is not refusing any kind of validation. Choice *B* is incorrect; the author's insistence is that poetry will not lose popularity. Choice *C* mimics the topic but compares two different genres, making it incorrect as the author makes no comparison in this passage.

5. B: The author's purpose is to disprove Gioia's article claiming that poetry is a dying art form that only survives in academic settings. In order to prove his argument, the author educates the reader about new developments in poetry, Choice *A*, and describes the brilliance of a specific modern poet, Choice *C*, but these serve as examples of a growing poetry trend that counters Gioia's argument. Choice *D* is incorrect because it contradicts the author's argument.

6. D: This question is difficult because the choices offer real reasons as to why the author includes the quote. However, the question specifically asks for the main reason for including the quote. The quote from a recently written poem shows that people are indeed writing, publishing, and performing poetry, Choice *B*. The quote also shows that people are still listening to poetry, Choice *C*. These things are true, and by their nature, serve to disprove Gioia's views, Choice *A*, which is the author's goal. However, Choice *D* is the most direct reason for including the quote, because the article analyzes the quote for its "complex themes" that "draw listeners and appreciation" right after it's given.

7. C: Extraneous most nearly means superfluous, or trivial. Choice *A*, indispensable, is incorrect because it means the opposite of extraneous. Choice *B*, bewildering, means confusing and is not relevant to the context of the sentence. Finally, Choice *D* is incorrect because, although the prefix of the word is the same, ex-, the word exuberant means elated or enthusiastic, which is irrelevant to the context of the sentence.

8. A: This is a challenging question because the author's purpose is somewhat open-ended. The author concludes by stating that the questions regarding human perception and observation can be approached from many angles. Thus, the author does not seem to be attempting to prove one thing or another. Choice *B* is incorrect because we cannot know for certain whether the electron experiment is the latest discovery in astroparticle physics because no date is given. Choice *C* is a broad generalization that does not reflect accurately on the writer's views. While the author does appear to reflect on opposing views of human understanding, Choice *D*, the best answer is Choice *A*.

9. C: The paragraph literally "presents a conundrum," explains the problem of partial understanding, and ends with more questions or inquiries. There is no solution offered in this paragraph, making Choices A and B incorrect. Choice *D* is incorrect because the paragraph does not begin with a definition.

10. D: Looking back in the text, the author describes that classical philosophy holds that understanding can be reached by careful observation. This will not work if they are overly invested or biased in their pursuit. Choices A, B, and C are in no way related and are completely unnecessary. A specific theory is not necessary to understanding, according to classical philosophy mentioned by the author.

11. B: Choices A and C are incorrect because such movement is not mentioned at all in the text. In the passage, the author says that electrons that were physically observed appeared to pass through one hole or another. Remember, the electrons that were observed doing this were described as acting like particles. Therefore, Choice *D* is incorrect. Recall that the plate actually recorded electrons passing through both holes simultaneously and hitting the plate.

This behavior, the electron activity that wasn't seen by humans, was characteristic of waves. Thus, Choice *B* is the correct answer.

12. C: Choice *A* mirrors the language in the beginning of the paragraph but is incorrect in its intent. Choice *B* is incorrect; the paragraph mentions nothing of not knowing the true nature of gravity. Choice *D* is incorrect as well. There is no mention of an "alternative solution" in this paragraph.

13. A: The important thing to keep in mind is that we must choose a scenario that best parallels, or is most similar to, the discovery of the experiment mentioned in the passage. The important aspects of the experiment can be summed up like so: humans directly observed one behavior of electrons and then through analyzing a tool (the plate that recorded electron hits), discovered that there was another electron behavior that could not be physically seen by human eyes. This summary best parallels the scenario in Choice *A*. Like Feynman, the colorblind person can observe one aspect of the world but through the special goggles (a tool), he is able to see a natural phenomenon that he could not physically see on his own. While Choice *D* is compelling, the x-ray helps humans see the broken bone, but it does not necessarily reveal that the bone is broken in the first place. The other choices do not parallel the scenario in question. Therefore, Choice *A* is the best choice.

14. B: The author would not agree that technology renders human observation irrelevant. Choice *A* is incorrect because much of the passage discusses how technology helps humans observe what cannot be seen with the naked eye; therefore, the author would agree with this statement. This line of reasoning is also why the author would agree with Choice *D*, making it incorrect as well. As indicated in the second paragraph, the author seems to think that humans create inventions and tools with the goal of studying phenomena more precisely. This indicates increased understanding as people recognize limitations and develop items to help bypass the limitations and learn. Therefore, Choice *C* is incorrect as well.

15. D: The author explains that Boethianism is a Medieval theological philosophy that attributes sin to temporary pleasure and righteousness with virtue and God's providence. Other than Choice *D*, the choices listed are all physical things. While these could still be divine rewards, Boethianism holds that the Applied reward for being virtuous is God's favor. It is also stressed in the article that physical pleasures cannot be taken into the afterlife. Therefore, the best Choice *Is* D, God's favor.

16. C: Choices A and B are generalized statements, and we have no evidence to support Choice *B*. Choice *D* is very compelling, but it looks at Boethianism in a way that the author does not. The author does not mention different levels of Boethianism when discussing the tales, only that the concept appears differently in different tales. Boethianism also doesn't focus on enlightenment.

17. D: Choice *A* is incorrect; while the text does mention thieves ravaging others' possessions, it is only meant as an example and not as the principle itself. Choice *B* is incorrect for the same reason as Choice *A*. Choice *C* is mentioned in the text and is part of the example that proves the principle, but it is not the principle itself. Choice *B* is incorrect for the same reason as A. Choice *C* is mentioned in the text and is part of the example that proves the principle, but it is also not the principle itself.

18. C: The word avarice most nearly means parsimoniousness, or an unwillingness to spend money. Choice *A* means evil or mischief and does not relate to the context of the sentence. Choice *B* is also incorrect, because pithiness means shortness or conciseness. Choice *D* is close because precariousness means danger or instability, which goes well with the context. However, we are told of the summoner's specific characteristic of greed, which makes Choice *C* the best answer.

19. D: Boethianism acknowledges desire as something that leads out of holiness, so Choice *A* is incorrect. Choice *B* is incorrect because in the passage, Boethianism is depicted as being wary of desire and anything that binds people to the physical world. Choice *C* can be eliminated because the author never says that desire indicates demonic possession.

20. A: The purpose is to inform the reader about what assault is and how it is committed. Choice *B* is incorrect because the passage does not state that assault is a lesser form of lethal force, only that an assault can use lethal force, or alternatively, lethal force can be utilized to counter a dangerous assault. Choice *C* is incorrect because the passage is informative and does not have a set agenda. Finally, Choice *D* is incorrect because although the author uses an example in order to explain assault, it is not indicated that this is the author's personal account.

21. C: If the man being attacked in an alley by another man with a knife used lethal force in self-defense, it would not be considered illegal. The presence of a deadly weapon indicates mal-intent and because the individual is isolated in an alley, lethal force in self-defense may be the only way to preserve his life. Choices A and B can be ruled out because in these situations no one is in danger of immediate death or bodily harm by someone else. Choice *D* is an assault and does exhibit intent to harm, but this situation isn't severe enough to merit lethal force; there is no intent to kill.

22. B: As discussed in the second passage, there are several forms of assault, like assault with a deadly weapon, verbal assault, or threatening posture or language. Choice *A* is incorrect because the author does not mention what the charges are on assaults; therefore, we cannot assume that they are more or less than unnecessary use of force charges. Choice *C* is incorrect because anyone is capable of assault; the author does not state that one group of people cannot commit assault. Choice *D* is incorrect because assault is never justified. Self-defense resulting in lethal force can be justified.

23. D: The statement in Choice *D* would most undermine the last part of the passage because it directly contradicts how the law evaluates the use of lethal force. Choices A and B are stated in the paragraph, so they do not undermine the explanation from the author. Choice *C* does not necessarily undermine the passage, but it does not support the passage either. It is more of an opinion that does not offer strength or weakness to the explanation.

24. C: Choice *C* is correct because it clearly establishes what both assault and lethal force are and gives the specific way in which the two concepts meet. Choice *A* is incorrect because lethal force doesn't necessarily result in assault. This is also why Choice *B* is incorrect. Not all assaults would necessarily be life-threatening to the point where lethal force is needed for self-defense. Choice *D* is compelling but ultimately incorrect; the statement touches on aspects of the two ideas but fails to present the concrete way in which the two are connected to each other.

25. A: Choice *D* is incorrect because while the passages utilize examples to help explain the concepts discussed, the author doesn't indicate that they are specific court cases. It's also clear that the passages don't open with examples, but instead, they begin by defining the terms addressed in each passage. This eliminates Choice *B* and ultimately reveals Choice *A* to be the correct answer. Choice *A* accurately outlines the way both passages are structured. Because the passages follow a nearly identical structure, Choice *C* can easily be ruled out.

26. C: Choices A and B are incorrect because it is clear in both passages that intent is a prevailing theme in both lethal force and assault. Choice *D* is compelling, but if a person uses lethal force to defend himself or herself, the intent of the defender is also examined in order to help determine if there was excessive force used. Choice *C* is correct because it states that intent is important for determining both lethal force and assault and that intent is used to gauge the severity of the issues. Remember, just as lethal force can escalate to excessive use of force, there are different kinds of assault. Intent dictates several different forms of assault.

27. B: The example is used to demonstrate a single example of two different types of assault and then adds in a third type of assault in its conclusion. The example mainly provides an instance of "threatening body language" and "provocative language" with the homeowner gesturing threats to his neighbor. It ends the example by adding a third type of assault: physical strikes. This example is used to show the variant nature of assaults. Choice *A* is incorrect because it doesn't mention the "physical strike" assault at the end and is not specific enough. Choice *C* is incorrect because the example does not say anything about the definition of lethal force or how it might be altered. Choice *D* is incorrect because the example mentions nothing about cause and effect.

28. A: While Choice *C*, contemplative might seem like an option because of the thoughtful nature of the text, Choice *A* is correct because the speaker expresses frustration over being asked to celebrate liberty that he and members of his race do not have. Choice *B* is incorrect because Frederick Douglass is drawing contrasts between two groups of people rather than being inclusive. He is neither nonchalant nor accepting of the circumstances which he describes.

29. C: Choice *C*, contented, is the only word that has the opposite meaning of obdurate.

30. B: While the speaker makes biblical references, it is not the main focus of the passage, thus eliminating Choice *A* as an answer. The passage also makes no mention of wealthy landowners and doesn't speak of any positive response to the historical events, so Choices C and D are not correct.

31. D: Choice *D* is the correct answer because it clearly references the disparity between slaves and free people in the United States.

32. D: It is an example of hyperbole; the physical distance between Frederick Douglass and his audience was not, in fact, immeasurable. However, it clearly demonstrated the differences in the lives and situations of free men and slaves in the United States. Choice *A* is incorrect because assonance is the repetition of sounds and commonly occurs in poetry. Choice *B* is incorrect because parallelism refers to two statements that correlate, or parallel each other, in some manner.

33. C: The speaker states, "Do you mean, citizens, to mock me, by asking me to speak today? If so there is a parallel to your conduct." The parallel in conduct that he speaks of is explained in the quote from the bible. The speaker is explaining that his invitation to speak at a celebration for freedom and independence is similar to the captives being asked to sing the songs of their homeland while being enslaved in another land. The quote was not included to connect on a religious level, to provide proof of injustices, or to request participation in joyous anthems.

34. B: It is apparent that Lincoln is referring to a period of time within the context of the passage because the sentence contains the words years and ago. Choices A, C, and D do not fit the language or context of the sentence and are therefore incorrect.

35. C: Lincoln's reference to "the brave men, living and dead, who struggled here" proves that he is referring to a battlefield. Choices A and B are incorrect, as a civil war is mentioned and not a war with France or a war in the Sahara Desert. Choice *D* is incorrect because it does not make sense to consecrate a President's ground instead of a battlefield ground for soldiers who died during the American Civil War.

36. D: Abraham Lincoln is a former president of the United States, and he referenced a "civil war" during his address.

37. A: The speaker is trying to convey that the audience should perpetuate the ideals of freedom that the soldiers died fighting for. Lincoln doesn't address any of the topics outlined in Choices B, C, or D. Therefore, Choice *A* is the correct answer.

38. D: Choice *D* is the correct answer because of the repetition of the word people at the end of the passage. Choice *A*, antimetabole, is the repetition of words in a succession. Choice *B*, antiphrasis, is a form of denial of an assertion in a text. Choice *C*, anaphora, is the repetition that occurs at the beginning of sentences.

39. A: Choice *A* is correct because Lincoln's intention was to memorialize the soldiers who had fallen as a result of war as well as celebrate those who had put their lives in danger for the sake of their country. Choices B and C are incorrect because Lincoln's speech was supposed to foster a sense of pride among the members of the audience while connecting them to the soldiers' experiences. Choice *D* is incorrect because Lincoln's comparison does not suggest that the dedication ceremony was inappropriate but rather that the soldiers' great sacrifice was worth remembering.

40. A: The word patronage most nearly means auspices, which means protection or support. Choice *B*, aberration, means abnormality and does not make sense within the context of the sentence. Choice *C*, acerbic, means sour or sharply critical, and it also does not make sense in the sentence. Choice *D*, adulation, is a positive word meaning praise, and thus does not fit with the word condescending in the sentence.

41. D: Working man is most closely aligned with Choice *D*, proletariat, which means working or middle class. Choice *A*, plebian, does suggest common people; however, this is a term that is specific to ancient Rome. Choice *B*, viscount, is a European title used to describe a specific degree of nobility. Choice *C*, entrepreneur, is a person who operates their own business.

42. C: In the context of the speech, the term working man most closely correlates with Choice *C*, a working man is someone who works for wages among the middle class. Choice *A* is not mentioned in the passage and is off-topic. Choice *B* may be true in some cases, but it does not reflect the sentiment described for the term working man in the passage. Choice *D* is not a definition, and the topics of the field, factory, and screen are not mentioned in the passage.

43. D: Enterprise most closely means cause. Choices A, B, and C are all related to the term enterprise. However, Dickens speaks of a cause here, not a company, courage, or a game. "He will stand by such an enterprise" is a call to stand by a cause to enable the working man to have a certain autonomy over his own economic standing. The very first paragraph ends with the statement that the working man shall ... have a share in the management of an institution which is designed for his benefit.

44. B: Recall from the first paragraph that the speaker is there to "accompany [the audience] ... through one of my little Christmas books," making him an author there to entertain the crowd with his own writing. The speech preceding the reading is the passage itself, and, as the tone indicates, it is a serious speech addressing the working man. Although the passage speaks of employers and employees, the speaker himself is not an employer of the audience, so Choice *A* is incorrect. Choice *C* is also incorrect, as the salutation is not used ironically, but sincerely, as the speech addresses the well-being of the crowd. Choice *D* is incorrect because the speech is not given by a politician, but by a writer.

45: B: Choice *A* is incorrect because that is the speaker's *first* desire, not his second. Choices *C* and *D* are tricky because the language of both of these is mentioned after the word *second*. However, the speaker doesn't get to the second wish until the next sentence. Choices *C* and *D* are merely prepositions preparing for the statement of the main clause, Choice B, for the working man to have a say in his institution, which is designed for his benefit.

46. C: In the final sentence of the first paragraph, it is stated that avarice can prevent a man from being necessitously poor, but it also makes him too timorous, or fearful, to be wealthy. Choice *A* is incorrect because avarice prevents a man from being poor. Choice *B* is incorrect because the passage states that oppression, not avarice, is the consequence of wealth. Choice *D* is incorrect because the passage does not state that avarice drives a person's desire to be wealthy.

47. D: Paine believes that the distinction that is beyond a natural or religious reason is between king and subjects. Choice *A* is incorrect because he states that the distinction between good and bad is made in heaven. Choice *B* is incorrect because he states that the distinction between male and female is natural. Choice *C* is incorrect because he does not mention anything about the distinction between humans and animals.

48. A: The passage states that the Heathens were the first to introduce government by kings into the world. Choice *B* is incorrect because the quiet lives of patriarchs came before the Heathens introduced this type of government, and Paine puts it in opposition to government by kings. Choice *C* is incorrect because it was Christians, not Heathens, who paid divine honors to living kings. Heathens honored deceased kings. Choice *D* is incorrect because, while equal rights of nature are mentioned in the paragraph, they are not mentioned in relation to the Heathens.

49. B: Paine doesn't say it is against the laws of nature, so Choice *A* is incorrect. He cites parts of scripture that he claims denounce monarchy, so Choices C and D are incorrect.

50. A: To be idolatrous is to worship someone or something other than God, in this case, kings. Choice *B* is incorrect because it is not defined as being deceitful. Choice *C* is incorrect because, while idolatry is considered a sin, it is an example of a sin, not a synonym for it. Choice *D* is incorrect because, while idolatry may have been considered illegal in some cultures, it is not a definition for the term.

51. A: The essential meaning of the passage is that the Almighty, God, disapproves of this type of government. Choice *B* is incorrect because, while heaven is mentioned, it is done so to suggest that the monarchical government is irreverent, not that heaven isn't promised. Choice *C* is incorrect because God's disapproval is mentioned, not his punishment. Choice *D* is incorrect because the passage refers to the Jewish monarchy, which required both belief in God and kings, and the tendency of monarchies to gloss over the anti-monarchical passages of scripture to support their form of government.

Practice Tests #2 - #20

To keep the size of this book manageable, save paper, and provide a digital test-taking experience, the 2nd - 20th practice tests can be found online. Scan the QR code or go to this link to access it:

testprepbooks.com/online387/mcat

SCAN ME

The first time you access the test, you will need to register as a “new user” and verify your email address.

If you have any issues, please email support@testprepbooks.com

Index

Dear MCAT Test Taker,

Thank you for purchasing this study guide for your MCAT exam. We hope that we exceeded your expectations.

Our goal in creating this study guide was to cover all of the topics that you will see on the test. We also strove to make our practice questions as similar as possible to what you will encounter on test day. With that being said, if you found something that you feel was not up to your standards, please send us an email and let us know.

We would also like to let you know about other books in our catalog that may interest you.

GRE

This can be found on Amazon: amazon.com/dp/1637757875

GMAT

amazon.com/dp/1637751613

We have study guides in a wide variety of fields. If the one you are looking for isn't listed above, then try searching for it on Amazon or send us an email.

Thanks Again and Happy Testing!
Product Development Team
support@testprepbooks.com

Online Resources

Included with your purchase are multiple online resources. This includes the practice tests in an interactive format and a convenient study timer to help you manage your time.

Scan the QR code or go to this link to access this content:

testprepbooks.com/online387/mcat

SCAN ME

The first time you access the page, you will need to register as a "new user" and verify your email address.

If you have any issues, please email support@testprepbooks.com.

Thank you for letting us be a part of your studying journey!

Made in United States
Cleveland, OH
07 November 2026

47770646R00161